COGNITIVE-BEHAVIORAL THERAPY FOR OCD AND ITS SUBTYPES

Also Available

FOR PROFESSIONALS

Assessment in Cognitive Therapy
Edited by Gary P. Brown and David A. Clark

*Cognitive Therapy of Anxiety Disorders:
Science and Practice*
David A. Clark and Aaron T. Beck

*Intrusive Thoughts in Clinical Disorders:
Theory, Research, and Treatment*
Edited by David A. Clark

FOR GENERAL READERS

*The Anxiety and Worry Workbook:
The Cognitive Behavioral Solution*
David A. Clark and Aaron T. Beck

*The Mood Repair Toolkit:
Proven Strategies to Prevent the Blues
from Turning into Depression*
David A. Clark

Cognitive-Behavioral Therapy for OCD and Its Subtypes

SECOND EDITION

DAVID A. CLARK

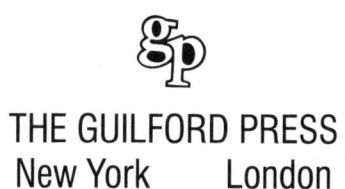

THE GUILFORD PRESS
New York   London

Copyright © 2020 The Guilford Press
A Division of Guilford Publications, Inc.
370 Seventh Avenue, Suite 1200, New York, NY 10001
www.guilford.com

All rights reserved

Except as noted, no part of this book may be reproduced, translated, stored in a retrieval system, or transmitted, in any form or by any means, electronic, mechanical, photocopying, microfilming, recording, or otherwise, without written permission from the publisher.

Printed in the United States of America

This book is printed on acid-free paper.

Last digit is print number: 9 8 7 6 5 4 3 2 1

LIMITED DUPLICATION LICENSE

These materials are intended for use only by qualified mental health professionals.

The publisher grants to individual purchasers of this book nonassignable permission to reproduce all materials for which photocopying permission is specifically granted in a footnote. This license is limited to you, the individual purchaser, for personal use or use with individual clients. This license does not grant the right to reproduce these materials for resale, redistribution, electronic display, or any other purposes (including but not limited to books, pamphlets, articles, video- or audiotapes, blogs, file-sharing sites, Internet or intranet sites, and handouts or slides for lectures, workshops, webinars, or therapy groups, whether or not a fee is charged). Permission to reproduce these materials for these and any other purposes must be obtained in writing from the Permissions Department of Guilford Publications.

The author has checked with sources believed to be reliable in his efforts to provide information that is complete and generally in accord with the standards of practice that are accepted at the time of publication. However, in view of the possibility of human error or changes in behavioral, mental health, or medical sciences, neither the author, nor the editor and publisher, nor any other party who has been involved in the preparation or publication of this work warrants that the information contained herein is in every respect accurate or complete, and they are not responsible for any errors or omissions or the results obtained from the use of such information. Readers are encouraged to confirm the information contained in this book with other sources.

Library of Congress Cataloging-in-Publication Data

Names: Clark, David A., 1954– author.
Title: Cognitive-behavioral therapy for OCD and its subtypes / David A. Clark.
Other titles: Cognitive-behavioral therapy for OCD
Description: Second edition. | New York : The Guilford Press, [2020] |
Revision of: Cognitive-behavioral therapy for OCD. 2004. | Includes bibliographical references and index.
Identifiers: LCCN 2019010915| ISBN 9781462541010 (paperback) | ISBN 9781462541027 (hardcover)
Subjects: LCSH: Cognitive therapy. | Obsessive–compulsive disorder. | BISAC: PSYCHOLOGY / Psychopathology / Compulsive Behavior. | MEDICAL / Psychiatry / General. | SOCIAL SCIENCE / Social Work.
Classification: LCC RC489.C63 C57 2020 | DDC 616.89/1425—dc23
LC record available at *https://lccn.loc.gov/2019010915*

About the Author

David A. Clark, PhD, Professor Emeritus in the Department of Psychology at the University of New Brunswick, Canada, has been a practicing clinical psychologist since 1985. He is a Fellow of the Canadian Psychological Association, Founding Fellow and Trainer Consultant of the Academy of Cognitive Therapy, and ad hoc consultant with the Beck Institute for Cognitive Behavior Therapy. Dr. Clark is a recipient of the Aaron T. Beck Award for Significant and Enduring Contributions to Cognitive Therapy. He was a founding member of the Obsessive Compulsive Cognitions Working Group and is a past associate editor of *Cognitive Therapy and Research*. Dr. Clark has published numerous research and clinical articles and offers professional training workshops worldwide on cognitive-behavioral therapy for obsessive–compulsive disorder, depression, and anxiety disorders. He is the author of several books for professionals and the general public, including *Cognitive Therapy of Anxiety Disorders* and *The Anxiety and Worry Workbook* (both with Aaron T. Beck) and *The Mood Repair Toolkit*.

Preface

It was 15 years ago that *Cognitive-Behavioral Therapy for OCD* was first published as a "comprehensive account of contemporary cognitive-behavioral theory, research, and treatment of OCD [obsessive–compulsive disorder]" (Clark, 2004, p. viii). At that time, psychological research on OCD experienced a rebirth as it emerged from an entrenched behavioral perspective and researchers began evaluating key aspects of the cognitive appraisal model of obsessions, as formulated by Salkovskis, Rachman, Freeston, and colleagues. Cognitive interventions derived from the cognitive appraisal model were integrated with the known effectiveness of exposure and response prevention (ERP) in the hope of expanding the breadth and durability of established treatment protocols. An international research collaboration, called the Obsessive Compulsive Cognitions Working Group (OCCWG), offered a coordinated program of research on the cognitive basis of OCD, as other prominent researchers argued that OCD was a heterogeneous disorder that would benefit from the development of more focused symptom-subtype interventions. In many respects, the years around 2004 were a heady time for the cognitive-behavioral therapy (CBT) perspective on OCD.

If the early 2000s represent the zenith of the CBT approach to OCD, what can be said of the subsequent years? Some might argue that progress has been limited and the CBT perspective has stagnated. Others would disagree, noting that several new findings have emerged about the cognitive basis of obsessions and compulsions, and there is now a better understanding of the role that cognitive strategies can play in the treatment of the disorder. It is within this context that a revision of *Cognitive-Behavioral Therapy for OCD* was undertaken. Its guiding objective was to drill into this question of the progress and the vitality of the CBT perspective, critically evaluating theory, research, and treatment developments over the last 15 years. After reading this second edition, you can decide if progress and innovation still characterize the CBT perspective on obsessions and compulsions.

Admittedly, when I first started the revision process in 2016, I assumed that little had changed in the last decade or so. The basic tenets of the cognitive appraisal model were well established and strategies such as cognitive restructuring and behavioral experiments were still the main ingredients in CBT for OCD. ERP remains the best empirically supported treatment for OCD. Of course, mindfulness-based therapy, acceptance and commitment therapy, and, more recently, compassion-focused therapy, were recent entrants for treatment of OCD, but their additive value is yet to be determined. As it turned out, my initial assumption was wrong. So much has changed in cognitive research and in the treatment of OCD that a complete rewrite was needed in order to capture all the theoretical developments, research findings, and treatment proposals that have emerged in the last 15 years. Because of this substantial growth in the understanding and treatment of the cognitive basis of OCD, this second edition of *Cognitive-Behavioral Therapy for OCD* bears little resemblance to the first edition.

Nevertheless, like its predecessor, the second edition begins with a summary of the psychopathology of OCD as well as a critical explication of the phenomenology of obsessions and compulsions. OCD is a difficult condition to treat because of its symptom heterogeneity, chronicity, and synchronous relation with personality characteristics. Before offering treatment, the mental health professional needs a working knowledge of the psychopathology of the disorder, as well as the theoretical and empirical basis of the cognitive and behavioral approach to OCD. The first part of the book provides this critical foundation, which is needed to treat OCD effectively. Therapists often fail in their treatment of OCD, not because of deficiencies in their therapy skills, but due to an insufficient understanding of the disorder. The second part of the book updates the reader on current OCD theory and research, including ERP. The third part of the book offers detailed, practical, step-by-step instruction on how to conduct CBT for OCD. This section of the book was extensively rewritten to strengthen its clinical tone and structure. It emphasizes therapy issues that are specific to OCD, addressing problems such as how to develop a therapeutic alliance, educate clients about the cognitive model, set treatment goals, and maintain engagement in the therapeutic process. The final section consists of four new chapters on OCD symptom subtypes. Each chapter replicates the general organization of the book, starting out with the phenomenology of the OCD subtype, then its cognitive formulation and research, and, finally, a consideration of specialized treatment strategies for each subtype.

More specifically, Chapters 1–3 present the clinical features of obsessions, compulsions, and their associated phenomena. Chapter 4, on ERP, presents practical guidance, recommendations, and resource tools for incorporating exposure-based strategies into the treatment protocol. A new section on inhibitory learning provides a more contemporary version of ERP. Chapter 5 presents the generic CBT model, along with a critical review of its key assumptions and hypotheses. Chapters 6–9 describe the fundamental components of CBT for OCD, with detailed clinical instruction and client-centered resource materials. The therapeutic relationship, cognitive case formulation, psychoeducation, goal setting, cognitive restructuring, and exposure-based behavioral experiments are explained in terms of their specific application to OCD. Finally, Chapters 10–13 discuss unique features of four symptom subtypes of OCD: physical and mental contamination, doubt and repeated checking, repugnant obsessions, and symmetry/order. These chapters present subtype-specific cognitive case formulations and treatment recommendations to enable therapists to offer more effective targeted CBT for these different symptom presentations.

The advances in the cognitive-behavioral perspective on OCD reported in this volume are the result of many talented, energetic, and highly prolific clinical researchers. It has been a privilege to work with many of these people as valued friends, colleagues, and coauthors. Included in this distinguished group are Jonathan Abramowitz, Amparo Belloch, Martine Bouvard, Meredith Coles, Guy Doron, Mark Freeston, Randy Frost, Gemma García-Soriano, Mujgan Inozu, Michael Kyrios, Richard Moulding, Christine Purdon, Adam Radomsky, Claudio Sica, Gregoris Simos, Gail Steketee, and Wing Wong. Their insights and ingenuity into OCD and its treatment permeate every chapter of this volume. We are all indebted to the pioneering work of Paul Emmelkamp, Edna Foa, Isaac Marks, and Paul Salkovskis, who laid the foundation for behavioral and then cognitive treatment of OCD. More recently, Jonathan Abramowitz, Marl Freeston, Kieron O'Connor, David Tolin, and Eric Rassin have made significant contributions in elucidating the cognitive basis of obsessions and compulsions. But it is Professor Stanley Rachman who has singlehandedly made the most important contributions to CBT research and treatment of OCD. If there is a "father of CBT for OCD," it is Professor Rachman. His brilliance, intellectual curiosity, and creativity pushed him further than his contemporaries in forging a new understanding of obsessive symptomatology. His penetrating analysis of obsessive–compulsive phenomenology, stimulating models of cognitive and behavioral mechanisms, and innovative treatment strategies have inspired a generation of OCD researchers and clinicians alike. I, too, am indebted to Professor Rachman for any understanding I may have about OCD. I was privileged to study under him as a graduate student at the Institute of Psychiatry in London in the early 1980s. I am grateful to both Professor Rachman and to my doctoral thesis supervisor, Dr. Padmal de Silva, for their kindness, understanding, and wisdom, which were critical in launching my 35-year quest to understand OCD. Professors Rachman and de Silva have been mentors to me, along with Dr. Aaron T. Beck, who taught me how to harness the synergy between research and practice and whose clinical wisdom and skill I continue to find enriching.

Writing this revision has been a much longer and more difficult process than I envisioned. The project might never have made it to completion without the encouragement, patience, and understanding of Jim Nageotte, Senior Editor at The Guilford Press. I am so grateful for Jim's advice and his incredible insight into preparing a clinical handbook on OCD. Those who have worked with Jim know he has this amazing ability to zero in on the heart of a matter. So, thank you, Jim, for your perseverance with this project. I also want to thank Jane Keislar, Senior Assistant Editor at Guilford, who demonstrated incredible tenacity and precision in detecting and rectifying the errors and inconsistencies in the manuscript. Her contribution was substantial in making sure the book achieved a high standard of accuracy and consistency. I am also grateful for the staff at Guilford, whose skill and professionalism contributed significantly to the eventual publication of this second edition: Laura Specht Patchkofsky, Oliver Sharpe, and Paul Gordon. Finally, but most importantly, I am deeply indebted to my partner of 41 years, Nancy Nason-Clark, an accomplished and highly regarded sociologist, whose patience, wisdom, and encouragement truly brought this project to completion.

Contents

PART I. The Nature of OCD

1. Diagnosis, Phenomenology, and Comorbidity — 3
2. Obsessions, Intrusions, and Their Correlates — 30
3. Compulsions, Neutralization, and Control — 50

PART II. Theory, Research, and Practice

4. Exposure and Response Prevention: Theory and Practice — 77
5. The Cognitive-Behavioral Model: Theory and Research — 108

PART III. Fundamentals of CBT for OCD

6. The Therapeutic Relationship — 137
7. Assessment and Case Formulation — 162
8. Goals, Education, and Cognitive Interventions — 195
9. Empirical Hypothesis-Testing Experiments — 232

PART IV. Subtype Treatment Protocols

10. Contamination OCD   257

11. Doubt, Checking, and Repeating   281

12. Harm, Sex, and Religious Obsessions   309

13. Symmetry, Ordering, and Arranging   339

References   363

Index   421

Purchasers of this book can download and print enlarged copies of the reproducible forms and handouts at *www.guilford.com/clark3-forms* for personal use or use with individual clients (see copyright page for details).

PART I
The Nature of OCD

CHAPTER 1

Diagnosis, Phenomenology, and Comorbidity

Obsessive–compulsive disorder (OCD) has held a special place in the annals of clinical psychology and psychiatry as one of the most puzzling, yet debilitating, of the emotional disorders. On the one hand, individuals with OCD are tormented by repetitive thoughts, images, or impulses about dreaded possibilities that they realize are exaggerated and highly improbable, and yet, on the other hand, they feel helpless to stop carrying out stereotypic rituals that reduce their distress or magically prevent a dreaded outcome.

The paradox of OCD can be seen in Louise, a 37-year-old mother with a fear of physical contamination. Her contamination fear began after an upsetting incident at a summer camp when she was 14 years old. An outbreak of lice occurred that required delousing to prevent a further spread of the infestation. Upon returning from camp, Louise became fearful of dirt and contamination at home and school and in public places. She started washing her hands repeatedly, took lengthy showers, and avoided touching anything that looked dirty. Now, decades later, Louise continues to be obsessed with cleanliness. Her obsessive fear has changed frequently with the passage of time. In the last 5 years, she has become obsessed with the fear of contracting cancer. She knows she can't "catch cancer," and yet whenever she comes in contact with something others have touched, she feels intensely anxious. The obsessive thought is "What if a person with cancer touched this object?" As well, the thought "That looks dirty" elicits fear because in her mind, dirt is associated with an increased risk of cancer. Louise is anxious most of the day due to dozens of thoughts about dirt and disease, despite tremendous effort to avoid potential contaminants and to keep her personal environment spotlessly clean.

Whenever she feels anxious, Louise cleans. She scrubs her hands to the point where they become cracked and bleed. She uses strong disinfectants throughout the house, and carries antibacterial wipes wherever she goes. Certain everyday activities like using the toilet, handling garbage, dealing with dirty laundry, preparing meals, and touching water faucets and doorknobs trigger her OCD. Despite her taking medication and having tried conventional forms of counseling, the contamination fears have continued unabated. Finally, the stress of the OCD was more than she could bear. Her family was losing patience with her excessive cleaning, and her husband was talking about a period of separation. In addition, Louise felt that she was losing a grip on her own mental health, having just been diagnosed with clinical depression. Feeling there was no way out, Louise began having suicidal thoughts, convinced her family would be better off without her.

Many individuals struggling with OCD have similar experiences to Louise's. OCD can ruin lives; tear families apart; and make highly intelligent, conscientious, and resourceful individuals victims to a bewildering onslaught of irrational thoughts and irresistible urges. OCD is associated with an array of negative emotions such as guilt, shame, and embarrassment, but the most common adverse emotions are fear and anxiety.

Anxiety and its core emotion, fear, are universal human experiences that play a central role in adaptation and survival. The primary function of fear is to signal a threat or impending danger (Barlow, 2002). The feeling of anxiousness associated with making a speech before a large audience or waiting for a job interview is understandable, given the potential for social disapproval and outright humiliation. But what if the fear concerns one's own thoughts? And what if the thoughts are about actions or circumstances that are highly improbable, if not impossible? In response to this intense anxiety, individuals learn that certain rituals or habitual ways of responding appear to bring temporary relief from their distress, even though the response may not be logically connected to the fear. The reduction in anxiety, then, strengthens the connection between the obsessional fear and the "neutralizing response," or compulsion, setting in motion a vicious cycle that we label *OCD*.

Until publication of the fifth edition of the *Diagnostic and Statistical Manual of Mental Disorders* (DSM-5; American Psychiatric Association [APA], 2013), OCD was considered an anxiety disorder. In DSM-5 it now appears in a separate diagnostic category called "obsessive–compulsive and related disorders." Here OCD is the prototypic disorder, along with other "spectrum conditions" like body dysmorphic disorder, hoarding disorder, trichotillomania, and excoriation disorder (i.e., skin picking). Considerable debate surrounded this reclassification, which is summarized in the following section. Despite this diagnostic change, the hallmark of the disorder remains the same: the presence of repetitive obsessions or compulsions that are severe enough to be time-consuming or to cause significant distress or interference in daily living (APA, 2013). Understanding and treating OCD can be one of the greatest challenges facing mental health practitioners, given the idiosyncratic, highly persistent, and irrational nature of the obsessional fear.

When confronted with a severe case of OCD, a clinician might assume that obsessive phenomena have no counterpart in normal human functioning. However, obsessions and compulsions can be found in most individuals to varying degrees. Who hasn't had an unwanted intrusive thought, image, or impulse that pops into the mind for no apparent reason? Examples include the urge to jump in front of an approaching train even though you are not suicidal, the thought of blurting out a rude or embarrassing comment to someone you have just met, or an annoying tune that keeps running through your head. And what about the superstitious, repetitive behaviors we perform to relieve anxiety? For example, consider the baseball player who taps the plate a certain number of times before the first pitch, or the routines a person may have when sitting down to take an exam.

Obsessions and compulsions can occur as normal as well as abnormal phenomena. When does an obsession or compulsion become pathological? And how can we effectively treat these conditions when they cause significant personal distress and interference in daily functioning? These are the two overarching questions that guide this book. I approach these issues with research on the cognitive basis of OCD. The emerging theory and research have given cognitive-behavioral therapists a greater understanding and effective treatments for obsessions, compulsions and their various subtypes.

DIAGNOSIS OF OCD

The essential features of OCD are the repeated occurrence of personally distressing or functionally impairing obsessions and/or compulsions (APA, 2013). *Obsessions* are unwanted, unacceptable, and repetitive intrusive thoughts, images, or urges that are resisted, difficult to control, and generally produce distress even though the person may recognize, to varying degrees, that the thoughts are excessive or senseless (Rachman, 1985). Thought content often focuses on troubling, repugnant, or even nonsensical themes about dirt and contamination; aggression; doubt; unacceptable sexual acts; religion; or orderliness, symmetry, and precision.

Compulsions are repetitive behaviors or mental acts associated with a subjective urgency whose aim is to prevent a dreaded outcome or reduce distress normally caused by an obsession (APA, 2013). A compulsion is generally accompanied by an especially strong urge to carry out the ritual, resulting in a diminished sense of voluntary control over the ritual (Rachman & Hodgson, 1980). Subjective resistance is often present, but the person eventually gives in to the overpowering urge to perform the ritual. Washing, checking, repeating specific behaviors or phrases, ordering (rearranging objects to restore balance or symmetry), and mental rituals (i.e., repeating certain superstitious words, phrases, or prayers) are the most common compulsions. Compulsive rituals are excessive, even senseless responses to the obsession, and tend to follow a strict self-imposed set of rules (APA, 2013).

DSM-5 Diagnosis of OCD

Since the publication of DSM-III (APA, 1980), OCD has been classified an anxiety disorder. Behavioral and cognitive-behavioral theory, research, and treatment accepted this classification, given the prominence of threat-based obsessions, anxiety reduction responses (i.e., compulsions), and avoidance behavior that also characterizes other types of anxiety disorders. Behavioral researchers emphasized that OCD has a symptom profile similar to generalized anxiety disorder (GAD), specific phobias, and hypochondriasis, which suggests the possibility of a common diathesis (e.g., Brown, 1998; de Silva, 1986).

Despite its controversial reclassification, DSM-5 offered only minor changes to the actual diagnostic criteria for OCD (see Abramowitz & Jacoby, 2014; Van Ameringen, Patterson, & Simpson, 2014). The term *impulse* was changed to *urge,* and *inappropriate* became *unwanted* in the definition of obsessions. Moreover, the DSM-IV criterion that obsessions and/or compulsions must at some point be recognized as excessive or senseless was dropped. This decision recognized that a range of insight into the excessiveness of obsessions and compulsions can be present, with over half of OCD sample participants expressing some belief in the reasonableness of their obsessional fears, and 4% certain that their obsessional fears are realistic (Foa et al., 1995).

DSM-5 also expanded the "poor insight" specifier to indicate that a person could have (1) "good or fair insight" into the unrealistic nature of his or her obsessions and compulsions, (2) "poor insight" signifying belief that the obsessional concerns are most likely realistic, or (3) "absent insight/delusional beliefs" when there is strong conviction in the veracity of the obsessional concern (APA, 2013). Again, the expansion of the insight specifier is an improvement because lack of insight is associated with poorer treatment response. Abramowitz and Jacoby (2014) noted that recognition that obsessional concerns can be delusional reduces the chance that individuals with severe OCD will be misdiagnosed with schizophrenia. Finally, a new specifier, "tic-related," was added to indicate whether the individual presently or in the past had a tic disorder. The justification for this specifier is that individuals with OCD and a history of tic disorder differ from those without a history in terms of symptoms, comorbidity, course, and family history (APA, 2013).

The decision to remove OCD from the anxiety disorders was controversial (see the DSM-5 Working Group recommendation; APA, 2012). Several review articles for and against the DSM-5 classification were published (see Abramowitz & Jacoby, 2014; Phillips et al., 2010; Stein et al., 2010; Storch, Abramowitz, & Goodman, 2008; Van Ameringen et al., 2014). Arguments in favor of reclassification included:

1. Evidence that OCD shares significant symptom similarity with body dysmorphic disorder (BDD) and hoarding disorder (HD), and some symptom similarity with trichotillomania (TTM) and excoriation (skin-picking) disorder.
2. OCD and the spectrum-related disorders have a common core symptom of repetitive behavior or compulsiveness that varies on a continuum with impulsivity (Hollander, 1996).
3. OCD and the spectrum disorders share similar clinical features such as age of onset, course, and family history, as well as high comorbidity rates within the diagnostic grouping.
4. The disorders share a common neural circuitry, with hyperactivation in the frontal–striatal region, in contrast to the anxiety disorders in which amygdala activation is prominent.
5. OCD and the spectrum disorders have a similar treatment response, especially to the selective serotonin reuptake inhibitors (SSRIs).

The main reason for grouping the spectrum disorders together with OCD was their supposed shared neurophysiological pathogenesis (see Phillips et al., 2010, for supportive argument). At the very least, the classification is predicated on the view that OCD has more in common with the spectrum disorders than it does with other anxiety disorders.

Several arguments were raised against separating OCD from the anxiety disorders (see Abramowitz & Jacoby, 2014; Stein et al., 2010; Storch et al., 2008).

1. The new focus on "compulsivity" as the core feature in OCD is a misconception because it ignores the functional nature of compulsions, which is the relief of obsessional anxiety. In addition, the DSM-5 approach fails to appreciate the role of cognition in the pathogenesis of OCD (Storch et al., 2008).
2. The new grouping assumes that impulsivity and compulsivity lie on the same continuum, and yet there is little empirical evidence to justify this assertion.
3. The presence of repetitive behavior can be seen in a variety of disorders and may be less pronounced in repugnant or "pure" obsessions. Therefore, this symptom characteristic lacks sufficient sensitivity or specificity to be a defining feature of a diagnostic grouping.
4. OCD does not have a more similar clinical course or higher comor-

bidity rates with the spectrum disorders compared to other anxiety disorders. In fact, OCD has a higher comorbid rate with some of the anxiety disorders than with the obsessive–compulsive spectrum disorders, except for BDD.
5. The empirical evidence for a distinct neural circuitry that is common within OCD and the spectrum disorders but distinct from other anxiety disorders is inconsistent and unreliable.
6. Treatment response in OCD and the spectrum disorders differs, again with the exception of BDD. For example, exposure and response prevention (ERP) is effective for OCD but not the other spectrum disorders, like TMM or excoriation disorder.

Given the compelling objections raised with the DSM-5 reclassification, this book continues with the assertion that OCD is an anxiety disorder. The basic DSM-5 diagnostic criteria for OCD can still be accepted without agreeing to its diagnostic segregation.

EPIDEMIOLOGY AND DEMOGRAPHY

Prevalence

Lifetime prevalence estimates for OCD vary across epidemiological studies because of methodological differences. The Epidemiologic Catchment Area (ECA) study reported a lifetime prevalence of 2.5% based on DSM-III criteria (Karno, Golding, Sorenson, & Burnam, 1988). Later the National Comorbidity Study Replication (NCS-R) found similar rates, with lifetime and 12-month prevalences estimated at 2.3% and 1.2%, respectively (Ruscio, Stein, Chiu, & Kessler, 2010). The German National Health Interview and Examination Survey found a 12-month prevalence rate of 0.7% (Adam, Meinlschmidt, Gloster, & Lieb, 2012). Two other epidemiological studies also reported a 0.7% 12-month prevalence rate (Andrews, Henderson, & Hall, 2001; Kringlen, Torgersen, & Cramer, 2001). Although there is some variation across studies, it is reasonable to conclude that the lifetime prevalence for OCD lies between 1 and 2% of the general population.

A much larger number of people experience subthreshold OCD, or isolated obsessive and compulsive symptoms. In the NCS-R, 28.2% of respondents reported experiencing obsessions or compulsions at some point in their life (Ruscio et al., 2010). In the German study, 4.5% reported a 12-month prevalence of subthreshold OCD, and 8.3% reported obsessive–compulsive symptoms (Adam et al., 2012). Although less severe and impairing than diagnosable OCD, these milder obsessive–compulsive states are significant in their own right. Presence of obsessive–compulsive symptoms confers greater risk for full-blown diagnosable OCD and is associated with higher rates of other mental disorders, greater functional impairment, and more health care utilization (Adam et al., 2012; Fryman et al., 2014; Ruscio et al., 2010). If OCD is considered along with these subclinical states, obsessions and compulsions are responsible for a greater mental health burden than might be assumed from prevalence of the disorder.

Gender, Age, and Onset

Most studies report a slightly higher incidence of OCD in women. In their review, Rasmussen and Eisen (1992) noted that 53% of their OCD sample was female, a gender difference confirmed in some epidemiological studies (Andrews et al., 2001; Karno & Golding, 1991; Kringlen et al., 2001; Ruscio et al., 2010) but not others (e.g., Adams et al., 2012). Men typically have an earlier age of onset and therefore begin treatment at a younger age (e.g., Lensi et al., 1996; Rasmussen & Eisen, 1992). However, it is unclear whether gender has any impact on the course of the disorder. There is some evidence of gender differences in symptom expression, with women displaying more washing and cleaning rituals and men reporting more sexual obsessions (Lensi et al., 1996; Rachman & Hodgson, 1980; Steketee, Grayson, & Foa, 1985).

Young adults between 18 and 24 years are at highest risk for developing OCD (Karno et al., 1988). The mean age of onset was 19½ years in the NCS-R (Ruscio et al., 2010). Sixty-five percent develop the disorder before age 25, with less than 5% reporting an initial onset after 40 years of age (Rachman & Hodgson, 1980; Rasmussen & Eisen, 1992). A substantial number of adults report onset in childhood or adolescence, and children and adolescents with severe OCD will continue to experience symptoms for many years (Rettew, Swedo, Leonard, Lenane, & Rapoport, 1992; Thomsen, 1995). Clearly, OCD is a disorder of the young, with evidence that rates may even decline with age (Karno & Golding, 1991; Ruscio et al., 2010). In the NCS-R, few new onsets were evident after the early 30s, with the average length of the disorder being 8¾ years (Ruscio et al., 2010).

It is hard to argue for a typical modal onset of the disorder. A substantial number of individuals experience a gradual onset of the disorder, whereas for others onset is acute, often in response to certain life experiences (Black, 1974; Lensi et al., 1996; Rachman & Hodgson, 1980). Half to two-thirds of persons with OCD report a significant life event prior to the onset of illness, such as the loss of a loved one, severe medical illness, or major financial problems (Lensi et al., 1996; Lo, 1967). A recent study using a semistructured interview to establish diagnosis and presence of a stressful life event found that 60.8% of an OCD sample reported the occurrence of a life event within the 12 months before illness onset (Rosso, Albert, Asinari, Bogetto, & Maina, 2012).

This relationship is also confirmed when single major life events are considered. For example, a significant number of women with OCD report initial onset during pregnancy (Neziroglu, Anemone, & Yaryura-Tobias, 1992). Abramowitz, Schwartz, and Moore (2003) concluded that a subset of women with OCD experience an onset or worsening of symptoms during pregnancy or the puerperium, but it is unclear whether this might be related to postpartum depression.

A recent systematic literature review concluded that there is no convincing evidence of an association between onset of OCD and environmental risk factors (Brander, Pérez-Vigil, Larrson, & Mataix-Cols, 2016). Potential risk factors were identified such as birth complications, reproductive cycle, and stressful life events, but the retrospective nature of most life event measures and the inconsistencies across studies preclude any firm conclusions about the environmental precipitates of OCD. Although life circumstances such as pregnancy may increase vulnerability to obsessive–compulsive symptoms, it is also important to remember that many individuals cannot identify an environmental trigger for their illness (Rasmussen & Tsuang, 1986).

Ethnicity, Marital Status, and Family Involvement

In the cross-national collaborative study (Weissman et al., 1994), prevalence, age of onset, and comorbidity were quite consistent across seven national sites (United States, Canada, Puerto Rico, Germany, Taiwan, Korea, and New Zealand). More recently the 12-month prevalence for OCD in Taiwan was 0.07% and in Singapore 1.1% (Huang et al., 2014; Subramanian, Abdin, Vaingankar, & Chong, 2012). These rates are substantially lower than the 0.7% 12-month prevalence in the NCS-R. In their review of epidemiological studies, Fontenelle, Mendlowicz, and Versiani (2006) concluded there are substantial differences in OCD rates across countries. Methodological variation across studies probably accounts for much of the difference, but intrinsic characteristics of the populations cannot be ruled out.

Differences in OCD prevalence can also be examined across racial/ethnic groups within countries. African Americans may have a lower lifetime prevalence of OCD (Karno et al., 1988), although the more recent National Survey of American Life found no difference in OCD prevalence rates in African American and African Caribbean populations compared to the European American population (Himle et al., 2008). In sum, it is not clear whether OCD is more prevalent in some racial/ethnic groups than in others. Methodological inconsistencies make it difficult to draw comparisons across studies. At the very least, we can conclude that OCD may vary across racial/ethnic groups, with the biggest differences associated with the symptom subtype most prevalent in a given group (Fontenelle, Mendlowicz, Marques, & Versiani, 2004).

Individuals with OCD are less likely to be married, tend to marry at an older age, and have a low fertility rate (Rachman, 1985). Rates of separation or divorce, marital dysfunction, and sexual dissatisfaction are common in people with OCD, but the rates do not appear greater when compared with other anxiety disorders or depression (Black, 1974; Coryell, 1981; Fontenelle & Hasler, 2008; Freund & Steketee, 1989; Karno et al., 1988; Rasmussen & Eisen, 1992).

Considerable stress is placed on family members living with an individual with severe OCD. Family members may be directly drawn into the illness either by trying to stop the symptoms or by cooperating with an individual's ritualistic behavior. Family members and relatives frequently make accommodations for the person's rituals, which in turn increase family stress and dysfunction (Calvocoressi et al., 1995). A higher rate of critical and rejecting comments may have a limited negative impact on symptom severity, and the level of depression and anxiety in family members influences how they respond to an individual's obsessions and compulsions (Amir, Freshman, & Foa, 2000). A meta-analysis concluded that greater obsessive–compulsive symptom severity was associated with more family accommodation, and that this relationship was not influenced by the presence of a comorbid disorder, gender, or age (Wu, McGuire, Martino, et al., 2016). Clearly, family members are caught in a dilemma. Regardless of whether they refuse to be drawn into ritualistic behavior or whether they accommodate to the rituals, they end up experiencing the distress of living with OCD. No doubt the relationship between symptom severity and family accommodation is bidirectional, causing a vicious cycle in which family members increase their efforts to deal with an escalation in clinical presentation.

Quality of Life and Suicidality

At one time, it was thought that individuals with OCD were more intelligent and attained a higher level of education than individuals with other psychiatric disorders (e.g., Black, 1974). Later research indicated that educational attainment in OCD is similar to that in other disorders but lower than in nonclinical groups (Andrews et al., 2001; Karno & Golding, 1991; Kringlen et al., 2001). Any evidence of higher scores on standardized intelligence tests is only slight and nonsignificant when compared with matched nonclinical controls (Rasmussen & Eisen, 1992).

OCD has a significant negative impact on social and occupational functioning. In a systematic review and meta-analysis of quality-of-life (QOL) research, individuals with OCD had significantly lower QOL scores in work, social, emotional, and family domains than healthy controls (Coluccia et al., 2016). However, when common indices of employment are used, it is unclear whether OCD is associated with worse employment outcomes compared to other psychiatric disorders. Generally, employment status and level of income did not differ when OCD was compared with other anxiety disorders (Antony, Downie, & Swinson, 1998; Karno et al., 1988), although contrary findings have been reported, with higher rates of unemployment and lower income in OCD relative to other emotional disorders (Steketee, Grayson, & Foa, 1987; Torres et al., 2006).

It is now recognized that elevated suicidality is a significant problem in OCD. Two large community studies found that 36–63% of individuals with an OCD diagnosis reported suicidal thoughts at some point during their life, and 11–26% reported lifetime suicide attempts (Torres, et al., 2006; Torres, Ramos-Cerqueria, Fontenelle, do Rosário, & Miguel, 2011). The presence of sexual/religious obsessions and comorbid major depression may increase suicidal risk. A meta-analysis based on 48 studies found a significant association between suicidality and OCD (Angelakis, Gooding, Tarrier, & Panagioti, 2015). Severity of obsessions as well as comorbid anxious and depressive symptoms predicted increased suicidality. A prospective study using the Danish population register revealed that OCD was associated with increased mortality rates even after controlling for depression, anxiety, and substance use disorders (Meier et al., 2016). Clearly, then, OCD poses considerable risk for those who suffer from this condition.

It is evident that OCD has a substantial detrimental impact on QOL and occupational attainment. Whether this negative impact is greater than the effects seen in other psychiatric disorders remains unclear. However, severe forms of the disorder can have devastating effects on individuals, who are often unable to carry out their usual work or social activities shortly after disorder onset (Pollitt, 1957). As well, clinicians must be concerned about increased suicidal risk in severe OCD that is comorbid for depression, substance use, and impulse-control disorders (Torres et al., 2011).

COURSE AND OUTCOME

Treatment Seeking

Most individuals with OCD delay seeking treatment for several years, and there can be considerable variability in treatment delay, from 2 to 7 years (Lensi et al., 1996; Rasmussen & Tsuang, 1986). In the Singapore Mental Health Study, the median treatment delay was 9 years, with 89.8% of those with a lifetime diagnosis of OCD never seeking treatment for their condition (Subramanian et al., 2012). However, severity of the disorder and presence of comorbidity may influence whether treatment is sought. In the NCS-R, 93% of individuals with severe OCD received treatment in the preceding year compared to 25.6% of the moderately severe cases (Ruscio et al., 2010). The German epidemiological study found treatment-seeking rates of 68.2% for those with diagnosable OCD, 36.3% for subthreshold OCD, and 36.6% for those with obsessive–compulsive symptoms (Adam et al., 2012). Moreover, 55.6% of individuals with comorbid OCD sought treatment compared to 13.9% of "pure" OCD cases (Torres et al., 2006).

Even when treatment utilization is high, less than one-third of individuals with severe OCD receive treatment specifically for OCD (Ruscio et al., 2010).

There are several conclusions that can be drawn from this research. First, individuals with OCD often do not seek treatment for years. Second, those with milder symptoms are less likely to seek treatment. And third, individuals with OCD and another comorbid condition, like major depression, are more likely to seek health care services. However, only a minority of individuals, even those with severe OCD, obtain specialized treatment for the disorder (Pollard, Henderson, Frank, & Margolis, 1989; Ruscio et al., 2010). This low level of treatment seeking is reminiscent of the dissemination problem that is evident in the treatment of psychological disorders more broadly (i.e., McHugh & Barlow, 2010). For those with OCD, the limited access to evidence-based treatment may be compounded by failure to even recognize that disorder-specific treatment is needed for obsessional states.

Natural Course and Outcome

Research on the natural course of any disorder is fraught with methodological challenges because follow-up periods spanning decades are required and any treatment during this time period will bias the natural trajectory of the disorder. Despite these hurdles, a few observations can be made about the natural course of OCD. In a longitudinal study that is remarkable because the follow-up period spans several decades ($M = 47$ years), Skoog and Skoog (1999) found that OCD tends to take a chronic course, with symptoms waxing and waning over the lifetime. Half of their OCD sample ($n = 122$) continued to experience clinically significant symptoms, and another one-third had subclinical features (although 83% showed improvement in the 40-year period). Complete recovery occurred in only 20% of the sample. These results are entirely consistent with other research showing that OCD episodes tend to be lengthy and that spontaneous remission of symptoms is low (Demal, Lenz, Mayrhofer, Zapotoczky, & Zitterl, 1993; Foa & Kozak, 1996; Karno & Golding, 1991). More recently a 5-year follow-up of treatment-seeking individuals with OCD revealed that only 17% achieved full remission and 59% of those who experienced partial or full remission relapsed (Eisen et al., 2013).

There have been attempts to characterize the typical course of OCD symptoms. Most individuals with OCD experience a chronic, continuous course with the disorder, although a minority (10%) shows deterioration over time. Others experience an intermittent course with obsessive–compulsive symptoms waxing and waning, possibly in response to stressful life experiences (Demal et al., 1993; Lensi et al., 1996; Rasmussen & Tsuang, 1986).

Although it is difficult to be definitive about the natural course of OCD, we can state that most individuals with the disorder experience a somewhat early but insidious onset in adolescence or early adulthood, with a mix of obsessive and compulsive symptoms that build during periods of stress and possibly subside during intervals of relative stability. This pattern of waxing and waning symptoms can continue over several years until symptom severity reaches a point where the person finally seeks treatment.

COMORBIDITY

Diagnostic comorbidity refers "to the co-occurrence of two or more current or lifetime mental disorders in the same individual" (Brown, Campbell, Lehman, Grisham, & Mancill, 2001, p. 585). Comorbidity is important because the presence of a coexisting disorder is usually associated with greater symptom severity, lower treatment response, and poorer prognosis (Bronisch & Hecht, 1990; Brown & Barlow, 1992). OCD has a high rate of diagnostic comorbidity, with half to three-quarters of individuals having at least one additional current disorder (Antony et al., 1998; Brown et al., 2001; Karno & Golding, 1991; see Yaryura-Tobias et al., 2000, for lower comorbidity rates). When lifetime comorbidity is considered, fewer than 15% of cases have a sole diagnosis of OCD (Brown et al., 2001; Crino & Andrews, 1996). In the NCS-R, 90% of individuals with lifetime OCD met diagnostic criteria for another lifetime disorder (Ruscio et al., 2010), and in the British National Psychiatric Morbidity Survey of 2000, 62% of individuals with OCD had one or more current comorbid disorder (Torres et al., 2006). The comorbidity rate was substantially higher than the rates seen in the "other neurotic disorders."

Comorbidity of OCD with other disorders is asymmetrical. Whereas additional diagnoses of depression or other anxiety disorders have a high rate of occurrence in OCD, obsessional disorder, as a co-occurring condition with major depression or other anxiety disorders, is less common, even when lifetime rates are considered (Antony et al., 1998; Brown et al., 2001; Crino & Andrews, 1996). Moreover, the temporal order of lifetime comorbidity may differ between disorders. Brown and colleagues (2001) found that comorbid anxiety disorders tended to temporally precede index cases of OCD, whereas comorbid depression tended to occur after the onset of an obsessional disorder. In the NCS-R, when OCD and anxiety disorders were comorbid, anxiety tended to occur first, whereas it was equally split on whether OCD or major depression occurred first (Ruscio et al., 2010). Once an obsessional episode is active, individuals are at elevated risk for anxiety, mood disorders, eating disturbance, and tic disorders for the duration of the episode (Yaryura-Tobias et al., 2000).

Depression

For decades, clinical researchers have recognized a close relationship between OCD and depression (e.g., Lewis, 1936; Rosenberg, 1968; Stengel, 1945). The co-occurrence of major depressive episode in persons with OCD is high, ranging from 30 to 50% (Bellodi, Sciuto, Diaferia, Ronchi, & Smeraldi, 1992; Brown, Moras, Zinbarg, & Barlow, 1993; Karno & Golding, 1991; Lensi et al., 1996). Lifetime prevalence rates are even higher (65–80%) (Brown et al., 2001; Crino & Andrews, 1996; Rasmussen & Eisen, 1992). More recent epidemiological studies confirm these early findings, with 25–50% of individuals with OCD having a current or lifetime comorbid depressive disorder (Huang et al., 2014; Ruscio et al., 2010; Subramanian et al., 2012; Torres et al., 2006). In most of the research depression is the most common comorbid condition, followed by GAD and substance use disorders. The NCS-R reported a slightly different comorbid pattern based on lifetime prevalence. Any anxiety disorder was most common (76%), followed by any mood disorder (63%), impulse-control disorder (56%), and any substance use disorder (39%) (Ruscio et al., 2010).

Although there is some inconsistency in whether major depression or OCD emerges first in comorbid conditions, the more usual pattern is that OCD leads to the development of a secondary depressive disorder (Demal et al., 1993; Rasmussen & Eisen, 1992; Rickelt et al., 2016; Subramanian et al., 2012; Welner, Reich, Robins, Fishman, & van Doren, 1976). In these studies, the progression from obsessive–compulsive symptoms to depression occurred three times more often than the reverse pattern. Likewise, Rickelt and colleagues (2016) found that 74% of their OCD sample had a secondary major depressive disorder. Although obsessive–compulsive symptoms and disorder can be found in diagnosable depressive disorders, it is less frequent than the incidence of depressive disorders in OCD samples (Kendell & Discipio, 1970; Lewis, 1936).

When depressive disorder is comorbid in OCD, it is associated with greater symptom severity, poorer QOL, and increased functional impairment. Comorbid major depression was associated with greater obsessive–compulsive symptom severity at 1-year follow-up in the Netherlands Obsessive Compulsive Disorder Association study (Rickelt et al., 2016). As well, Huppert and colleagues found that comorbid depression accounted for much of the variance in the poor QOL and impaired functioning found in individuals with OCD (Huppert, Simpson, Nissenson, Liebowitz, & Foa, 2009).

Depression may have a greater negative effect on obsessions than compulsions (Ricciardi & McNally, 1995). McNally, Mair, Mugno, and Riemann (2017) performed a Bayesian network analysis on obsessive–compulsive and depressive symptoms in 408 treatment-seeking individuals with OCD. They found that degree of interference caused by obsessions and compulsions, as well as the level of distress associated with obsessions, were responsible for depression comorbidity. Furthermore, depressive symptoms such as guilt, anhedonia, and suicidality occurred when sad mood was activated by distress associated with obsessions. These findings suggest that treating obsessional distress first may help prevent escalation of sad mood and the subsequent development of depression (McNally et al., 2017). Other research has indicated that individuals with OCD and comorbid major depression have a greater propensity to misinterpret the significance of unwanted intrusive thoughts (Abramowitz, Storch, Keeley, & Cordell, 2007). Thus, dysfunctional cognitive processing could be another mediator between obsessive–compulsive symptom severity and depression.

Individuals with OCD and comorbid major depression can achieve clinically significant treatment gains, although the posttreatment symptom level is significantly greater than for those without concurrent depression (e.g., Abramowitz & Foa, 2000). In their meta-analysis of CBT for OCD, Olatunji, Davis, Powers, and Smits (2013) found that depressive symptom severity was not associated with a decrease in treatment effect sizes. Other reviewers also have concluded that the presence of comorbid major depression has no significant association with treatment outcome (Knopp, Knowles, Bee, Lovell, & Bower, 2013). However, it may be that level of depression severity determines its impact on treatment. Abramowitz (2004) concluded that severe depression does reduce treatment response and so recommended that cognitive therapy be introduced to address pertinent issues in severely depressed cases of OCD. Despite some inconsistencies across reviews, the most parsimonious conclusion is that severe levels of depressive symptoms will negatively affect treatment response, whereas mild to moderate depression may not substantially influence outcome (Abramowitz, Franklin, Street, Kozak, & Foa, 2000; Keeley, Storch, Merlo, & Geffken, 2008).

Anxiety Disorders

The relationship between OCD and the anxiety disorders has been hotly debated with the DSM-5 reclassification of the disorder. Early studies found that social anxiety disorder had the highest comorbidity rate with OCD (35–41%), with specific phobias (17–21%) having the next highest rate of co-occurrence. Results are more mixed concerning panic disorder, with some studies showing moderately high comorbidity rates (29%), whereas others report relatively low rates of co-occurrence (12%); it is still unclear whether GAD co-occurs rarely (7%) or, at the very least, somewhat less frequently (12–22%) (see Antony et al., 1998; Brown et al., 1993, 2001; Crino & Andrews, 1996).

More recent epidemiological studies have reported more inconsistency in the comorbidity rates for anxiety. In the NCS-R (Ruscio et al., 2010), lifetime prevalence was highest for social anxiety (43.5%), followed by specific phobia (42.7%), separation anxiety disorder (37.1%), panic disorder (20%), and GAD (8.3%). However, in the British epidemiological study, which was based on ICD-10 diagnoses, GAD had a comorbid rate of 31.4%, panic disorder/agoraphobia 22.1%, social anxiety disorder 17.3%, and specific phobia 15.1% (Torres et al., 2006). The German epidemiological study was more consistent with the NCS-R findings, except that GAD had a higher rate (21.1%) and panic attacks were present in 34% of the OCD sample (Adam et al., 2012). A Swiss population-based study reported lifetime comorbidities of 50% for GAD, 40% for social anxiety, 20% for simple phobia, and 16.7% for panic disorder (Fineberg et al., 2013). Torres and colleagues (2016) found that social anxiety disorder (34.6%), GAD (34.3%), and specific phobia (31.4%) were the most common comorbid conditions after major depression (56.4%) in a large Brazilian OCD clinical study. Separation anxiety disorder can also be seen in OCD, with a lifetime prevalence of 27.2% as well as heightened personal dysfunction and poorer treatment response (Franz et al., 2015).

It is noteworthy that comorbidity rates increase with greater obsessive–compulsive severity, and the co-occurrence of anxiety with OCD is associated with greater distress and psychosocial impairment (Fineberg et al., 2013; Hofmeijer-Sevink et al., 2013). Obsessions and compulsions often co-occur with other anxiety symptoms, so that the more anxiety exhibited by an individual, the greater the negative impact on functioning (Welkowitz, Struening, Pittman, Guardino, & Welkowitz, 2000). Increased severity of comorbid anxious symptoms is also a significant predictor of suicidality in OCD (Angelakis et al., 2015).

Although other anxiety disorders are frequently found in persons with OCD, obsessions and compulsions are rarely evident when other anxiety disorders are the principal diagnosis. Brown and colleagues (1993), for example, found that OCD rarely occurred (2%) when GAD was the principal diagnosis. This asymmetry was also evident at the symptom level, with 41% of the OCD sample reporting worry but only 15% of those with primary GAD had obsessions. This trend was confirmed in a recent study of 57 individuals with GAD and 58 with panic disorder (Camuri et al., 2014). Only 7% of the GAD sample had co-occurring OCD, and the rate was even lower in panic disorder (1.7%).

Anxious symptoms and disorders are common in OCD, and when present they are associated with greater personal distress, symptom severity, and impaired psychosocial functioning. Although the findings are not entirely consistent, GAD, social anxiety, specific phobias, and to a lesser extent, panic and separation anxiety disorders may be present. From a conceptual perspective, the comorbidity data are consistent with those who consider OCD an anxiety disorder. Clearly, individualized case formulations and treatment goal setting may require a broader perspective that takes into consideration the presence of other anxiety disorders and symptoms.

Obsessive–Compulsive Spectrum Disorders

Two key questions in the relationship between the obsessive–compulsive spectrum disorders (OCSD) and OCD concern their comorbidity rates and whether they have a shared phenotype or clinical presentation. In DSM-5 the primary OCSDs are BDD, TTM, excoriation (skin-picking) disorder (SPD), and HD (APA, 2013). Recently the ICD-11 Working Group on Obsessive–Compulsive and Related Disorders proposed an expanded diagnostic grouping in which hypochondriasis and olfactory reference disorder would be added to DSM-5 OCSDs (Stein et al., 2016). The argument is similar to that previously advanced by the DSM-5 working group (APA, 2012).

For OCD, the OCSD comorbidity rate is much lower than one might expect for disorders within the same diagnostic category, and less than the prevalence of anxiety disorders and symptoms. In OCD samples the lifetime prevalence of comorbid BDD ranges from 8.7 to 15%, for TTM from 5.3 to 11%, for SPD from 17 to 31%, and for HD or compulsive buying from 7 to 11% (Bienvenu et al., 2012; Costa et al., 2012; Lochner et al., 2014; Torres et al., 2016). Concurrent rate for HD is around 10% (Chakraborty et al., 2012). However, the comorbidity rate of obsessive–compulsive symptoms and disorder is much lower in those with a principal OCSD diagnosis. In TTM approximately 5% of individuals have comorbid OCD (Lochner et al., 2012) and in HD, only a small percentage of individuals have OCD symptoms (Hall, Tolin, Frost, & Steketee, 2013). The rate of OCD is higher (31–35%) in individuals with early-onset BDD (Bjornsson et al., 2013). Except for BDD, the comorbidity rates for certain anxiety disorders, like social anxiety, specific phobias, and GAD, are substantially higher than the rates for OCSDs. Thus, the pattern of comorbidity evident in OCD does not support the contention that obsessional disorders have a closer association with the OCSDs than with the anxiety disorders.

Advocates for a distinct OCD and related disorders classification argue that these conditions have a common core symptom presentation (APA, 2012; Stein et al., 2016). In their review, Phillips and colleagues (2010) concluded that OCD and BDD have the closest symptom similarity, TTM some symptom overlap, but less symptom similarity with HD. A direct clinical comparison of an SPD sample with an OCD group revealed few symptom similarities and no overlap in prevalence among first-degree relatives (Grant, Odlaug, & Kim, 2010). A multimodal modeling analysis of OCD and OCSD self-report symptom measures based on 6,310 individual twins from the U.K. Adult Twin Registry revealed a nonspecific genetic vulnerability factor in which OCD loaded with BDD and HD, and to a lesser extent, with TTM and SPD (Monzani, Rijsdijk, Harris, & Mataix-Cols, 2014). A second disorder-specific genetic vulnerability factor emerged that included only TTM and SPD, whereas OCD, BDD, and HD also evidenced disorder-specific influences. The researchers concluded that environmental risk factors tend to be disorder-specific. Finally, a recent logistic regression analysis of obsessive–compulsive symptom dimensions and the OCSDs revealed that the aggression and hoarding subscales of the dimensional Yale–Brown Obsessive–Compulsive Scale (YBOCS) were related to SPD, whereas the sexual/religious dimension was related to BDD (Torres et al., 2016). It is possible, then, that specific obsessive–compulsive symptoms are related to OCSDs.

As noted, the introduction of a distinct OCD and related disorders classification category in DSM-5 continues to be a controversial decision. The relationship between OCD and the OCSDs is not at all clear. In terms of prevalence and symptom similarity, OCD appears to have the closest association with BDD. Hoarding symptoms and disorder are much less prevalent in OCD than originally thought (Hall et al., 2013), and may have a higher correlation with obsessive–compulsive personality disorder (OCPD) traits (Samuels et al., 2008). TTM and SPD may have minimal association with OCD. For the minority of individuals with OCD and hoarding or BDD symptoms, the co-occurrence of OCSD pathology predicts greater symptom severity, impaired functioning, and poorer treatment response (Costa et al., 2012; Knopp et al., 2013). Given their negative impact, practitioners are well advised to assess for OCSD pathology in their clients with OCD.

Tic Disorders

Relatively high rates of tics or tic disorders, including Tourette syndrome, have been found in individuals, especially children and adolescents, with OCD (Goldsmith, Shapira, Phillips, & McElroy, 1998; March & Mulle, 1998). In a sample of 239 adults with OCD, 19% had a lifetime history of motor and/or phonic tics (Holzer et al., 1994). Thirty to 40% of adults with Tourette syndrome experience obsessive and compulsive symptoms (Leckman, 1993). In fact, one of the largest clinical studies based on a sample of 1,374 individuals with Tourette syndrome found a lifetime prevalence of 50% for OCD (Hirschtritt et al., 2015). Other studies have confirmed an elevated co-occurrence of tic disorders in OCD, with lifetime prevalence rates ranging from 12.5% for Tourette syndrome alone to 28% for any tic disorder (Lochner et al., 2014; Torres et al., 2016). DSM-5 now includes a "tic-related" specifier to identify individuals with OCD and a comorbid tic disorder. There is considerable evidence that OCD with a lifetime history of chronic tic disorder, especially in children and adolescents, has a different symptom presentation, family history, and possibly a poorer response to SSRI treatment (Leckman et al., 2010). Clinicians treating children and adolescents with OCD should be particularly cognizant that tic-related symptoms could influence the clinical presentation and course of the disorder.

Psychosis

Researchers have been particularly interested in the lifetime co-occurrence of OCD with psychosis because of its etiological implications. Early psychiatric writing proposed a relationship between obsessional thinking and the thought disturbance seen in schizophrenia (for discussion, see Lewis, 1936; Stengel, 1945). However, only a minority of individuals with OCD (15–20%) show any symptoms of psychosis, and these are usually in the form of poor insight or lack of resistance to the obsession (Insel & Akiskal, 1986). A small number of individuals with OCD have obsessional ideation that meets the criteria for delusion, but the number of individuals with OCD who progress to schizophrenia is no greater than the number of those with other anxiety disorders (Rachman & Hodgson, 1980; Stein & Hollander, 1993). Torres and colleagues (2006) found that only 2.6% of their OCD sample met ICD-10 criteria for schizophrenia, whereas Adam and colleagues (2012) found that 39% of their sample reported possible psychotic symptoms.

Substance Use Disorders

Substance use disorders (SUDs), especially alcohol use disorder, are found in OCD samples. In the NCS-R, 38.6% of those with OCD had a lifetime comorbid SUD, with alcohol (24%) higher than drug (14%) dependence (Ruscio et al., 2010). However, large clinical studies have reported lower comorbidity rates for SUDs. A large Dutch clinical study found that only 13.6% of the OCD sample had a lifetime prevalence of any SUD (Hofmeijer-Sevink et al., 2013). In the Singapore Mental Health Study 5.1% of the OCD sample had lifetime alcohol abuse and 2.1% lifetime prevalence for alcohol dependence (Subramanian et al., 2012). Likewise, Fineberg and colleagues (2013) reported a low prevalence of comorbid lifetime diagnoses of drug and alcohol misuse in their OCD sample. A Danish epidemiological study found that comorbidity for SUDs was actually lower than for other psychiatric conditions (Toftdahl, Nordentoft, & Hjorthøj, 2016).

Other studies have found SUD comorbidity rates that are similar to the NCS-R. In the British National Psychiatric Morbidity Survey of 2000, 34% of individuals with OCD had a comorbid drinking problem (Torres et al., 2006). A Dutch epidemiological study found that 54.6% of men and 23.5% of women with OCD had a lifetime prevalence of an SUD (Blom et al., 2011). The OCD group had significantly higher risk for an SUD than those without a psychiatric disorder, and men with OCD had a higher risk of SUD than those with other psychiatric conditions. However, OCD may have a stronger effect in heightening risk for a comorbid SUD in women.

The heightened risk of SUDs in OCD is not surprising given their similar phenomenology. Compulsivity, a core feature of OCD that is now emphasized in DSM-5, involves a sense of urgency and diminished voluntary control in which a repetitive, self-defeating behavioral or mental ritual is performed to reduce anxiety or distress, prevent a dreaded outcome, and/or undo or put right an unwanted state (APA, 2013; Denys, 2011; Rachman & Hodgson, 1980). For this reason OCD has been viewed as a "behavioral addiction," with compulsivity a clinical feature that also has been implicated in alcohol and drug addictions more generally (i.e., Koob & Le Moal, 2005). A common neurocircuitry has been implicated in the compulsivity of OCD and addictions, a circuitry that is characterized by impaired reward and punishment processing in the ventral striatum, reduced self-regulation due to attenuation in the ventromedial prefrontal region, and imbalances between the ventral and dorsal frontal–striatal areas (Figee et al., 2015).

The relationship between OCD and the SUDs exhibits considerable variability. For example, elevated substance abuse in OCD is primarily related to alcohol rather than drugs, as mentioned (e.g., Ruscio et al., 2010; Torres et al., 2006). Men with OCD have significantly higher rates of comorbid SUDs than women with OCD, although the effect of obsessionality on SUD is much greater in women (Blom et al., 2011). There is also evidence that the heightened prevalence of SUDs can be attributed to individuals with less severe obsessive–compulsive symptoms. As the obsessive–compulsive symptom severity increases, past and current alcohol or drug abuse becomes less likely (Cuzen, Stein, Lochner, & Fineberg, 2014).

Despite inconsistencies across studies and the many unanswered questions about the relationship between OCD and SUDs, it is important that clinicians ask questions about past and current alcohol and drug use when assessing individuals for OCD. Presence of alcohol or drug abuse in any psychiatric condition is associated with adverse outcomes and more difficult response to treatment (i.e., Drake, Mueser, Brunette, & McHugo, 2004; Toftdahl et al., 2016).

OCPD and the Personality Disorders

A final comorbidity issue that deserves mention is the relationship between OCD and the personality disorders, especially OCPD, which is an enduring tendency to be excessively concerned with organization, perfectionism, and control while eschewing flexibility and openness to experience (see also DSM-5; APA, 2013).

The concept of OCPD is rooted in Freud's notion of the anal personality, characterized by a tendency to be parsimonious, obstinate, and orderly (Freud, 1908/1959). Originally, the obsessional personality or anal character was considered the premorbid personality for OCD, and some early studies suggested a strong link between the presence of OCD symptoms and obsessional personality traits (Ingram, 1961b; Kline, 1968; Sandler & Hazari, 1960).

Empirical studies conducted in the 1970s and 1980s challenged the conventional psychoanalytic view that posited an etiological link between OCPD and OCD. Findings at that time indicated that obsessional personality characteristics were quite distinct from obsessive–compulsive symptoms, and most individuals with OCD did not have a premorbid obsessional personality (for reviews, see Pollak, 1979; Rachman & Hodgson, 1980). Despite a high personality disorder comorbidity rate, the most common personality disorders in OCD were the dependent and avoidant types, with OCPD being less prevalent than one might expect (see the review by Summerfeldt, Huta, & Swinson, 1998). Thus, behavioral researchers such as Rachman and Hodgson (1980) concluded that OCPD was less relevant to OCD than originally proposed by the psychoanalytic school.

More recently, several OCD researchers have reexamined whether OCPD might be an important factor in OCD. Contrary to earlier studies, OCPD emerged as the most prevalent personality disorder in several OCD samples. For example, a study of 72 individuals with OCD found that 32.4% had comorbid OCPD, followed by avoidant (11.3%) and narcissistic (6.9%) personality disorders (Samuels et al., 2000). Another study of 420 outpatients with OCD reported that 9% had comorbid OCPD, 7.6% dependent personality disorder, 5.6% borderline personality disorder, and 4.6% avoidant personality disorder (Denys, Tenney, van Megen, de Geus, & Westenberg, 2004). And in a meta-analysis of personality disorder research in the anxiety disorders, OCPD had the highest prevalence in the OCD samples, followed by avoidant and dependent personality disorders (Friborg, Martinussen, Kaiser, Øvergård, & Rosenvinge, 2013). These findings have been replicated in the most recent comorbidity studies (e.g., Bulli, Melli, Cavalletti, Stopani, & Carraresi, 2016; Melca, Yücel, Mendlowicz, de Oliveira-Souza, & Fontenelle, 2015).

When based on more rigorous diagnostic interviews, the comorbid prevalence rate for OCPD may be even higher than expected. Gordon, Salkovskis, Oldfield, and Carter (2013) found that 45% of their OCD sample met DSM-IV criteria for OCPD compared to a 14.7% comorbidity rate in the panic disorder group. In addition, those with comorbid OCPD had higher alcohol consumption, greater symptom severity, and more depressive symptoms.

OCPD may exhibit a stronger association with certain obsessive–compulsive symptoms, such as doubting and checking, than others like washing (Gibbs & Oltmanns, 1995; Tallis, Rosen, & Shafran, 1996). Studies that dismantled OCPD found that comorbidity may be due primarily to hoarding, perfectionism, and preoccupation with details rather than other DSM-IV criteria such as rigidity, inflexible morality, excessive devotion to work, etc. (Eisen et al., 2006; see also Gordon et al., 2013, for similar findings). Moreover, Coles and associates concluded that individuals with OCD and OCPD represent a specific subtype of OCD with earlier age of onset, higher rates comorbid anxiety and avoidant personality disorders, greater frequency of certain obsessive–compulsive symptoms, and more impaired functioning (Coles, Pinto, Mancebo, Rasmussen, & Eisen, 2008). As expected, the presence of comorbid personality disorders is associated with poorer treatment outcome in OCD (Keeley et al., 2008; Thiel et al., 2013).

Although the empirical research does not support the view that OCPD is a personality determinant of OCD, its importance may have been understated in earlier behavioral research. Rasmussen and Eisen's (1992) conclusions about OCPD remain pertinent: (1) OCPD occurs in many people who never develop a psychiatric disorder, (2) the personality constellation often occurs in non-OCD psychiatric conditions, and (3) 55–75% of individuals with OCD do not have OCPD. However, the presence of OCPD in those with OCD may constitute a distinct subgroup that experiences greater clinical severity and impaired functioning, as well as poorer treatment response. Therefore, clinicians treating patients with OCD should routinely assess for OCPD traits and modify their treatment protocols to deal with perfectionism, meticulousness, and other compulsive traits that might have a negative impact on the course of the disorder and its treatment.

SYMPTOM SUBTYPES

OCD is a heterogeneous disorder with a varied symptom presentation. Although considered a unified diagnostic construct, individuals with OCD can have completely distinct symptom presentations—a problem that challenges the validity and clinical utility of the diagnosis (Bloch, Landeros-Weisenberger, Rosario, Pittenger, & Leckman, 2008). This issue raises the possibility that diagnostic clarity and treatment effectiveness might be improved if OCD could be broken into more homogeneous subtypes. Given this possibility, specific CBT protocols have been developed for contamination/washing (Rachman, 2006), doubt/checking (Rachman, 2002), and repugnant obsessions (Rachman, 2003). The subtype approach has a long history in OCD, beginning with early clinical studies on differences in compulsive behavior, then progressing to multivariate analyses of symptom checklists, and most recently, the search for underlying psychological processes that might differentiate various types of OCD (Calamari, 2005).

Early Research

Research on subtyping began with systematic clinical observation and experimentation on differences in compulsions. Rachman and Hodgson (1980) compared the clinical presentation of compulsive cleaning and checking. Cleaning compulsions had a stronger phobic component involving escape (i.e., reduction of fear associated with a perceived contaminant), whereas checking was more often associated with doubting and indecision accompanied by active avoidance behavior (i.e., checking prevents some future negative outcome). Checking rituals took longer to complete, had a slow onset, evoked more internal resistance, and were more often accompanied by feelings of anger or tension than were cleaning compulsions. In addition, individuals with compulsive checking had more difficulty obtaining the required certainty or assurance that the possible negative future event had been averted. Steketee and colleagues (1985) also found significant differences in symptoms and fear structure in individuals with cleaning versus checking compulsions.

Some individuals with OCD have obsessional ruminations without overt compulsions (Akhtar, Wig, Varma, Pershad, & Verma, 1975; Ingram, 1961a; Rachman, 1985; Rasmussen & Tsuang, 1986; Welner et al., 1976). The prevalence of this OCD subtype might be as high as 20% (Freeston & Ladouceur, 1997a), although Foa, Steketee, and Ozarow (1985) speculated that most individuals with "pure obsessions" exhibit mental compulsions. This was borne out in the DSM-IV field trial in which only 2.1% of the OCD sample had obsessions without compulsions (Foa et al., 1995). Because overt and covert (mental) compulsions/neutralization exhibits the same role and function in OCD, it is still not clear whether obsessional rumination should be considered distinct from other OCD subtypes.

Rasmussen and Eisen (1992, 1998) conducted one of the largest clinical studies on symptom subtyping based on more than 1,000 Americans with OCD. The most common obsessions were fear of contamination (50%) and pathological doubt (42%), whereas washing/cleaning (50%) and checking (61%) were the most common compulsions. Religious/blasphemous (10%) obsessions and hoarding (18%) were less common.

This early research on OCD subtyping had a profound impact on how practitioners dealt with obsessive–compulsive symptom heterogeneity. Most experts in OCD research and treatment believe that the disorder comprises five symptom dimensions: contamination/cleaning, symmetry/order/repeating/counting, hoarding, harm (aggression) obsessions and checking, and sexual/religious obsessions (Mataix-Cols, Pertusa, & Leckman, 2007). However, there are several problems with this approach. First, it assumes that individuals with OCD have one primary obsessive or compulsive symptom, when in reality most individuals have multiple obsessions and compulsions (e.g., Akhtar et al., 1975) that transcend subtype categories. Second, most individuals with OCD show substantial change in their obsessive–compulsive symptoms over time (Skoog & Skoog, 1999). The cross-sectional nature of most subtype research ignores the changing nature of obsessive–compulsive symptoms. And third, the early subtype research failed to show that these categories met key criteria for establishing distinct and valid psychiatric subtypes (Rowsell & Francis, 2015). Given these difficulties, researchers turned to multivariate analysis of symptom checklists in a search for coherent and reliable symptom patterns.

Multivariate Symptom Dimensions

The dimensional perspective does not assume that individuals can be categorized into specific symptom subtypes. Instead, distinct symptom dimensions are identified on which individuals differ to varying degrees. These dimensions are usually identified through factor or cluster analysis of obsessive–compulsive symptom measures. In recent years most of this research has relied on multivariate structural analysis of the obsessions and compulsions symptom checklist of the Yale–Brown Obsessive–Compulsive Scale (YBOCS; Goodman et al., 1989a, 1989b)

Four symptom dimensions often emerged in early structural analyses of the YBOCS Symptom Checklist. These symptom dimensions were labeled (1) aggressive, sexual, religious, somatic obsessions and checking compulsions; (2) symmetry, exactness obsessions and counting, and ordering compulsions; (3) dirt, contamination obsessions, and cleaning compulsions; and (4) hoarding (Baer, 1994; Leckman et al., 1997; Summerfeldt, Richter, Antony, & Swinson, 1999). A review of 12 YBOCS factor-analytic studies confirmed that four symptom dimensions accounted for most of the symptom variance in OCD: symmetry/ordering, hoarding, contamination/cleaning, and obsessions/checking (Mataix-Cols, do Rosario-Campos, & Leckman, 2005). Furthermore, the symptom domains showed some evidence of temporal stability, as well as distinct patterns of comorbidity, neural correlates, and treatment response. A later meta-analysis performed on 21 YOBCS factor-analytic studies essentially replicated this solution (Bloch et al., 2008). The authors concluded that these four dimensions account for most of the obsessive–compulsive symptom heterogeneity, although there is some uncertainty about where to place somatic and miscellaneous obsessions and checking compulsions.

There have been numerous reports of failure to replicate the four-factor symptom structure (e.g., Summerfeldt et al., 1999). Calamari, Wiegartz, and Janeck (1999) performed a cluster analysis on the YBOCS Symptom Checklist and identified five patient subgroups: harming, hoarding, contamination, certainty, and obsessions. However, an attempted replication failed to support the five-cluster solution, with a seven-group taxonomy proving more interpretable (Calamari et al., 2004). The authors noted that some clusters, such as contamination and harming, were more stable, whereas others, such as obsessions, symmetry, and certainty, were less consistent. In their taxonomic analysis of OCD symptoms and cognitions, Haslam, Williams, Kyrios, McKay, and Taylor (2005) found that only an obsessional subtype with beliefs about the importance and control of thoughts met criteria as a distinct taxon, whereas inflated responsibility, perfectionism, checking, and contamination subtypes were more dimensional in nature.

Although numerous methodological problems are apparent in the subtype research, there is sufficient empirical evidence to indicate that reliable and valid symptom subtypes have been identified, with potential clinical utility for OCD research and treatment. In their review McKay and colleagues (2004) concluded that four symptom subtypes have consistently emerged as the primary dimensions of OCD: contamination/washing, checking, hoarding, and symmetry/ordering. Sookman, Abramowitz, Calamari, Wilhelm, and McKay (2005) recommended that specialized CBT protocols be developed for specific symptom subtypes to enhance treatment effectiveness. Radomsky and Taylor (2005) questioned whether symptom subtyping might be improved by considering the functions of symptoms as well as associated psychological processes, such as the cognitive aspects of OCD. Others have argued that subtyping might be more successful if researchers took a dimensional rather than categorical approach (e.g., Clark, 2005; Mataix-Cols et al., 2005).

The empirical and clinical utility of symptom-based subtyping has been bolstered by an expanding research base. More recently, confirmatory factor analysis using the Dimensional Obsessive–Compulsive Scale (DOCS; Abramowitz et al., 2010) discovered that the symptom heterogeneity of OCD is best captured by a general obsessive–compulsive symptom factor that coexists with four specific symptom-based dimensions: contamination, responsibility for harm, unacceptable obsessional thoughts, and order/symmetry (Olatunji, Ebesutani, & Abramowitz, 2017). In the original psychometric study of the DOCS, Abramowitz and colleagues (2010) used exploratory and confirmatory factor analyses on OCD, anxiety disorder, and nonclinical samples to support the four-dimensional structure of the DOCS. The four symptom dimensions were replicable across samples, had acceptable levels of convergent and discriminant validity, and were sensitive to treatment effects. Distinct genetic correlates have been found for washing, unacceptable or forbidden obsessions, checking, and order/symmetry (López-Solà et al., 2016).

Symptom-based OCD subtypes may have a differential response to treatment. Most research has found that certain symptom dimensions, such as hoarding and, to a lesser extent, unacceptable obsessions without overt compulsions, have a poorer response to treatment (Keeley et al., 2008; Mataix-Cols et al., 2005; Sookman et al., 2005), although others have found no difference in treatment response across symptom dimensions (Chase, Wetterneck, Bartsch, Leonard, & Riemann, 2015). Except for hoarding, which is now a distinct disorder in DSM-5, Knopp and colleagues (2013) concluded in their treatment review that the association between obsessive–compulsive symptom dimensions and treatment outcome is unreliable.

In one of the most recent critical reviews of OCD subtyping, Rowsell and Francis (2015) concluded that most of the symptom-based subtypes lacked validity. Although no subtype met all six guidelines proposed by Robins and Guze (1970) for establishing validity, the authors concluded that the autonomous versus reactive classification of obsessions offered by

Lee and Kwon (2003) was the most valid, meeting five out of six criteria. This bifurcated classification is not exclusively based on symptoms because cognitive phenomena are also included in defining their dimensions.

Alternative Subtyping

As noted previously, some have argued that compulsivity is the core symptom feature in OCD. Gillan and Sahakian (2015) proposed the *habit hypothesis* of OCD, in which compulsions are the core feature of the disorder and obsessions a mere byproduct. In this conceptualization, compulsions reflect a neurobiologically based disruption in goal-directed behavior and automatic habits that is manifest as excessive habit learning. Rodgers and colleagues created two subtypes based on the notion of compulsivity: a pure compulsive and a mixed obsessive–compulsive group (Rodgers et al., 2015). The subtypes were derived from three representative Swiss community samples, with the pure compulsions group consisting of individuals with compulsions but no obsessions and the mixed group with obsessive thoughts with or without compulsions. Within those diagnosed with OCD, the mixed subtype tended to be significantly more prevalent, although 26–49% fell into the compulsion-only group. Moreover, the mixed subtype had more childhood adversity, familial burden, and higher comorbidity with other disorders.

Subtyping based on presence or absence of compulsions is reminiscent of earlier behavioral distinctions (e.g., washers vs. checkers). In clinical samples, pure compulsions may be a rare clinical presentation. In the DSM-IV field trial, less than 1% of individuals with OCD had predominantly compulsions, as based on obsession and compulsion severity scores on the YBOCS (Foa et al., 1995). However, when differentiation was based on what bothered individuals most, 50% said both obsessions and compulsions, 20% reported mainly compulsions, and 30% indicated mainly obsessions. A retrospective study of 1,086 individuals who received inpatient or outpatient treatment for OCD found that 94.4% endorsed both obsessions and compulsions on the YBOCS (Leonard & Riemann, 2012)

Clearly, parsing out those with compulsions only may not be helpful, given its low prevalence in OCD samples. As well, it may be that "pure compulsions" represents an earlier stage in the development of OCD (Rodgers et al., 2015), or these individuals may lack insight into their OCD symptoms (Leonard & Riemann, 2012). Other researchers have suggested that OCD subtyping might benefit from a consideration of the cognitive features of the disorder (Radomsky & Taylor, 2005). Most of this research has been based on the six maladaptive OCD-related beliefs (i.e., inflated responsibility, overestimated threat, importance of thought, control of thoughts, perfectionism, and intolerance of uncertainty) proposed by the Obsessive Compulsive Cognitions Working Group (OCCWG, 1997, 2001).

However, initial attempts at identifying reliable and valid OCD subtypes based on dysfunctional beliefs have not been encouraging. In their taxonomic analysis, Haslam and colleagues (2005) concluded that inflated responsibility, overestimated threat, and perfectionism were more dimensional in nature, and only the importance of thought beliefs and obsessional symptoms emerged as taxons that were potential candidates for subtyping. Some researchers have advanced a simple bifurcated categorization into high and low obsessive–compulsive belief groups (Taylor et al., 2006), although there was failure to replicate this two-cluster classification in another study (Calamari et al., 2006). Although findings have been mixed, there is reason to conclude that responsibility and threat beliefs are associated with contamination/washing; importance and control of thoughts with harm obsessions; and perfectionism and certainty beliefs with order, symmetry, and precision (Julien, O'Connor, Aardema, & Todorov, 2006; Tolin, Brady, & Hannan, 2008).

Other attempts to derive a subtype classification of OCD based on neuropsychological differences, patterns of comorbidity, or course of the disorder have failed to offer reliable and valid differentiation of OCD (for reviews, see McKay et al., 2004; Rowsell & Francis, 2015). Despite inconsistencies in the OCD subtype research, the symptom heterogeneity of OCD is undeniable, and so the search for a valid subtype classification for OCD continues. In light of these considerations, the last four chapters of the book present treatment protocols for the four symptom subtypes showing the most reliable empirical support: contamination/washing, doubt/checking, harm/sex/religion obsessions, and symmetry/order.

CONCLUSION

OCD is a complicated disorder that strikes individuals during their youth and then persists, often for a lifetime, with an intermittent worsening of symptoms that can have severe and fairly generalized negative effects on daily living and personal attainment. Although individuals are often aware of the irrationality of their fears and the futility of their rituals, they seem powerless to overcome their obsessionality. There are several treatment implications that can be drawn from the phenomenology of OCD.

- Although DSM-5 considers OCD diagnostically distinct from the anxiety disorders, obsessional states have a shared symptom presentation, high comorbidity, common psychological processes, and similar treatment response to other anxiety conditions. Therefore, the cognitive-behavioral perspective continues to consider OCD a variant of the anxiety disorders.
- Chronicity and possible reluctance to seek treatment can be

expected, especially if obsessive–compulsive symptom severity is in the mild to moderate range.
- Therapists should explore the negative impact of OCD on QOL, family relations, occupational attainment, and emotional functioning to strengthen the client's readiness motivation for treatment.
- During treatment, suicide potential must be continually monitored, especially in cases of severe OCD and/or comorbid depression and anxiety disorders.
- Assessment should include the impact of major life events on obsessive–compulsive symptom severity. As well, therapists should be mindful that symptom improvement could be due to reduction in life stress rather than to genuine treatment response.
- Because depressive symptoms are common, a thorough evaluation of depression must be included when assessing OCD. If depression is severe, treatment protocols may require modification to deal with heightened negativity, low motivation, and hopelessness.
- Clinicians can expect that many individuals with OCD will also have social anxiety, phobias, separation anxiety, pathological worry (i.e., GAD), and/or panic attacks. Therefore, assessment must be broadly based to ensure that comorbid anxiety is not overlooked in the case conceptualization.
- When treating adolescents and young adults with OCD, clinicians should be cognizant of a possible comorbid history of BDD and tic disorder. As well, a progression from obsessive–compulsive symptoms to psychosis is rare but still possible.
- Clinicians should ask about past and current use of alcohol, especially for individuals with mild to moderate obsessive–compulsive symptoms.
- Personality features should be considered when treating OCD, with a particular focus on OCPD traits such as perfectionism, preoccupation with detail, excessive concern with control, and rigidity. Some refinement in treatment may be needed to take into account personality features that have a negative impact on treatment effectiveness.
- Clinicians should identify the primary obsession and compulsion in each client in order to determine which CBT symptom protocol would be most appropriate for a particular client.

The foundation of any theory, research, or treatment of OCD begins with a solid understanding of obsessions and compulsions. However, distinguishing this phenomenology from other pathological experiences can be difficult because of the multiplicity of common features. The next two chapters address this challenge, offering an overview of the latest research into the nature of obsessions, compulsions, and their correlates.

CHAPTER 2

Obsessions, Intrusions, and Their Correlates

When individuals present with unwanted, persistent, and repetitive negative thoughts, it can be difficult to determine if the cognitive disturbance is an obsession or some other form of maladaptive thought like worry, negative automatic thoughts, or rumination. This difficulty can be seen in the following examples: (1) a man with HIV is preoccupied with whether he has put others at risk of contracting the disease; (2) a woman experiences intense anxiety that her spouse will be involved in a deadly accident each time he travels; (3) a teenager repeatedly scans her body for signs of illness for fear she'll vomit; and (4) a student is constantly distracted by faint background noise whenever she studies. OCD is the principal diagnosis in each case, but the individuals' negative repetitive thoughts involved a mix of obsessive thinking, worry, rumination, and self-criticalness. Determining which type of cognitive disturbance is most relevant depends on the context and functional characteristics of the thought process.

This chapter explores the nature of obsessive thinking. The critical defining features of obsessional phenomena are presented, as well as differences between obsessions and normal unwanted intrusive thoughts. The problem of overvalued ideation and delusional thought content is contrasted with obsessional ruminations. In addition, the similarities and differences among obsessions, worry, and negative automatic thoughts are discussed. Throughout, an emphasis is placed on identifying the critical features of obsessive thinking that must be considered when developing a cognitive case formulation for OCD.

OBSESSIONAL CONTENT

Multiplicity

Most individuals with OCD experience multiple obsessions, making it important that clinicians select the most problematic obsession for treatment. Early studies indicated that approximately half to three-quarters of individuals with OCD have multiple obsessions (Akhtar et al., 1975; Rasmussen & Eisen, 1998). An Iranian study found that 99% of adults with OCD had more than one obsession (Ghassemzadeh et al., 2002), and 88% of a pediatric OCD sample presented with multiple current obsessions and compulsions (Bernstein, Victor, Nelson, & Lee, 2013). In fact, multiple obsessions and compulsions are so common that respondents are asked to select the three primary obsessions and compulsions when completing the YBOCS Symptom Checklist (Goodman et al., 1989a, 1989b).

Temporal Instability

Not only do most individuals with OCD have multiple obsessions, but also the primary obsessional content can change over time (Skoog & Skoog, 1999). As well, obsessional symptoms emerge years before individuals meet diagnostic criteria for the full disorder. In a retrospective study involving a small sample of individuals with OCD, all reported several years of obsessive–compulsive symptoms without significant distress or impairment (Coles, Hart, & Schofield, 2012). Interestingly, increase in stress, the desire for things to feel "just right," and greater attention to one's thoughts were significant contributors to escalating the symptoms to a full-blown OCD disorder. Table 2.1 provides examples of the most prominent obsessional content encountered in clinical practice.

Obsessional content is highly individualistic and shaped by personal experiences, sociocultural influences, and critical life incidents. Moreover, there appear to be gender differences in obsessional content, with men reporting more sexual, symmetry, and exactness obsessions, and women reporting more intrusive thoughts or obsessions of dirt, aggression, and sexual victimization (Byers, Purdon, & Clark, 1998; Lensi et al., 1996). Within OCD samples, contamination obsessions and washing compulsions may be higher in women, whereas sexual/religious obsessions are elevated in men, at least in Eastern countries (Cherian et al., 2014).

Cultural Influences

The most significant impact of culture may be in the predominance of particular obsessional content. Most of the cross-cultural research concludes that contamination, harm/aggression, and pathological doubt are the most

TABLE 2.1. Clinical Examples of Different Types of Obsessions

Type of obsession	Clinical example
Dirt/contamination	• "Maybe I've contaminated myself by touching these library books." • "The clothes I'm wearing touched the floor, so I'm contaminated." • "I'm sitting in a public place that is contaminated by other people's germs, so I could get sick."
Harm/injury to self/others	• "Have I accidentally killed someone?" • "There's an image of taking a knife and stabbing the person next to me." • "I'm having repugnant thoughts of losing control and sexually assaulting a woman." • "I have the thought that my two best friends could be murdered." • "I'm plagued by recurrent questions of whether I was molested by babysitters when I was 4 years old." • "Maybe I locked someone in the freezer by mistake." • "I have the premonition that harm will come to my family if I don't complete a task that I'm doing at the time of the intrusive thought." • "Did I accidentally run over someone with the car?"
Pathological doubt	• "Did I touch these items in the store and damage them?" • "Did I make a mistake, or did I do this task completely?" • "Maybe I didn't complete the application honestly and accurately before I mailed it." • "Did I turn the stove burners completely off?"
Symmetry/exactness	• "If I am using the right side of my body too much, I must compensate and use the left side more often." • "The number 14 is unlucky and must be avoided." • "I must avoid the words *power, world,* and *harvest* because they remind me of the past and this will upset me." • "I don't understand completely what I just read."
Unacceptable sex	• "Did I deliberately touch a child for sexual purposes?" • "Am I sexually attracted to children?" • [A young heterosexual woman is anxious that she might be sexually aroused by women.] • [A married man has intrusive thoughts of oral or anal sex with other men.]
Religious	• [A woman has frequent intrusive thoughts of cursing God or of sexual slang while reading the Bible.] • [The phrase *god damn* occurs whenever the person has a religious or moral thought.] • "Did I displease God?" or "I must have displeased God today." • "I have not made the right decision that is honoring to God and so the Spirit of God has left me and I am condemned to hell."
Somatic/health concerns	• "I have repeated images of vomiting." • "I have recurrent thoughts that I'm getting sick."

prevalent themes across different countries (e.g., Ghassemzadeh et al., 2002; Girishchandra & Khanna, 2001; for a review, see Sasson et al., 1997). However, significant differences can be found in other types of obsessions. For example, religious obsessions and concerns about impurity are far more common in Eastern religious cultures than in the West (e.g., Cherian et al., 2014; Girishchandra & Khanna, 2001; Okasha, Saad, Khalil, Dawla, & Yehia, 1994). In their review of OCD samples drawn from several countries, Fontenelle and colleagues (2004) concluded there was a preponderance of aggression and religious obsessions in the Brazilian and Middle Eastern samples. A later epidemiological study across six European countries found some differences, with harm and religious/sexual obsessions higher in France and somatic obsessions higher in Italy (Fullana et al., 2010). The Dutch sample had significantly lower rates on most symptom dimensions. A multinational nonclinical study of unwanted intrusive thoughts across 11 countries revealed significant differences in the most prevalent intrusive thought content, with the largest differences involving sex, religion, and harm intrusions (Radomsky, Alcolado, et al., 2014).

Trauma-Related Obsessions

Personal life experiences and negative emotional states also influence the content of obsessional ideation. Preoccupation with aggression may be evident in OCD with a comorbid depressive disorder (Rachman & Hodgson, 1980; see also Fullana et al., 2010). The onset of obsessions may be preceded by certain traumatic or critical incidents that are thematically related to the content of the obsession (de Silva & Marks, 1999; Rhéaume, Freeston, Léger, & Ladouceur, 1998). This is evident in the case described by de Silva and Marks (1999), in which a woman developed a compulsion to pray in order to avoid further harm to herself or her mother after she had been robbed at knife point.

Several studies have found an association between traumatic life events and obsessive–compulsive symptoms, although this may be accounted for, in part, by comorbid posttraumatic stress disorder (PTSD) symptoms (Morina et al., 2016). In a series of case studies of trauma-related OCD, symptoms were functionally related such that increases in OCD-specific symptoms decreased PTSD-specific symptoms (Gershuny, Baer, Radomsky, Wilson, & Jenike, 2003). Cromer, Schmidt, and Murphy (2007) also reported a unique significant relationship between traumatic life events and OCD symptom severity, especially obsessions/checking and symmetry/ordering. Noting considerable symptom overlap and commonality in the CBT models of OCD and PTSD, Dykshoorn (2014) concluded in her review that the "impact of trauma on OCD is irrefutable" (p. 526). She described a posttraumatic OCD subgroup that should respond to conventional CBT as long as it is directed at facilitating reinterpretation of trauma-related intrusive thoughts. However, as noted in Chapter 1, Brander and colleagues (2016) concluded in their systematic review that the etiological significance of environmental factors in OCD remains uncertain. At the very least, this research indicates that life experiences, especially more severe negative events or traumas, can have an impact on clinical course and should be taken into account when planning treatment.

Obsessional Imagery

Most often obsessions are experienced as thoughts, with obsessive images (7%) and impulses (17%) reported less frequently (Akhtar et al., 1975). Rachman (2007) noted that obsessional imagery (1) has content similar to obsessive thoughts, (2) emerges fully formed and is highly consistent across situations, (3) is vivid but brief, and (4) is considered highly uncontrollable. Preliminary analysis suggests that recurring repugnant images can produce feelings of mental contamination (Rachman, 2007).

In one study that specifically assessed the presence of mental imagery, 81% of the OCD sample reported that imagery was associated with their obsessive–compulsive symptoms (Speckens, Hackmann, Ehlers, & Cuthbert, 2007). The recurrent images had a strong visual quality, and 34% focused on an earlier adverse event. Individuals who experienced mental images had more obsessive–compulsive symptoms and anxiety, engaged in more mental neutralizing, and had higher endorsement of responsibility beliefs. The authors speculated that imaginal reliving and cognitive restructuring of imagery appraisals might enhance CBT for obsessional imagery.

De Silva (1986) provided the most thorough analysis of obsessional imagery. He concluded that obsessional phenomena in the imagery modality are sufficiently different from obsessional thoughts that a different etiology and treatment modifications may be required. However, so little research has investigated obsessional imagery that most clinicians end up utilizing the same interventions that are used with obsessive thoughts.

CORE FEATURES OF OBSESSIONS

For centuries obsessions were considered distorted religious experiences until the advent of medical theories in the 19th century. Esquirol was probably the first to describe a case of OCD in 1838, although the term *obsession* is attributed to Morel in 1866 (Black, 1974). In 1878 German neurologist Karl Westphal offered one of the first comprehensive definitions of obsessions, which emphasized the emergence into consciousness of ideas that are against the will, difficult to control or suppress, but are recognized by the person as abnormal and uncharacteristic of him- or herself (Black, 1974; Rosenberg, 1968).

Contemporary definitions of obsessions emphasize, to varying degrees, the four core features of obsessional phenomena summarized in Table 2.2. None of these features are necessary or sufficient for defining a thought process as obsessive, but together they identify features of repetitive thought that determine its obsessive quality.

Intrusiveness

A fundamental characteristic of obsessions is their intrusive quality. Although often triggered by external stimuli, obsessions nevertheless intrude into conscious awareness against a person's will. It's this involuntary quality that is particularly distressing to individuals with OCD who are already concerned about loss of control over their mental faculties. The intrusive quality of obsessions is inherent to all stimulus-independent or self-generated cognitive activity like mind wandering, task-irrelevant thoughts, daydreams, and so on (Christoff, 2012; Killingsworth & Gilbert, 2010; Smallwood, 2013). Moreover, unwanted thoughts, like obsessions, have a distinct neural basis that is characterized by lower connectivity in the right dorsolateral prefrontal cortex and heightened activity in the left striatum (Kühn, Vanderhasselt, De Raedt, & Gallinat, 2014). As a product of unexpected, spontaneous cognitive activity, obsessions interrupt ongoing activity by capturing a disproportionate amount of limited attentional resource. One clinical implication of intrusiveness is that many individuals with OCD often tolerate an obsession when generated voluntarily in a therapy session but then experience the same obsession as intolerable when it is experienced as a sudden mental intrusion in the natural environment.

TABLE 2.2. The Defining Features of Obsessions

Defining features	Explanation
Intrusiveness	The thought, image, or impulse repeatedly enters consciousness in an unintended, involuntary manner; that is, it occurs against one's will.
Unacceptability	The extent that a repetitive intrusive thought is considered unwanted or undesired or engenders disapproval.
Subjective resistance	A strong urge to resist, suppress, dismiss, or prevent the obsession through avoidance, mental control strategies, or compulsive rituals.
Perceived uncontrollability	An evaluation of diminished control over the obsession that is considered unacceptable and threatening.

Unacceptability

Another important characteristic of unwanted mental intrusions or obsessions is their personal unacceptability, undesirability, or perceived disapproval (e.g., England & Dickerson, 1988). This characteristic involves the personal meaning attributed to the unwanted intrusive thought. An intrusion could be unacceptable because (1) it threatens or is incongruent with a person's core values, (2) its very occurrence diminishes self-worth, or (3) it is associated with high subjective distress. In their original study on unwanted intrusive thoughts, Parkinson and Rachman (1981a) found that intrusions deemed unacceptable were more distressing and difficult to control. Freeston and Ladouceur (1993) showed that appraisals of intrusions as low probability but high disapproval were associated with a greater use of maladaptive escape/avoidance control strategies. Also, OCD research on the self suggests that obsessions may be distressing because they threaten values that are inherent to the person's self-view (see Ahern & Kyrios, 2016; Doron & Kyrios, 2005; García-Soriano & Belloch, 2012). Thus, significant incongruence or threats to self-worth are another reason for evaluating the degree of unacceptability.

Resistance

In DSM-5, efforts to ignore, suppress, or neutralize recurrent and persistent thoughts are a central feature of obsessions (APA, 2013). This attribute, called *resistance,* is what differentiated clinical obsessions from normal intrusive thoughts in the Rachman and de Silva (1978) study. Although the degree of resistance against the obsession varies, individuals with OCD are highly motivated to ignore, suppress, or neutralize the distressing thought. The desire to rid one's mind of the obsession is fueled by the belief that highly undesirable consequences will occur to self, or others, if the obsession is not successfully terminated. Other research indicates that individuals with OCD have significantly higher ratings on the importance of controlling the obsession than non-OCD clinical and nonclinical groups (García-Soriano, Roncero, Perpiña, & Belloch, 2014; Morillo, Belloch, & García-Soriano, 2007). As well, individuals' most upsetting obsession is associated with higher ratings of importance and control of thoughts than the least upsetting obsession (Rowa, Purdon, Summerfeldt, & Antony, 2005). Overall, perceived importance and degree of resistance are important characteristics of the obsessive experience.

Perceived Uncontrollability

Despite strong motivation to resist, individuals with OCD invariably perceive that their efforts at control are short-lived and inadequate at best.

This leads to a heightened sense of subjective uncontrollability over the obsession. Numerous studies on both clinical and nonclinical samples have shown a strong association between frequency, distress, and perceived uncontrollability of unwanted intrusive thoughts and obsessions (e.g., Clark & de Silva, 1985; García-Soriano & Belloch, 2013; Morillo et al., 2007; Purdon & Clark, 1994a; Rachman & de Silva, 1978). However, it would appear that individuals with OCD do not exhibit an actual decrement in their ability to control their obsessions (Janeck & Calamari, 1999; Purdon, Rowa, & Antony, 2005; for a review, see Magee, Harden, & Teachman, 2012). Thus, the most relevant characteristic for obsessions is the perception of uncontrollability rather than actual mental control ability.

The four core features of obsessions (Table 2.2) are dimensions on which specific obsessional content will vary in degree or intensity. Thus, obsessions differ in the composition or relative contribution of each characteristic, although we would expect most obsessions to show all four attributes to varying degrees. These constructs are useful in distinguishing obsessions from other types of negative cognition, as well as in distinguishing normal from abnormal obsessions.

OBSESSIONS AND UNWANTED INTRUSIVE THOUGHTS

DSM-5 (APA, 2013) takes a categorical perspective on OCD, which means that individuals either meet diagnostic criteria or they do not. In 1978, Stanley Rachman and Padmal de Silva published a controversial study that challenged this categorical conceptualization of obsessions. In two studies, they compared nonclinical individuals and those with OCD to determine whether both groups experienced unwanted, obsessive-like intrusive thoughts, images, and impulses. The results were striking. They found that 84% of their nonclinical participants reported unwanted cognitive intrusions that were qualitatively similar in form and content to clinical obsessions. Not surprisingly, clinical obsessions were rated as more frequent, intense, and uncontrollable, and more likely associated with neutralizing responses, than were the unwanted intrusions of the nonclinical participants. In subsequent years, other researchers have replicated these findings (e.g., Calamari & Janeck, 1997; García-Soriano & Belloch, 2013; Morillo et al., 2007).

Numerous studies have found that most individuals (80–90%) experience intrusive, obsessive-like thoughts, images, or impulses (e.g., Clark & de Silva, 1985; Freeston, Ladouceur, Thibodeau, & Gagnon, 1991; Parkinson & Rachman, 1981a; Purdon & Clark, 1993; Radomsky, Alcolado, et al., 2014; Salkovskis & Harrison, 1984). The cognitive phenomena investigated in these studies have been labeled *unwanted intrusive thoughts*. They are defined as thoughts, images, or impulses that (1) interrupt ongoing activity, (2) are recognized as having an internal origin, and (3) are difficult to control (Rachman, 1981). Unwanted intrusive thoughts are often triggered by a person's current concerns and situations, including stressful experiences (e.g., Horowitz, 1975; Parkinson & Rachman, 1981b). As a result, unwanted cognitive intrusions are a transdiagnostic phenomenon that can be found in other clinical states, such as depression (Brewin, Hunter, Carroll, & Tata, 1996; Wahl et al., 2011), PTSD (Michael, Ehlers, Halligan, & Clark, 2005), eating disorders (García-Soriano et al., 2014), serious medical illness (Whitaker, Watson, & Brewin, 2009), and generalized anxiety (Gross & Eifert, 1990). However, certain segments of the population, like incarcerated individuals with elevated psychopathy, may be less likely to report unwanted intrusive thoughts (O'Neill, Nenzel, & Caldwell, 2009).

Evidence of "normal obsessions" in the general population is a key construct in CBT theories of OCD. From the cognitive perspective, normal unwanted intrusive thoughts develop into pathological obsessions when individuals misinterpret the intrusions as a significant personal threat that must be neutralized (Rachman, 2003; Salkovskis, 1985). In recent years, several researchers have challenged this continuity assumption of the CBT perspective. Julien, O'Connor, and Aardema (2009) found that most of the intrusions in their nonclinical sample were directly related to an environment trigger, whereas the intrusions in the OCD participants more often had indirect links to the environmental context. In a later study, intrusions judged as relevant to OCD were more likely to lack a reality basis, whereas the non-OCD-relevant intrusions were more likely rated as ego-syntonic and have links to the here and now (Audet, Aardema, & Moulding, 2016). Others have argued for a qualitative difference in the content of normal and abnormal obsessions (Rassin, Cougle, & Muris, 2007; Rassin & Muris, 2006). Despite these objections, there is considerable evidence that the obsessive themes most common in OCD also are frequently seen in the unwanted intrusions of nonclinical individuals (i.e., Rachman & Hodgson, 1980; Radomsky, Alcolado, et al., 2014)

The continuity of normal and abnormal obsessions also is consistent with a dimensional perspective on OCD more generally. CBT models adhere to the view that clinical and nonclinical differences in obsessive–compulsive symptoms are a matter of degree rather than kind. Support for the dimensionality of OCD is evident in community-based studies that report rates of 2–20% of subthreshold OCD (for review, see Gibbs, 1996). Other research also found elevated levels of obsessive and compulsive symptoms in the general population that is greater than the prevalence of diagnosable OCD (Fineberg et al., 2013; Nestadt, Samuels, Romanoski, Folstein, & McHugh, 1994; Stein, Forde, Anderson, & Walker, 1997; Subramanian et al., 2012; Welkowitz, Struening, Pittman, Guardino, & Welkowitz, 2000). Individuals with an OCD disorder often report a gradual onset, during which they experience years of subthreshold obsessive–compulsive symptoms (Coles et al., 2012; Pinto, Mancebo, Eisne, Pagano, & Rasmussen, 2006).

There is considerable empirical evidence, then, for a continuity perspective on obsessions. Distressing intrusive thoughts are upsetting phenomena for most people, whether or not they suffer from an obsessional disorder (see Clark, 2018; also Forrester, Wilson, & Salkovskis, 2002). The critical difference between normal and abnormal obsessions lies in how the mental intrusion is evaluated and responded to, rather than in the content or occurrence of specific types of cognition (Gibbs, 1996). Table 2.3 presents various dimensions that can be used to determine the clinical status of unwanted intrusive cognition.

These differential features are based on research that directly compared individuals with OCD and nonclinical participants (Calamari & Janeck, 1997; Garcia-Sorianó & Belloch, 2013; Julien et al., 2009; Morillo et al., 2007; Rachman & de Silva, 1978). Clinicians can use the table as a checklist to determine whether an individual's experience of repetitive negative thought meets the threshold for clinical obsessions and is therefore appropriate for the CBT protocols presented in subsequent chapters. Of course, obsessions must be differentiated from other types of repetitive thinking that require a different treatment approach, such as delusions, worry, and rumination.

TABLE 2.3. Criteria for Distinguishing between Normal and Abnormal Obsessions

Normal obsessions	Abnormal obsessions
Less frequent	More frequent
Less unacceptable/distressing	More unacceptable/distressing
Little associated guilt	Significant feelings of guilt
Less resistance to the intrusion	Strong resistance to the intrusion
Some perceived control	Diminished perceived control over the obsession
Considered meaningless, irrelevant to the self	Considered highly meaningful, threatening important core values of the self (ego-dystonic)
Brief intrusions that fail to dominate conscious awareness	Time-consuming intrusions that dominate conscious awareness
Less concern with thought control	Heightened concern with thought control
Less emphasis on neutralizing distress	Strong focus on neutralizing distress associated with the obsession
Less interference in daily living	Significant interference in daily living

INSIGHT, OVERVALUED IDEATION, AND DELUSIONS

The Insight Continuum

Many early writers assumed that an individual's insight into the excessive or unreasonable nature of the obsession was its defining feature (e.g., Jaspers, 1963; Schneider, 1925, as cited in Black, 1974). However, contemporary research indicates that insight is not a necessary criterion for obsessions. In the DSM-IV field trial for OCD, only 13% of the sample were certain that their feared consequences would not occur (i.e., had insight into the unreasonableness of their obsessions), whereas 26% were mostly certain that the consequences would occur, and 4% were completely certain that the feared consequences would occur (Foa et al., 1995). It is estimated that 15–36% of individuals with OCD have poor insight (see Alonso et al., 2008). This variability is captured by the DSM-5 specifier that distinguishes between good, poor, or absent insight–delusional beliefs.

Most individuals with OCD recognize the excessive nature of their obsessions. Frequently, a person with OCD will exclaim, "I know this is so silly, but I get really upset if I think the light switch is not completely off." But what about the person with OCD who really believes that a light switch not "absolutely off" could cause an electrical fire? In this case the person might not consider his or her obsessive doubt and repeated light-switch checking unreasonable.

It is well known that insight into one's obsessions is situation bound, with insight highest in nonthreatening but lower in threatening situations (Kozak & Foa, 1994; Steketee & Shapiro, 1995). If the person is not around children, for example, the intrusive thought of child molestation seems truly absurd. However, when in the presence of children, the obsessive thought can be quite convincing, given its persistence and associated distress. Thus, insight is a dynamic construct that fluctuates over time and across situations.

Poor insight into the excessive nature of one's obsessions and compulsions has important clinical implications. Several studies found that individuals with poor insight have greater obsessive–compulsive symptom severity, higher comorbidity, longer illness duration, and earlier age of onset (Alonso et al., 2008; Catapano et al., 2010; Jakuboski et al., 2011; Türksoy, Tükel, Özdemir, & Karali, 2002). Poor insight may be associated with weaker treatment response, although the outcome research is inconsistent (Alonso et al., 2008; Catapano et al., 2010). Moreover, insight into the senselessness of obsessive–compulsive symptoms is broadly distributed and varies along a continuum. Poor insight might be more evident in religious or harming obsessions (Tolin, Abramowitz, Kozak, & Foa, 2001), and it may have more impact on the treatment of compulsions than obsessions (Neziroglu, Stevens, McKay, & Yaryura-Tobia, 2001).

Considerable interest has focused on those individuals who exhibit a fairly constant and unwavering conviction in the reasonableness of the obsession fear. For these individuals, the obsession may have developed into an overvalued idea (OVI) or possibly even a delusion. Insel and Akiskal (1986) originally proposed that OCD can vary along a continuum of insight from obsessions to overvalued ideation to psychotic-like delusions. For the latter condition, they suggested the term *obsessive–compulsive psychosis.*

Overvalued Ideation

Wernicke first introduced the term *overvalued ideation (OVI)* in 1900 to refer to a solitary belief that a person feels justified in holding and that strongly determines the person's behavior (see Kozak & Foa, 1994). Jaspers (1963) noted that OVIs also involve strong personal identification and fairly intense affect. However, it was Foa's (1979) research on behavioral treatment failure in OCD that reignited interest in OVI and its relevance to OCD. She found that 4 of the 10 individuals with OCD who did not respond successfully to behavior therapy believed that their obsessive thoughts or fears were realistic and that their compulsive behavior actually prevented the occurrence of the perceived negative consequences associated with the obsession.

At first, research on OVI was hampered by poor conceptualization and inadequate measurement. The relationship of OVI to concepts such as insight, judgment, belief, and delusions has not been well articulated (see discussion by Neziroglu & Stevens, 2002). The most widely accepted view is that OVIs are "strongly held unreasonable beliefs that are not as firmly held as delusional ideas" (Kozak & Foa, 1994, p. 344). Thus, the main difference between obsessions, OVIs, and delusions is how firmly the erroneous idea is held (i.e., the strength or fixity of belief). Veale (2002) offered a broader cognitive-behavioral perspective on OVI that emphasizes not only strength of belief but also excessive identification or importance of the value (idea) for the self and the degree of rigidity or inflexibility of the idealized value.

Two clinician-administered rating scales were developed to provide a standardized measure of OVI: the Brown Assessment of Beliefs Scale (Eisen et al., 1998) and the Overvalued Ideas Scale (Neziroglu, McKay, Yaryura-Tobias, Stevens, & Todaro, 1999). The Overvalued Ideas Scale has good internal consistency, test–retest stability, and convergent and discriminant validity (Neziroglu et al., 1999), although both measures are highly correlated (Shimshoni, Reuven, Dar, & Hermesh, 2011). Later studies have used these measures to provide a more accurate assessment of the impact of OVI on treatment response (e.g., Alonso et al., 2008; Catapano et al., 2010).

Some studies have found that high OVI was associated with reduced treatment response (Basoglu, Lax, Kasvikis, & Marks, 1988; Foa, 1979; Foa, Abramowitz, Franklin, & Kozak, 1999; Neziroglu et al., 2001), whereas others did not find that it predicted poor outcome (Lelliott, Noshirvani, Basoglu, Marks, & Monteiro, 1988). In the Neziroglu and colleagues (2001) study, scores on the Overvalued Ideation Scale were correlated with residual gains in compulsions but not obsessions. However, there is evidence that OCD with OVI can be successfully treated with cognitive and behavioral therapy (Lelliott et al., 1988; Salkovskis & Warwick, 1985) or medication (O'Dwyer & Marks, 2000).

Further research is needed to determine the extent that lack of insight or OVI is a poor prognostic indicator for OCD. It may be that better outcome is achieved with longer treatment (Catapano et al., 2010) and interventions tailored to the individual's strong belief in obsessional concerns. At the very least, clinicians should assess level of insight and introduce cognitive intervention that targets the maladaptive beliefs that characterize poor insight.

Delusions

Delusions are "fixed beliefs that are not amenable to change in light of conflicting evidence" (APA, 2013, p. 87). DSM-5 emphasizes that the main distinction between a strongly held belief (i.e., OVI) and a delusion is the degree of conviction held in the delusion even when confronted with clear contradictory evidence of its validity (APA, 2013).

Early writings proposed a link between OCD and schizophrenia spectrum disorders (Enright, 1996; Insel & Akiskal, 1986; Stengel, 1945). As noted previously, development of schizophrenia is no more likely than the rate seen in other emotional disorders (Rachman & Hodgson, 1980; Stein & Hollander, 1993; Torres et al., 2006). However, psychotic symptoms are more prevalent in OCD samples (Adam et al., 2012), although these usually present as poor insight and strong conviction in the veracity of the obsessional fear (Kozak & Foa, 1994; see also Welner et al., 1976).

Given their relevance to OCD, it is important to differentiate OVI from delusions. In their review, Eisen, Phillips, and Rasmussen (1999) concluded that obsessions, OVI, and delusions occur on a continuum of insight, with delusional OCD being extremely rare. However, individuals with OCD and high OVI may exhibit cognitive dysfunction that has similar characteristics to that seen in schizophrenia (Kitis et al., 2007), although others suggest that high conviction in OCD does not show the same reasoning bias evident in delusional disorder (Jacobsen, Freeman, & Salkovskis, 2012). Furthermore, in the rare instances that delusions are present in OCD, it may be that comorbid depression and schizotypal personality disorder have contributed to their development (Fear, Sharp, & Healy, 2000).

Despite some inconsistencies in the research literature, clinicians are still faced with the challenge of differentiating poor insight, OVI, and delusions when developing an individualized case formulation and treatment plan. A delusional disorder may be suspected when

- Belief in the obsession is held with such firm conviction that it is entirely unresponsive to clear contradictory evidence.
- The obsession has a bizarre, implausible quality that is disconnected from ordinary life experience.
- There is less distress associated with repeated occurrences of the obsession (i.e., delusion).

DIFFERENTIATING WORRY, RUMINATION, AND OBSESSIONS

Repetitiveness is a prominent feature of many types of cognition such as worry, rumination, planning, problem solving, perseverative cognition, and the like (Watkins, 2008). Considered a transdiagnostic concept, repetitive thought is "the process of thinking attentively, repetitively, or frequently about oneself and one's world" (Segerstrom, Stanton, Alden, & Shortridge, 2003, p. 909). Watkins (2008) noted that repetitive thought can be constructive or unconstructive, with the latter prominent in negative emotional states. Worry and rumination are two forms of negative repetitive thought that are well researched as core cognitive features of anxiety and depression, respectively. Although involving different content and temporal orientation, worry and rumination share many of the same appraisal, goal disruption, and mental control processes (Segerstrom, Tsao, Alden, & Craske, 2000; Watkins, Moulds, & Mackintosh, 2005). Therefore, it is important to consider both rumination and worry when differentiating obsessions from other types of negative cognition.

Watkins (2008) did not include obsessive thinking in his taxonomy of unconstructive repetitive thought. Possibly the intrusive and nonvolitional nature of obsessions led to their exclusion. However, there are many similarities between repetitive negative thought and obsessions such as their high frequency, uncontrollability, negative content, self-relevance, and disruption of goals concerning safety, security, or certainty (see Ehring & Watkins, 2008). As well, individuals with OCD experience elevated levels of worry and rumination (Calleo, Hart, Björgvinsson, & Stanley, 2010; Wahl et al., 2011; see also Ehring & Watkins, 2008). Clearly, clinicians must be able to distinguish obsessions, worry, and rumination to construct an accurate case formulation.

Worry

The human capacity to generate mental representations of various possible future threats is the basis of worry (Borkovec, 1994). Worry is "a persistent, repetitive, and uncontrollable chain of thinking that mainly focuses on the uncertainty of some future negative or threatening outcome in which the person rehearses various problem-solving solutions but fails to reduce the heightened sense of uncertainty about the possible threat" (Clark & Beck, 2010, p. 235). Worry is a verbal–linguistic form of mentation that is focused on actual or potential nonattainment of goals in important life domains (Borkovec, 1994; Eysenck, 1992; Wells & Matthews, 1994). It deals with real or imagined threat to a wide range of personal and social concerns related to the safety, security, and vitality of the individual. Normal daily experiences are often represented in worry content (Wells, 2005). Consequently, worry is associated with increased anxiety and a sense of uncontrollability.

Although adaptive worry is characterized by problem solving that leads to an effective response to a difficult life situation (Mathews, 1990), it is pathological worry that is more relevant to OCD. Its main features are:

- Pervasiveness
- Time-consuming protractedness
- Uncontrollability
- Selective threat bias
- Focus on minor matters or remote but significant personal threats
- Restricted autonomic reactivity

Consequently, it is pathological worry that is associated with heightened anxiety and distress, and is the cardinal feature of GAD.

Pathological worry is prominent in OCD, as indicated by the prevalence of comorbid GAD (Adam et al., 2012; Fineberg et al., 2013) and the prominence of worry symptoms (Brown et al., 1993). Moreover, measures of obsessive–compulsive symptoms and worry are correlated in both clinical and nonclinical samples (Calleo et al., 2010; Freeston, Ladouceur, et al., 1994; Macatee et al., 2016; van Rijsoort, Emmelkamp, & Vervaeke, 2001). To complicate matters, OCD and GAD share several underlying cognitive processes, such as deficits in inhibitory control of responses, threat overestimation, intolerance of uncertainty, low attentional control, and negative intrusive thoughts (Brown, Dowdall, Côté, & Barlow, 1994; Fergus & Wu, 2010; Gentes & Rusico, 2011; Macatee et al., 2016; Nota, Schubert, & Coles, 2016; Turner, Beidel, & Stanley, 1992; Wells, 2005). How, then, can these cognitive phenomena be differentiated so that a precise case formulation is developed? Table 2.4 presents several characteristics that distinguish obsessions from worry.

TABLE 2.4. **Differential Features of Obsessions and Worry**

Obsessions	Worry
Content is contrary to, or at least uncharacteristic of, valued domains of self-representation.	Content is highly congruent with or characteristic of core self-relevant concerns.
Occurs in varied forms as distinct thoughts, images, or urges.	Occurs primarily as a chain of thinking.
Often it is the repetitiveness of the thought occurrence that is most distressing.	The primary source of distress is the imagined negative outcome of a real-life situation.
Strong evidence of thought–action fusion.	Less evidence of thought–action fusion.
Greater perceived responsibility for the thought.	Possibly less perceived responsibility for the thought.
Negative affect linked to intrusion content.	Strong negative affect related to the real-life worry concern.
Strongly resisted (i.e., mental control effort)	Moderately resisted
Highly intrusive and unwanted	Moderately intrusive and unwanted
Moderate subjective uncontrollability	High subjective uncontrollability
Strong belief in the importance and control (suppression) of thought	Moderate belief in importance and control of thought
High likelihood of associated neutralization	Moderate likelihood of associated neutralization
Interpreted as highly unacceptable	Interpreted as moderately unacceptable
More likely viewed as implausible (e.g., bizarre, senseless)	Quite plausible although exaggerated
Less amenable to rational disputation	Somewhat amenable to rational disputation

Note. Based on research comparing obsessions and worry (i.e., Calleo et al., 2010; Clark & Claybourn, 1997; Coles, Mennin, & Heimberg, 2001; Fergus & Wu, 2010; Langlois, Freeston, & Ladouceur, 2000a, 2000b; Wells & Morrison, 1994; see also Ehring & Watkins, 2008; Wells, 2005).

Not only do worry and obsessions share many similarities, but individuals with OCD can worry about their obsessional concerns (e.g., "What if my OCD gets worse and I can't function?") as well as about the same types of life concerns that preoccupy non-OCD pathological worriers (e.g., "What if I lose my job and have to declare bankruptcy?"). To complicate matters, many of the differences between obsessions and worry are a matter of degree rather than kind. And yet, a different treatment protocol is needed for obsessions and worry, so correctly identifying each form of pathological thinking is important to treatment integrity.

To illustrate the difference between obsessions and worry, consider Louise, the case example in Chapter 1. Louise had physical contamination OCD and so several times a day she had the obsessive thought "Have I become contaminated by touching something dirty?" In addition, Louise struggled with worry about her OCD, often having worry episodes focused on whether her OCD could get so bad that she could no longer work or look after her family. Although both types of maladaptive thinking are relevant to physical contamination OCD, the thought processes are quite different. When Louise had the obsession about contamination, the thought was experienced as a distinct mental intrusion, often triggered by an external stimulus, but clearly unwanted and distressing. The thought itself was inconsistent with Louise's self-view as a cautious, responsible person who avoids risk and seeks safety and security for herself and others. The very existence of such thinking was a highly threatening experience that indicated she really might be contaminated. There was a strong urge to repel the thought and neutralize the feeling of anxiety and perceived uncertainty.

Louise experienced her worry about the consequences of OCD quite differently. The worry came as a chain of thought in which she considered all the ways in which OCD could get worse and impair her ability to function. Her focus was not so much on the worry thought itself, but rather on what life would be like if she ceased to function at home and work. She felt a mounting sense of anxiety and sadness as she thought what would happen to her family if she became more incapacitated by her obsessions and compulsions. Her thinking felt uncontrollable as she jumped from one related stream of thought to the next, all the while focused on how she was failing her family. She searched for solutions, for ways to avoid this impending calamity, but nothing worthwhile came to mind. She became convinced that she was a pathetic wife and mother, and could only see future misery and heartache for her family—heartache she had caused but was powerless to change. For Louise these worry episodes were activated by long-standing core beliefs of being weak, helpless, and vulnerable, and now the worry was more evidence of the seriousness of her predicament.

Rumination

Rumination is a type of self-focused, repetitive thought involving an attempt to make sense of a past upsetting event or solve a problem that is creating a perceived discrepancy between a desired goal and one's current state (Watkins, 2016). Watkins notes that rumination is a normal thought process that is usually quite brief but triggered by unresolved concerns or unattained goals. It persists until a desired goal is attained or abandoned. Some examples of normal rumination are:

- Thinking back to an important meeting and wondering whether you appeared competent and well prepared or insecure and inept.
- Trying to understand the cause and consequence of a recent cancer diagnosis.
- Thinking about being forced to take early retirement.
- Wondering why your adult daughter is so cold and distant toward you.
- Trying to understand why your OCD has gotten worse and what this means for the future.

Watkins (2016) stated that rumination often involves shifting between trying to solve a problem that is perceived as a setback and efforts to evaluate the meaning of the problem. He noted that rumination becomes excessive when (1) important life goals are difficult to attain and hard to abandon and (2) problem-solving skills are inadequate for goal attainment. Depression researchers have taken the most interest in rumination, in large part due to the pioneering work of Nolen-Hoeksema (1991). Numerous studies have shown that rumination is associated with an increase in depressive states (e.g., Nolen-Hoeksema, 2000; Riso et al., 2003; Spasojević & Alloy, 2001), and it is a mediator between stressful life events and depression (Michl, McLaughlin, Shepherd, & Nolen-Hoeksema, 2013; Nolen-Hoeksema, Parker, & Larson, 1994).

Excessive rumination is often present in OCD. Since most individuals with OCD experience a depressive episode and concurrent depressive symptoms are prevalent, maladaptive rumination can be expected. Moreover, there is considerable overlap in the cognitive processes involved in rumination and obsessions, so distinguishing between the two is an important clinical issue.

It is worth noting that some writers refer to obsessions without compulsions as "pure obsessions" or *obsessional rumination* (i.e., Clark & Guyitt, 2008). However, in this context the term *rumination* has a different meaning from its use in the depression literature. In his discussion paper, de Silva (2003) commented that an obsession cannot be rumination, and so concluded that "an obsessional rumination is a compulsive cognitive activity that is carried out in response to an obsessional thought" (p. 198). He provided several clinical examples of this type of phenomena, mainly dealing with existential questions like "Is there life after death?"; "What is the meaning of life?"; "Am I genetically flawed?"; and so on.

In one of the few studies to directly compare obsessions and rumination, Wahl and colleagues (2011) investigated both phenomena in OCD versus major depressive disorder. The OCD sample reported frequent and distressing rumination, but obsessions were much less frequent in the depressed group. Moreover, there were differences in how both types of negative cognition were experienced, with ruminations more past-oriented and realistic, and obsessions more visual, irrational, and associated with a greater urge to act. Rumination, of course, is very similar to worry, with the main difference being in their temporal orientation. Worry is future-oriented whereas rumination focuses on past experiences (Watkins, 2016). Many of the distinctions listed in Table 2.4 can be used to differentiate obsessions from rumination.

The following example illustrates how rumination might occur in a person with religious obsessions. Imagine that the primary obsession is "Have I offended God?" Each time the person makes a decision, the obsession returns and she thinks, "Have I made a wrong choice that displeases God?" At the same time, the individual feels tormented by memories of a difficult childhood. Her father was cold, rejecting, and critical. She spends hours thinking back to her childhood, distraught over her father's uncaring attitude and wondering why he didn't seem to love her. Although one might be tempted to draw similarities between thoughts of "offending God" and the distressing memories of her childhood, the first is clearly an obsession, whereas the latter is an example of rumination. In this case, the therapist will need to adopt different strategies to modify the religious obsession and the rumination about the client's childhood.

CONCLUSION

CBT for OCD places considerable emphasis on the treatment of obsessions. Thus, a thorough understanding of obsessive thought is a prerequisite for effective treatment. And yet, obsessions are highly varied in form and content, having both common and distinct features with other types of repetitive negative thought that are also experienced by individuals with OCD. Several points raised in this chapter should be incorporated into cognitive case conceptualization and treatment planning:

- Most individuals with OCD have multiple obsessions that change over time and are influenced by culture, personal experiences, and significant life events. It is important that clinicians select the *primary obsession* currently responsible for the greatest amount of distress and functional impairment, at the same recognizing this could change with time and different life circumstances.
- Assessment should include a screen for past traumatic experiences and their role in the etiology and maintenance of obsessions. If traumatic obsessions are present, trauma-focused interventions should be integrated into the CBT protocol.
- Obsessive thinking is characterized by intrusiveness, unacceptability, resistance, and uncontrollability. It becomes pathological when there is increased frequency and distress, greater disconnect from

reality, greater interference in daily living, a stronger urge to neutralize, and it is increasingly time-consuming.
- Level of insight into the excessiveness of the obsession is one indicator of treatment readiness. Adjustments to the cognitive treatment ingredients will be needed to take into account the presence of poor insight.
- Standardized measures can be used to identify OVI and the possibility of delusional disorder in extreme cases. If OVI is present, expect a longer course of treatment and include cognitive restructuring that addresses maladaptive beliefs about the veridicality of the obsession.
- During assessment and case formulation, consider whether worry and rumination are significant features in the clinical presentation. If different types of repetitive negative thought are present (e.g., obsessions, worry, rumination), therapists must be able to distinguish between them.

For the past two decades, CBT has placed greater emphasis on obsessions than on compulsions. The latter were considered a response to the obsessions and already effectively treated with ERP. It was the obsessions that seemed less responsive to standard behavior therapy, especially obsessions without overt compulsions (Rachman, 1983). The introduction of cognitive therapy into standard ERP was intended to address behavior therapy's weaker effects on obsessions. However, the pendulum may have swung too far, prompting several researchers to argue for greater attention to compulsions (Bucarelli & Purdon, 2015; Wahl, Salkovskis, & Cotter, 2008). The next chapter is devoted to compulsions and related processes as major contributors to the pathogenesis of OCD.

CHAPTER 3

Compulsions, Neutralization, and Control

Any response to an obsession can become a compulsion if it occurs repeatedly in order to neutralize the obsession, reduce distress, or prevent/undo its feared outcome. Consider the following examples:

- A woman scrubs her hands vigorously dozens of times daily with abrasive detergents because she feels dirty and contaminated by toxic chemicals.
- A man spends hours reading and rereading outdated supermarket flyers for fear that he has missed an item or not fully understood what he's read.
- A student can't stop studying until he achieves the "feeling of knowing."
- An engineer spends hours each week searching the Internet and other sources for evidence of the end of the world.
- A woman can't stop asking her family and close friends whether she looks sick even though she knows they find her relentless questions frustrating.

Compulsions, or its more technical term *neutralization,* are just as important in the pathogenesis of OCD as obsessions and so deserve equal attention in any CBT of OCD. The novice therapist might assume that compulsions are easier to treat than obsessions, but nothing could be further from the truth. There is a paradox to compulsivity in OCD that makes treatment challenging. On the one hand, individuals experience irresistible urges to perform rituals (i.e., compulsions) that cause substantial interference and impairment in daily living, and yet, they most often realize these actions are irrational, even senseless. This is evident in the 52-year-old government official who had repeated thoughts of being responsible for fatal accidents happening to others and so felt compelled to check newspapers and other sources to determine whether he had inadvertently harmed someone. In another example, a 41-year-old homemaker had an irresistible urge to check her freezer to ensure that no one was locked inside, even though she realized this was a silly idea. Often individuals with OCD are frustrated that they keep giving into these self-defeating compulsions when they know they're nonsensical.

This chapter focuses on compulsions and its correlates. The nature and function of various types of responses to obsessions are discussed, including compulsive rituals, avoidance behavior, covert neutralization, cognitive avoidance, and excessive reassurance seeking. Research on the "stop criteria" used to determine when a compulsive cycle ceases is considered. The chapter concludes with a discussion of thought suppression and the importance of mental control in OCD. Throughout the chapter clinical recommendations and resource materials are provided that therapists can use to more fully assess neutralization and control when treating individuals with OCD.

BEHAVIORAL COMPULSIONS

Compulsions are "perseverative, repetitive actions that are excessive and inappropriate to a situation" (Berlin & Hollander, 2014, p. 62). This is a broad definition that recognizes that compulsions can range from higher-order cognitive responses, like praying or mentally rehearsing what was just spoken, to simple motor responses like tapping repeatedly, checking, or washing (Berlin & Hollander, 2014). Berlin and Hollander (2014) consider compulsivity a transdiagnostic construct that is evident to varying degrees in several disorders, including autism, pathological gambling, and attention-deficit/hyperactivity disorder (ADHD). Compulsions such as checking and reassurance seeking are apparent in GAD and hypochondriasis (Fallon, Javitch, Hollander, & Liebowitz, 1991; Schut, Castonguay, & Borkovec, 2001). However, it is in OCD where compulsions are most prominent and play a definitive role in the phenomenology of the disorder.

Compulsions are found in the general population. Many nonclinical individuals report that they sometimes or often perform ritualistic behaviors involving (1) checking; (2) cleaning, washing, and ordering; (3) "magical" protective behaviors; or (4) avoidance of certain objects (Muris, Merckelbach, & Clavan, 1997). Moreover, certain population subgroups, such as postpartum women, report a higher incidence of compulsive symptoms even among those who do not meet criteria for OCD (Miller, Hoxha, Wisner, & Gossett, 2015). As well, compulsion induction procedures in healthy participants can produce cognitive and emotional changes that are relevant to obsessive–compulsive behaviors (e.g., Deacon & Maack, 2008; Radomsky, Dugas, Alcolado, & Lavoie, 2014; Radmonsky, Gilchrist, & Dussault, 2006; for a review, see Abramowitz et al., 2014), although the effects may be weaker than in OCD samples (de Putter, Van Yper, & Koster, 2017). Phenomenologically, clinical compulsions occur with greater frequency and intensity, elicit more resistance and discomfort, and are more often executed in response to a distressing thought or negative mood state.

Defining Features

There are several characteristics of OCD compulsions that distinguish them from other types of perseverative responses. Form 3.1* presents a checklist that can be used to distinguish OCD compulsions from other forms of perseverative response. The features listed in this checklist are derived from several sources on the characteristics of clinical compulsions (e.g., Berlin & Hollander, 2014; Chamberlain, Fineberg, Blackwell, Robbins, & Sahakian, 2006; Rachman & Shafran, 1998). It is expected that compulsions will exhibit many of these characteristics to varying degrees, with the more features checked increasing the likelihood that the response meets clinical criteria. The following illustrative example of order and rearranging compulsions highlights the clinical utility of the checklist.

Let's assume that a neat and tidy person, whom we'll call Charles, had the reputation of being fastidious at work. He prided himself on having high standards, though he was often criticized for being too slow and pedantic. Charles valued order and balance in his life, and had great difficulty tolerating any form of confusion, irregularity, or mess in his personal living space. He was constantly tidying up at home to the point that he could never sit still, relax, or enjoy life. Also, he was spending so much time organizing his work that he was failing to meet important deadlines. Of course, being neat and well organized is a positive attribute, so determining whether the behavior is a compulsion can be challenging.

During the assessment the clinician could begin by asking Charles about his "tidying" experience, keeping in mind the various statements in Form 3.1. Charles reported a strong urge to tidy anything that looked messy or out of place. He couldn't relax until he felt everything was "just right" (i.e., a form of neutralization). Most often he considered his concern for neatness to be reasonable but recognized that at times it got excessive and uncontrollable. Threat avoidance was not associated with the behavior, but the tidying had become repetitive, such that Charles often performed the same actions over and over. He tried to stop himself "straightening up" books, magazines, and other items, but it was difficult to resist. Clearly, Charles's

---

*All forms and handouts appear at the ends of chapters.

tidying behavior met several criteria for clinical compulsions listed in Form 3.1. He had (1) a strong urge to engage in the behavior, (2) a desire to feel "just right" that served a neutralization function, (3) varying insight into its unreasonableness, (4) a highly repetitive and stereotypic response profile, (5) impaired response inhibition, and (6) cognitive inflexibility.

The essence of a clinical compulsion is the intense urge to perform the response, which serves a harm avoidance function, compared to the reward-seeking function and feelings of pleasure associated with impulse disorders such as kleptomania, pathological gambling, compulsive sexuality, and so on (Berlin & Hollander, 2014; Fineberg et al., 2014). The classic example of a compulsion is the urge to repeatedly clean in response to an obsessive fear of contamination, which persists until the person experiences a significant decline in subjective anxiety. Once anxiety has declined to an acceptable level, the individual ceases to engage in the compulsive washing ritual (Rachman & Hodgson, 1980). In neutral situations when the obsessional fear is not present, the individual may consider the compulsion excessive and unreasonable. This insight may provoke subjective resistance so that the individual delays, extends, or postpones acting on the compulsion when fearful, but eventually the urge to carry out the compulsion becomes so strong that the individual gives in to the urge (Rachman & Shafran, 1998). Many individuals with OCD eventually give up their struggle against the compulsion, showing only slight or no resistance (Foa et al., 1995; Stern & Cobb, 1978).

Most often an obsession elicits a negative state such as fear, anxiety, guilt, or disgust, which is then alleviated to a certain extent by the compulsive ritual (Rachman & Hodgson, 1980). Thus, obsessions and compulsions are functionally related in most cases (Akhtar et al., 1975; Foa et al., 1995; Leonard & Riemann, 2012). This functionality is supported empirically with factor-analytic studies indicating that obsessions and compulsions load on the same factors (e.g., Bloch et al., 2008; Olatunji et al., 2017; Summerfeldt et al., 1999). Although clinicians tend to treat obsessions and compulsions as distinct symptom dimensions, it is important to realize that they have considerable commonality and functional interconnectedness.

MENTAL COMPULSIONS

Mental compulsions—also called *covert compulsions, cognitive compulsions,* or *covert/cognitive neutralization*—are internal, repetitive responses most often triggered by an obsession and associated with a strongly felt urge to think through some aspect of the obsession or its details (de Silva, 2003). Mental compulsions have the same function as overt compulsions when they occur in response to an obsession. However, there are instances in which the mental compulsion is not associated with an obsession but occurs independently as a repetitive existential or unsolvable issue that the person feels compelled to ponder (de Silva, 2003). Research on mental compulsions includes (e.g., Abramowitz, Franklin, Schwartz, & Furr, 2003; Williams, Farris, et al., 2011):

- Mental repetition of words, images, or numbers
- Repetition of special prayers, songs, or phrases
- Mental counting
- Mental list making
- Mental reviewing, questioning, or analyzing

The following examples illustrate the two types of mental compulsions. The first is a woman who experienced frequent, unwanted, and distressing intrusive thoughts like "At this moment, am I experiencing reality or just a perception of reality? If I am just having a visual perception, how can I know I am real or that what I see and experience is real?" In response to this obsessive doubt, the client would engage in long, repetitive, and futile efforts to review her experience, looking for proof of reality and analyzing the logic of her thinking. In this case she mentally repeated her questions, and her process of analyzing constituted a form of mental compulsion triggered by her obsessive doubt about reality.

In the second case, a middle-age professional felt drawn to any information on death. She would search the Internet and listen into conversations that dealt with death, wanting to know every detail of how the person had died. She was also consumed by a compulsion to read about the end of civilization and to image what it would be like to live through the apocalypse. An obsession was not associated with this repetitive mental activity, nor did the client feel distressed by her morbid fascination. Instead, she reported an overwhelming urge to read everything she could on death and end of the world as we know it.

Mental compulsions may be more common in OCD than might be assumed. In a sample of 225 adults with OCD, 12.9% reported that a mental ritual was their primary compulsion, and 20.4% indicated that a mental compulsion was one of their current symptoms (Sibrava, Boisseau, Mancebo, Eisen, & Rasmussen, 2011). Only 50.7% reported no history of mental rituals. Similarly, a multicenter sample of 1,001 Brazilians with OCD found that 56.7% reported a mental compulsion (Shavitt et al., 2014). Mental compulsions are more often evident with repugnant obsessions and the order/symmetry subtype (Abramowitz, Franklin, et al., 2003; Williams, Farris, et al., 2011). They may be more evident in comorbid borderline personality disorder, have greater chronicity and symptom severity, and be performed more automatically (Melca et al., 2015; Sibrava et al., 2011; Starcevic et al., 2011). Abramowitz, Franklin, and colleagues (2003), however, found no significant difference in CBT outcome between those with mental compulsions compared to other symptom themes.

EXCESSIVE REASSURANCE SEEKING

Excessive reassurance seeking (ERS) was first considered a vulnerability factor in depression (e.g., Joiner & Metalsky, 2001) and a key construct in Coyne's (1976) interpersonal theory of the disorder. However, ERS is also a common response strategy found with distressing obsessions (Kobori & Salkovskis, 2013). Freeston and Ladouceur (1997b) found that 41% of their OCD sample used direct reassurance seeking or transference of responsibility to others in response to their obsessions.

There are several important differences between the ERS associated with depression and ERS in OCD. For depression, reassurance seeking is an attempt to gain a sense of self-worth and assurance that others truly care for the person (Timmons & Joiner, 2008). The excessive nature of the depressed person's reassurance seeking leads to a host of unintended consequences, such as rejection, dejection, and hopelessness, which in turn intensify the depressive state.

ERS in OCD focuses on a perceived threat and its associated distress. As well, the reassurance seeking in OCD is often more stereotypic than in depression. Rachman (2002) described ERS as a *checking compulsion by proxy,* in which the person repeatedly seeks the same reassurance from others, often looking for the same specific answer to obtain relief from anxiety, discomfort, and a heightened sense of responsibility for harm associated with the obsession (see also Salkovskis & Kobori, 2015). Salkovskis (1985; Salkovskis, Forrester, & Richards, 1998; Salkovskis & Kobori, 2015) considered ERS a form of specialized neutralization in which seeking the opinion of others reduces (or diffuses) the individual's sense of responsibility for harm by sharing, or even transferring, it to those providing the reassurance. As well as diffusing a heightened sense of responsibility, ERS may function to reduce threat uncertainty (Kobori, Salkovskis, Read, Lounes, & Wong, 2012), or it can be used as a "stop criteria" for confirming that a compulsion has been executed thoroughly and correctly. As well, ERS in OCD can be subtler than in depression, with individuals seeking certain behaviors or situations that they then interpret as reassuring (Salkovskis, 1985).

On occasion ERS is the primary neutralization response to an obsession. In the following example, a middle-age man reported a frequent and highly distressing sexual obsession. Several times throughout the day, the man had the unwanted thought "I wonder if my wife enjoyed sexual intercourse more with a former boyfriend than with me?" Often this thought was accompanied by a sexual image of his wife and the boyfriend, whom the client knew as an acquaintance. The client recognized the absurdity of the obsession because the sexual liaison had taken place 15 years ago, a couple of years before the man and his wife even started dating.

To deal with his distressing thought, the client asked his wife over and over whether sex with the "boyfriend" was better than with him. His reassurance seeking often took an angry and accusatory tone, quizzing his wife on her "immorality" and whether she now felt guilty and remorseful for her "infidelity." His interrogations could be lengthy and frequently brought her to tears of frustration. Nothing she said could satisfy his relentless interrogation. The man could not resist his destructive questioning whenever the obsession arose, even though he knew it was causing great emotional harm to his wife and threatening their marriage. Rarely did her response produce anything more than a fleeting sense of relief, and so he would often continue the badgering until she became so emotionally distraught that she had to escape. (This could also be understood as example of pathological jealousy [Leahy, 2018].) This case illustrates several important points from an ERS perspective:

1. Most often, ERS produces only transient relief from anxiety and discomfort caused by the obsession.
2. Individuals who rely on ERS often seek a specific response, even if vaguely articulated, that they believe will diminish the obsessional concern.
3. The compulsive urge associated with ERSs can be as strong as for any compulsion.
4. ERS can have a significant negative emotional effect on family, friends, and caregivers from whom the reassurance is sought.

Empirical research has shed new light on the function of ERS in OCD. It is more frequent and intense in OCD than in other anxiety disorders, with self-reassurance being especially common (Kobori & Salkovskis, 2013; Kobori, Sawamiya, Iyo, & Shimizu, 2015). Individuals with OCD seek reassurance to reduce anxiety, prevent anticipated harm, and achieve a sense of certainty (Korbori et al., 2012; Parrish & Radomsky, 2010; Rector, Kamkar, Cassin, Ayearst, & Laposa, 2011). However, only short-term relief is achieved, with elevated reassurance seeking associated with a greater return of anxiety and a stronger urge to seek more reassurance (Salkovskis & Kobori, 2015). A qualitative study of caregivers who provide reassurance to OCD sufferers reported that caregivers found the experience frustrating but felt that they had to give into the requests for reassurance, even though they knew it was counterproductive in the long term (Halldorsson, Salkovskis, Kobori, & Pagdin, 2016).

ERS is a maladaptive neutralization strategy that needs to be included in the cognitive case conceptualization and targeted for treatment. Its deleterious effects should be explained in the psychoeducational phase, and family members may need to be coached on how to respond to reassurance-seeking requests. Therapists also must be vigilant for subtle efforts by the client to extract reassurance in the therapy session.

AVOIDANCE

Avoidance involves any effort or activity intended to avert a perceived internal or external trigger of the obsession and its associated distress. It is often the first choice of action that individuals with OCD use to manage their obsessive–compulsive symptoms. Although avoidance is evident in all anxiety disorders, it is particularly prominent in OCD subtypes with a strong phobic element, such as compulsive washing and cleaning (Rachman & Hodgson, 1980). Because of an intense fear of dirt or disease contamination, individuals with compulsive washing often take extreme care to avoid any situation that might bring them in contact with perceived contaminants (e.g., public areas, close physical contact with others, hospitals or clinics). Only when avoidance fails do they attempt to "escape" from their anxiety by compulsive cleaning. Avoidance is thought to contribute to the salience of obsessions by preventing prolonged exposure to obsessional fears. Moreover, avoidance can be considered a safety behavior that deprives individuals of the opportunity to experience disconfirming evidence against the threatening nature of the obsession (Salkovskis, 1996). In CBT avoidance is addressed through graded exposure assignments and hypothesis-testing experiments. Often individuals with OCD are unaware of the subtle ways they avoid perceived threats, so therapists may need to directly observe clients' responses in a variety of obsessive–compulsive-relevant situations.

NEUTRALIZATION

Defining Neutralization

Neutralization refers to any coping response to an obsession, including compulsive rituals (i.e., Bocci & Gordon, 2007). Similarly, Salkovskis and Westbrook (1989) considered neutralization as anything a person does intentionally or effortfully in response to the obsession. Freeston and Ladouceur (1997b) offered a more elaborated definition, stating that neutralization is "any voluntary, effortful cognitive or behavioral act that is directed at removing, preventing, or attenuating the thought or the associated discomfort" (Freeston & Ladouceur, 1997b, p. 344). Rachman and associates opted for a narrower conceptualization of the construct, distinguishing neutralization from compulsions, thought suppression, and cognitive reappraisal (Rachman & Shafran, 1998; Rachman, Shafran, Mitchell,

Trant, & Teachman, 1996). According to this view, the key differences between neutralization and compulsions are:

- The primary aim of neutralization is to reduce, remove, cancel out, undo, or put right the anticipated or current negative effect of the obsession.
- Though usually covert, neutralizing strategies are functionally equivalent to overt compulsions.
- Neutralization is an attempt to compensate or eliminate, that is, undo, the effects of the obsession, and not to evaluate or change the meaning of the obsession.

In recent years, OCD researchers have referred to neutralization in its broader sense by considering it to refer to any overt or covert response to the obsession, including compulsions (e.g., Ahern, Kyrios, & Meyers, 2015; Belloch, Carrió, Cabedo, & García-Soriano, 2015; Radomsky, Alcolado, et al., 2014).

An array of coping responses is included under the rubric of *neutralization*. In addition to overt compulsive rituals, reassurance seeking, self-punishment, worry, distraction, thought suppression, cognitive reappraisal, mental checking, rationalization, thought stopping, thought replacement, and self-questioning are considered neutralization strategies (Belloch et al., 2015; Freeston & Ladouceur, 1997b; Radomsky, Alcolado, et al., 2014). Individuals with OCD report a significantly greater use of overt compulsions, mental checking, thought stopping, self-questioning, worry, self-punishment, and reappraisal than nonclinical control groups (Abramowitz, Whiteside, Kalsy, & Tolin, 2003; Amir, Cashman, & Foa, 1997; Ladouceur et al., 2000). Interestingly, Levine and Warman (2016) found that individuals were more likely to recommend unhelpful response strategies with more distressing intrusive thoughts. And yet, Freeston and Ladouceur (1997b) found that only a third of the cognitive strategies and one-quarter of the behavioral responses used by individuals with OCD to cope with obsessions are compulsive rituals and other types of classic obsessive–compulsive neutralization. More often individuals with OCD respond to an obsession with the same mental control strategies common in nonclinical individuals, including behavioral distraction, trying to convince oneself that the thought is not important, thought replacement, talking about it, doing nothing, rationalization, and the like. Although many of these strategies may appear adaptive, they are problematic responses because their aim is to counter the negative effects of the obsession, thereby enhancing the obsession's meaning and significance (i.e., Freeston & Ladouceur, 1997b; Rachman, 1998).

Form 3.2 provides a checklist of compulsions and other forms of neutralization that are often found in OCD. When assessing OCD, clinicians can use the checklist to ensure that they conduct an extensive inquiry into the various types of neutralizing strategies associated with an obsession.

Determinants of Neutralization

In CBT, neutralization is considered an important factor in the etiology and persistence of OCD (Salkovskis, 1985, Salkovskis et al., 1998; Rachman, 1998). Several cognitive and emotional processes have been implicated in the pathogenesis of compulsive responses and other forms of neutralization. This research provides an important evaluation of the CBT theory of OCD as well as highlighting the critical factors responsible for the obsessional person's inexplicable reliance on maladaptive neutralization.

Anxiety/Distress Reduction

Early behavioral accounts of OCD posited that compulsions are a form of active avoidance that persists because they offer a temporary reduction in anxiety or distress associated with the obsession (Emmelkamp, 1982; Rachman & Hodgson, 1980). There is considerable experimental evidence in support of the anxiety reduction hypothesis. Clinical experiments on OCD indicate that provocation of an obsession causes a steep rise in anxiety, with performance of a compulsion resulting in a quicker decline in anxiety than a delay in the compulsion (for reviews, see Rachman & Hodgson, 1980; Rachman & Shafran, 1998). Moreover, covert neutralization appears to function in the same manner, with a decline in subjective discomfort when an image is produced that cancels the effects of the obsession (Marks et al., 2000). A similar effect was found when OCD participants were instructed to form a neutralizing thought when listening to their unwanted intrusive thought (Salkovskis, Thorpe, Wahl, Wroe, & Forrester, 2003). Those in the neutralizing condition experienced an immediate decrease in discomfort while listening to the intrusion but an increase in discomfort when again exposed to the intrusion 15 minutes later, compared to a comparison group instructed to count backward.

Other forms of neutralization also appear to reduce anxiety or distress. In analogue and clinical samples, neutralization leads to a significant reduction in anxiety associated with an unacceptable intrusive thought or obsession, but more discomfort and a greater urge to neutralize occur after a 30-minute delay (i.e., Ahern et al., 2015; Rachman et al., 1996; Salkovskis, Westbrook, Davis, Jeavons, & Gledhill, 1997). Others have replicated these findings, with neutralization causing an immediate reduction in anxiety and urge to neutralize, although distraction and spontaneous decay can have the same effect over a longer time period (e.g., Bocci & Gordon, 2007; van den Hout, Kindt, Weiland, & Peters, 2002; van den Hout, van Pol, & Peters, 2001). However, any response, such as distraction or waiting, can lead to some reduction in anxiety, and evidence is less consistent that neutralization causes a rebound in anxiety during subsequent exposure to the obsession. Also, some individuals, especially those with compulsive checking, experience an elevation in their anxiety and discomfort when performing a compulsion (Carr, 1974; Rachman & Hodgson, 1980; more recently, Bucarelli & Purdon, 2015). These findings have led many CBT researchers to consider other processes that may contribute to the persistence of compulsions.

Safety Seeking

Closely akin to the anxiety reduction hypothesis is the view that neutralization serves a safety-seeking function. Safety seeking is any overt or covert "action intended to detect, avoid or escape a feared outcome" (Deacon & Maack, 2008, p. 537). According to Salkovskis and Millar (2016), safety seeking occurs in OCD in order to reduce the perceived likelihood of an imagined threat and an inflated sense of personal responsibility associated with the obsession. Thus, a person washes in response to a fear of contamination in order to reduce the perceived likelihood of contamination and being responsible for causing such harm to self and/or others. Salkovskis and Millar argue that at first the washing response may be considered reasonable and logical, but as the safety-seeking response builds in frequency and intensity, it can become less reasonable and more irrational to the person. As well, anxiety reduction is not considered a necessary motive in safety seeking. Rather, the key element is a change in the perceived likelihood of the obsessional fear. However, in the long term, compulsions are an ineffective way to obtain a sense of safety. This is because the very act of neutralizing shields the individual from disconfirming evidence that neutralization did not prevent a feared event from occurring or that it was not responsible for reductions in subjective discomfort (Rachman, 1998; Salkovskis, 1996). As a result, the person with OCD fails to comprehend the ineffectiveness of the compulsion in attaining an enduring sense of safety or reduced threat.

There is experimental evidence that compulsions and other forms of neutralization have a safety-seeking function. Deacon and Maack (2008) found that undergraduates instructed to engage in contamination-related safety behavior for 1 week experienced a significant increase in threat overestimation, contamination fear symptoms, and avoidant responses during a contamination-related behavioral avoidance test. In the original thought–action fusion induction study, neutralization was associated with a significant decline in probability estimates that an accident really would occur within the next 24 hours (Rachman et al., 1996). However, using the same induction procedure, Bocci and Gordon (2007) found an increase rather than decrease in threat estimates shortly after individuals engaged in spontaneous neutralizing. As well, Bucarelli and Purdon (2016) conducted an analogue stove-checking procedure and eye-tracking measures with an OCD- and non-OCD-anxious group. They found that longer check duration predicted greater posttask harm severity and probability ratings, which calls into question the safety-seeking function of the compulsion. There is little doubt that safety seeking probably motivates neutralization, although its influence may be more nuanced in producing different short- and long-term effects.

Perceived Responsibility

Responsibility appraisals play a central role in Salkovskis's (1985, 1989a, 1999) cognitive-behavioral account of OCD. Unwanted intrusive thoughts escalate into obsessions when individuals believe they may be responsible for harm or its prevention to self or others, as indicated by the mental intrusion. This faulty interpretation of responsibility causes an increase in the intrusion's discomfort and elicits a neutralizing response. Thus, perceived threat and heightened appraisals of responsibility motivate individuals to engage in neutralizing responses. Salkovskis (1999) predicts that compulsions and other forms of neutralization will cause an immediate discharge of responsibility for the obsession, but that responsibility and threat appraisals will increase in the long term.

Several studies have investigated the relationship between responsibility appraisals and neutralization. Bocci and Gordon (2007) found that spontaneous neutralization was associated with an increase in responsibility ratings in a nonclinical thought–action fusion induction study. Rachman and colleagues (1996) found that neutralization caused an immediate decline in responsibility, followed by an increase 20 minutes later. Taylor and Purdon (2016) found that higher trait responsibility was associated with longer hand washing after a contamination induction task in a student sample. However, the responsibility manipulation had less impact on washing parameters. Belloch and colleagues (2015) showed that increased tendency to use covert neutralization strategies was associated with increased responsibility appraisals in an OCD sample. Together, these findings indicate that responsibility appraisals may play a role in the persistence of compulsions. However, it is likely that responsibility overlaps with threat appraisals and other aspects of the safety-seeking function to motivate neutralization.

"Not Just Right" Experiences

Another motive for engaging in compulsive behavior has been labeled the *"not just right" experience (NJRE)*. Some individuals with OCD perform a compulsive ritual until they achieve a certain sensory-based state described as a "just right" feeling, or a sense of completeness (Ferrão et al., 2012; Leckman et al., 2000). NJREs are defined as "the subjective sense that something isn't just as it should be, an unsettled feeling because something in the individual or in the world around them is not right" (Sica et al., 2015, p. 73). This sensory-based criterion is ill-suited for judging when neutralizing is complete because the person is using a vague, indeterminable criterion for completion (Richards, 1995).

As discussed more extensively in Chapter 13, NJREs are especially relevant for order and rearranging compulsions (Rasmussen & Eisen, 1992; Summerfeldt et al., 1999). Coles and Ravid (2016) found that number and severity of NJREs were more highly correlated with ordering/arranging than with other obsessive–compulsive symptoms. Sica and colleagues (2015) also found a specific association between NJREs and ordering and mental neutralizing, although the correlation with washing symptoms was also elevated. Ferrão and colleagues (2012) found that 65% of their OCD sample reported that some type of sensory experience (e.g., NJRE) preceded the compulsion, with the frequency and severity of the NJRE associated with symmetry/order/arranging and washing compulsions.

Correlational studies have shown a significant relationship between NJREs and compulsions, especially order/rearranging but also checking and washing symptoms (Coles, Frost, Heimberg, & Rhéaume, 2003; Coles & Ravid, 2016; Sica et al., 2015), and individuals with OCD score higher on NJRE measures than those with other anxiety disorders or with nonclinical controls (Coles & Ravid, 2016; Ghisi, Chiri, Marchetti, Sanavio, & Sica, 2010). However, NJREs are evident to some extent in other diagnostic conditions, including GAD, TTM, and eating disorders (Fergus, 2014; Sica et al., 2015). In a CBT trial, Coles and Ravid (2016) found that amount of change in NJREs correlated with a decrease in overall obsessive–compulsive symptoms, although not specifically with order/rearranging symptoms.

There is also evidence that NJREs can influence the persistence of compulsions. In one of the first studies to utilize an NJRE laboratory-based induction, the production of an NJRE resulted in increased distress and an urge to arrange disorganized objects (Coles, Heimberg, Frost, & Steketee, 2005). Based on a semistructured interview, Wahl and colleagues (2008) found that individuals with compulsive washing used more internal feelings of rightness as a criterion for stopping their compulsion compared to individuals with other obsessional problems or healthy controls. A subsequent interview-based study on compulsive checking again showed that feelings of rightness were more important in terminating a check for those with OCD than for the anxious or healthy controls (Salkovskis, Millar, Gregory, & Wahl, 2017). In an OCD diary study, compulsions that were deemed "less effective in achieving the desired outcome" were considered less likely to have achieved the "just right feeling" (Bucarelli & Purdon, 2015). There is considerable empirical evidence, then, that sensory experience can be an important contributor to the persistence of compulsions, especially order and rearranging.

Intolerance of Uncertainty

Intolerance of uncertainty (IU) is a cognitive construct originally proposed for the etiology and persistence of worry and GAD (Dugas, Gagnon, Ladouceur, & Freeston, 1998). It is "the excessive tendency of an individual to consider it unacceptable that a negative event may occur, however small the probability of its occurrence" (Dugas, Gosselin, & Ladouceur, 2001, p. 552). Various studies have shown that IU is highly correlated with worry and anxiety as well as with obsessive–compulsive symptoms (e.g., Buhr & Dugas, 2002; Dugas et al., 2001; Fergus & Wu, 2010; Laposa, Collimore, Hawley, & Rector, 2015; Tolin, Abramowitz, Brigidi, & Foa, 2003). It is a transdiagnostic construct that is probably linked to negative affect or the common experience of repetitive negative thought (Gentes & Ruscio, 2011).

Rachman (2002) proposed that the search for certainty is one of the self-perpetuating mechanisms responsible for checking compulsions. The individual continues to check in an effort to attain a desired level of certainty that an imagined harm to self or others has been averted. From this account, a predisposition toward IU would amplify the individual's quest for certainty or safety from harm. Whereas Dugas and colleagues (1998) defined IU in reference to worry and GAD, others, such as the OCCWG, offered a slightly different view of IU derived from the OCD literature. IU was conceptualized as an enduring set of beliefs involving (1) the necessity of attaining certainty, (2) the inability to cope with unpredictable change, and (3) the difficulty dealing with ambiguous situations (OCCWG, 1997). In a review of factor-analytic studies of the 27-item Intolerance of Uncertainty Scale (IUS; Freeston, Rhéaume, Letarte, Dugas, & Ladouceur, 1994), it was concluded that the IUS consists of two latent factors: a "desire for predictability" dimension in which uncertainty is a negative experience and knowing what the future holds is preferable, and an "uncertainty paralysis" dimension that refers to being unable to function in uncertain situations (Birrell, Meares, Wilkinson, & Freeston, 2011). The OCCWG definition of IU is weighted toward the "uncertainty paralysis" dimension, whereas the Dugas and colleagues (2001) construct is more inclined toward the "desire for predictability" dimension. In a meta-analysis of IU studies, Gentes and Ruscio (2011) found that both aspects of IU were related to GAD, OCD, and major depression, although IU was more strongly associated with GAD symptoms when the GAD-specific definition was used. Thus, it may be that certain aspects of IU, such as "uncertainty paralysis," is more relevant for OCD than other aspects, although Fourtounas and Thomas (2016) found that "desire for predictability" and "uncertainty paralysis" were equally associated with checking in a university student sample.

There is empirical evidence that IU is a factor in the persistence of neutralization. A nonclinical study based on self-report measures found that NJREs mediated the relationship between IU and checking behavior (Bottesi, Ghisi, Sica, & Freeston, 2017). The authors suggest that an inability to tolerate uncertainty may cause individuals to check repeatedly, until they attain a sense of certainty and "just right" feeling. Likewise, Bucarelli and Purdon (2015) found that compulsions deemed uncertain in effectiveness were characterized by a greater number of repetitions and less certainty than compulsions considered to have been done properly. In an experimental study, individuals with subclinical obsessive–compulsive symptoms responded with more checking behavior to a mildly uncertain induction task than did non-obsessive–compulsive participants (Toffolo, van den Hout, Hooge, Engelhard, & Cath, 2013). These findings were partially replicated in a subsequent study, although uncertainty was unrelated to increased checking behavior (Toffolo, van den Hout, Engelhard, Hooge, & Cath, 2014).

Distress Tolerance

A final construct in the persistence of neutralization is *distress tolerance* (DT), which is "the capacity to experience and withstand negative psychological states" (Simons & Gaher, 2005, p. 83). It has two dimensions: (1) the perceived ability to withstand negative states and (2) the act of tolerating distressing internal states elicited by a stressor, such as a pain tolerance test (Zvolensky, Vujanovic, Bernstein, & Leyro, 2010). DT has been considered an emotion regulation construct involved in the pathogenesis of various psychological disorders, including OCD (Leyro, Zvolensky, & Bernstein, 2010). Zvolensky and colleagues (2010) presented a hierarchical model in which DT is comprised of several lower-order constructs, such as tolerance of uncertainty, ambiguity, frustration, negative emotion, and physical discomfort.

There is evidence that poor DT is more closely associated with obsessions than with compulsions (e.g., Blakey, Jacoby, Reuman, & Abramowitz, 2016; Laposa et al., 2015; Macatee, Capron, Schmidt, & Cougle, 2013). In two prospective nonclinical studies, low DT predicted obsessive but not compulsive symptoms (Cougle, Timpano, Fitch, & Hawkins, 2011), but possibly more so under conditions of heightened stress (Macatee et al., 2013). However, low DT has less specificity to obsessionality than other constructs, such as IU, and has emerged as a general factor across several anxiety disorders (Michel, Rowa, Young, & McCabe, 2016).

Empirical evidence that low DT contributes to neutralization is mixed. When given the opportunity to neutralize after a thought–action fusion induction, students who neutralized reported significantly lower DT and greater responsibility beliefs (Cougle, Timpano, et al., 2011). Using a pain tolerance test, Hezel, Riemann, and McNally (2012) found that individuals with OCD endured physical pain significantly longer than healthy participants. Macatee and Cougle (2015) found that a brief computerized intervention reduced self-reported distress intolerance (DI) in a high DI analogue group, which led to a lower urge to neutralize but not to actual neutralization behavior.

In sum, it is unclear whether low DT plays a unique role in the persistence of compulsions. The association of low DT with obsessional symptoms appears more robust. It may be that poor DT is a general factor that is expressed through more specific lower-order constructs such as IU.

Clinical Application

It is obvious that the factors responsible for the etiology and maintenance of neutralization more generally are complex and somewhat idiosyncratic to each person with OCD. To assist in the assessment of neutralization, Form 3.3 is a worksheet for rating the relevance of each motive for neutralization. A separate worksheet should be completed for each neutralization response reported by the client. This information is important to the cognitive case formulation and in designing the response prevention component of CBT.

STOP RULES

Knowing the determinants of an individual's compulsions is only part of the story. It is also important to understand why individuals with OCD have difficulty stopping their compulsive rituals. Salkovskis and colleagues consider this a decision-making problem in which individuals with OCD use an internally based, counterproductive "stop criteria" to decide when they have done enough washing, checking, counting, and so on (Wahl et al., 2008). The researchers note that the subjective internal state used to decide when to stop a compulsion can involve the achievement of a specific mood state, a sense of completeness, a "just right feeling," or some combination. However, internal states are more difficult to evaluate than external, sensory-based criteria, and so the obsessional person may end up relying on multiple criteria because of the importance attributed to making the "correct" decision to stop (Wahl et al., 2008). This state of affairs constitutes what is called an *elevated evidence requirement*, making the decision to cease a compulsive act more difficult (Salkovskis, 1999; see also Salkovskis & Millar, 2016). Tallis and Eysenck (1994) first introduced the concept of elevated evidence requirement as one of the factors that may account for poor problem solving in individuals with chronic worry.

Research into stop rules in OCD is partly influenced by Szechtman and Woody's (2004) security motivation theory of OCD. This model proposes that compulsions continue until the individual attains an internal state of a "feeling of knowing" called *yedasentience*. This internal state is not simply the absence of anxiety but rather a "satiety signal" indicating that a compulsive ritual can stop because yedasentience has been achieved (see Chapter 11 for further discussion).

Several studies indicate that individuals with OCD use different criteria than non-OCD individuals when deciding when to stop checking. In one study, individuals with obsessional checking needed more criteria to determine when to stop checking and relied more on "feelings of rightness" than did non-OCD-anxious controls (Salkovskis, Millar, Gregory, & Wahl, 2017), whereas in a second study obsessional washers used more subjective stop criteria than did controls (Wahl et al., 2008). Bucarelli and Purdon (2015) found that evidence requirements increased with more repetitions of compulsive responses that were considered uncertain.

When formulating a CBT plan for compulsions, biases and distortions in stop criteria must be taken into account. The following questions could be incorporated into the clinical assessment interview to determine a person's decision-making requirements for terminating a compulsion.

- To what extent does the client rely exclusively on subjective criteria to decide when to terminate the compulsion (e.g., a certain internal feeling state)? Are more objective external criteria ever considered?
- List the various ways in which the client knows when to stop a compulsion. Are elevated evidence requirements present?
- What role does change in mood play in the client's deciding when to stop the compulsion?
- Do the stop criteria vary across different situations or contexts? For example, does the presence of others influence the evidence requirements needed for termination?
- How committed is the client to the stop criteria? Is there any evidence of a willingness to consider using externally based stop rules?

THE ROLE OF MENTAL CONTROL

Theoretical Considerations

Given the distressing and repetitive nature of obsessions and the irresistible urge associated with compulsions, it is little wonder that individuals with OCD perceive a loss of control. Compulsions and other forms of neutralization could be viewed as efforts to regain a sense of control over unwanted thoughts, feelings, and behavior. In their seminal account of OCD, Rachman and Hodgson (1980) speculated that individuals with OCD experience a state of helplessness, and the compulsive behavior can be viewed as a type of *compensatory rebound* in which the repetitive act "is an attempt to assert control over a more manageable situation after having experienced helplessness in other, more important situations" (p. 394).

The importance of control gained further prominence in later CBT formulations. Salkovskis (1999), for example, argues that neutralization is a counterproductive attempt to reduce obsessional intrusions and decrease their associated perceived responsibility. Compulsions and other forms of neutralization reflect the obsessional person's trying "too hard to exert control over [his or her] own cognitive function, over the occurrence of thoughts" (Salkovskis, Richards, & Forrester, 1995, p. 284). Rachman (2003) noted that individuals with OCD often use thought suppression when an unwanted intrusive thought is considered a highly significant personal threat. When these mental control efforts fail, the person will often resort to neutralization responses. The OCCWG (1997) also proposed that beliefs in the importance of controlling unwanted thoughts is a cognitive vulnerability factor in the pathogenesis of obsessions and compulsions.

Clark and Purdon (1993) presented a cognitive perspective on obsessions that emphasized the importance of control. They proposed that preexisting dysfunctional beliefs about mental control lead obsession-prone individuals to exert excessive effort to control or suppress an unwanted intrusive thought. Inevitably, these control efforts fail, which the vulnerable individual misinterprets as a sign of weakness and escalating personal threat. Not only does the failure of mental control contribute to the increased frequency and salience of the intrusion, but it also might encourage reliance on more dysfunctional strategies, such as a compulsive ritual or other neutralization, in an effort to regain some semblance of control over the obsession. This cognitive perspective was more fully discussed in the first edition of this book (Clark, 2004), in which maladaptive appraisals of failed mental control and heightened mental control efforts were considered critical factors in the escalation of obsessive–compulsive symptomatology.

Two decades later Salkovskis and Millar (2016) offered a strong critique of the Clark and Purdon (1993) paper. They noted that it's not necessary to shift CBT theory toward a greater emphasis on control beliefs because thought control is subsumed within Salkovskis's conceptualization of responsibility. They also note that dysfunctional mental control beliefs may not be universal in OCD. As well, Salkovskis and Millar contend that Clark and Purdon consider failed thought control the key factor in the etiology of obsessions and not overt or covert neutralizing rituals. From their perspective poor thought control is a consequence of erroneous responsibility appraisals that contribute to the pathogenesis of obsessions by fueling further negative appraisals of the unwanted intrusions. They conclude that thought control strategies are "safety-seeking behaviors, along with mental arguments and other types of neutralizing reactions and compulsions"

(p. 6). In their rebuttal, Clark and Purdon note that Salkovskis and Millar offer a sweeping definition of responsibility that may offer less heuristic value than differentiating various obsessive–compulsive belief dimensions. Also, they note that emphasizing the role of mental control effort and its failure in the persistence of obsessive–compulsive symptomatology is warranted, given the nuanced findings in the empirical literature. In their critical review of CBT theories for OCD, Cougle and Lee (2014) note that reliance on maladaptive mental control strategies could be a consequence of high obsession frequency rather than a contributor to obsession frequency and failure to disconfirm obsessional beliefs.

EMPIRICAL RESEARCH

There is considerable evidence that individuals with OCD perceive that their unwanted obsessive intrusive thoughts are uncontrollable and that better control over such thoughts is important to reduce the frequency and distress of obsessions (e.g., Bouvard, Fournet, Denis, Sixdenier, & Clark, 2017; García-Soriano & Belloch, 2013; García-Soriano et al., 2014; Janeck & Calamari, 1999; OCCWG, 2003, 2005; Purdon et al., 2005; Tolin, Worhunsky, & Maltby, 2006). Even though individuals with OCD may try longer and harder to control their obsessions, in the end they rate themselves as significantly less effective in their mental control efforts than do nonclinical individuals (Ladouceur et al., 2000). However, when it comes to thought suppression, individuals with OCD are indistinguishable from nonclinical samples in their ability to control unwanted thoughts (Janeck & Calamari, 1999; Purdon et al., 2005; for a review, see Magee et al., 2012). And yet, there is evidence that personal intrusive thoughts are harder to replace for individuals with OCD, and that greater difficulty in thought replacement is associated with more obsessive–compulsive symptoms (Ólafsson et al., 2014). Magee and colleagues (2012) suggest that heightened motivation to suppress unwanted thoughts and faulty appraisals of thought control failure may be aspects of mental control worth considering in psychopathological states.

Although the exact parameters of mental control relevant to OCD may be unclear, there can be little doubt that concerns about control weigh heavily in the pathogenesis OCD. Freeston and Ladouceur (1997b) found that individuals with OCD used a broad range of coping responses to their obsession but perceived that their efforts were less efficient than nonclinical individuals. More recently, an OCD treatment study found that participants who reported a greater use of covert coping responses (i.e., neutralization, thought stopping, self-criticism, thought suppression) also reported higher ratings on importance to control their obsessions (Belloch et al., 2015). However, Bucarelli and Purdon (2015) failed to find any relationship between importance of control beliefs and completion of a compulsion. Purdon (2017) reported on more recent diary and interview studies in which persistence of compulsions was related to attainment of an internal sense of certainty, rightness, or satisfaction. Although perceived control was not measured, the internal stop criteria found in these studies are consistent with the need to establish a sense of personal mental control.

To date there is insufficient research on mental control to determine its role in the persistence of compulsions. Do individuals with OCD persist with their compulsive rituals and other forms of neutralization until they perceive a return to some semblance of acceptable mental control? How does need for control differ from other factors in the persistence of compulsions, such as inflated sense of responsibility, NJREs, IU, safety seeking, distress reduction, and the like? Which parameters of mental control might be most critical in the persistence of compulsions: degree of control effort, perceived success, appraisals of control failure, beliefs about control, or reliance on ineffective control strategies? To make progress on answering these questions, researchers will need to broaden their scope so that mental control is not equated solely with thought suppression. In OCD, people utilize a variety of strategies to deal with obsessions, and direct thought suppression may be one of the least important.

CONCLUSION

Cognitive-behavioral theory and therapy recognizes that the individual's response to his or her obsessional concerns is a key factor in the pathogenesis of OCD. Cognitive-behavioral therapists must target these maladaptive "coping strategies" to effectively treat obsessive–compulsive symptoms. In most cases, individuals will exhibit repetitive, stereotypic overt or covert compulsive rituals that function to neutralize the perceived negative consequence of the obsession or its associated distress. In this chapter several features of OCD neutralization were considered that should be included in the CBT case formulation.

- Compulsions and neutralization responses occur along a normal–abnormal continuum, which means that clinicians must determine whether a frequent, recurring response to an obsession meets compulsivity criteria.
- Repetitive behavior that serves a harm reduction function is more likely a compulsion, whereas repetitive, irresistible behaviors characteristic of impulse-control disorder are reward seeking and associated with pleasure.
- Mental compulsions may also be present and will necessitate a modification in the case formulation and treatment plan.

- ERS and avoidance are prominent maladaptive response strategies in OCD. Cognitive restructuring and graded response prevention are important treatment approaches for ERS, whereas planned systematic exposure will be needed for avoidance of external and internal triggers of obsessional concerns.
- Cognitive-behavioral theory of OCD conceptualizes responses to an obsession as efforts to neutralize its untoward effects. A broad array of maladaptive and even adaptive coping responses falls within the neutralization category. Assessment of the presence and function of these coping responses is an important aspect of the case formulation.
- Several factors may be responsible for the persistence of neutralization responses—safety-seeking, inflated responsibility appraisals, NJREs, IU, DT, and anxiety reduction—although Purdon (2017) recently questioned whether anxiety reduction is a critical determinant of compulsions. Cognitive case formulation and treatment must determine the role played by these constructs in the person's OCD.
- Individuals with OCD find it more difficult to decide when to stop a compulsive ritual because they seek an elevated level of internally based evidence to determine completion of a response. Thus, one goal of CBT is to help clients shift to a more externally based criteria and to tolerate a greater degree of uncertainty (i.e., lower evidence requirement) that a response to the obsession is satisfactory.
- Clinicians should consider that neutralization may be driven by a need to reestablish a sense of control over one's mental processes. Beliefs about mental control as well as fear of losing control are constructs that could contribute to the persistence of compulsions, although the empirical support for this contention is limited at this time.

The chapters in Part I focused on diagnostic issues, clinical features, and the varied phenomenology of obsessions and compulsions. OCD has one of the most heterogeneous, complicated, and multifaceted symptom presentation of the emotional disorders. The more we learn about the pathogenesis of this disorder, the more idiosyncratic its phenotypic expression from one case to the next. After decades of research, there is no one process that is common to all types of OCD. Instead many different psychological processes are relevant, with none either necessary or sufficient for the persistence of the disorder. Despite these challenges, clinical researchers have continued to offer new insights into the disorder. The next two chapters delve into behavioral and cognitive theories of OCD. Together, the two chapters provide the necessary conceptual framework needed to offer effective CBT for OCD.

FORM 3.1. **Clinical Compulsions Checklist**

Instructions: The following statements represent the core features of clinical compulsions. In the space provided, write the response you are evaluating for compulsiveness. Then check the statements that describe your client's experience with the response.

Response: _____

- ☐ There is a strong urge to engage in the response.
- ☐ The primary function of the response is to neutralize key aspects of the obsession; that is, to prevent, undo, or correct an anticipated negative consequence or to reduce subjective distress.
- ☐ The individual has some insight into the excessiveness or unreasonableness of the response, although this may vary over time.
- ☐ The primary motivation of the response is threat/harm reduction or avoidance.
- ☐ The response is repetitive and performed in a stereotypic or habitual manner.
- ☐ Impaired behavioral response inhibition is evident with the response.
- ☐ The individual exhibits considerable cognitive inflexibility during the response.

From *Cognitive-Behavioral Therapy for OCD and Its Subtypes, Second Edition*, by David A. Clark. Copyright © 2020 The Guilford Press. Permission to photocopy this material is granted to purchasers of this book for personal use or use with individual clients (see copyright page for details). Purchasers can download enlarged versions of this material (see the box at the end of the table of contents).

FORM 3.2. Checklist of Neutralization Strategies Associated with OCD

Instructions: Place a checkmark beside the neutralization strategies that the client employs to reduce obsessional thinking and its associated distress. This checklist can be used later in the assessment to provide a more complete formulation of the client's neutralization profile.

☐ Behavioral compulsion (e.g., washing, checking, redoing, repeating)
☐ Mental compulsion (e.g., repetition of words, phrases, prayers, counting)
☐ Thought replacement
☐ Analyze the meaning of the obsession
☐ Engage in direct mental suppression (e.g., thought stopping, thought suppression)
☐ Avoid triggers of the obsession
☐ Seek reassurance from others
☐ Rationalize (i.e., try to convince oneself the obsession is not important)
☐ Behavioral distraction (i.e., engage in a competing activity)
☐ Self-reassurance (i.e., tell oneself everything will be fine)
☐ Become verbally or physically aggressive to self or others
☐ Try to relax
☐ Engage in minor self-harm (e.g., slap, pinch, scratch, hit oneself)
☐ Worry about the obsession and its effects
☐ Make self-critical remarks for having the obsession
☐ Counter with a positive or pleasant thought, image, or memory
☐ Engage in mindful, nonjudgmental acceptance
☐ Cry or use other form of emotional venting
☐ Withdraw, isolate self from others

From *Cognitive-Behavioral Therapy for OCD and Its Subtypes, Second Edition*, by David A. Clark. Copyright © 2020 The Guilford Press. Permission to photocopy this material is granted to purchasers of this book for personal use or use with individual clients (see copyright page for details). Purchasers can download enlarged versions of this material (see the box at the end of the table of contents).

FORM 3.3. Determinants of Neutralization Rating Scale

Instructions: Below are five questions about the importance that various motives may play in the persistence of a compulsion or other forms of neutralization. Write down the compulsion or other neutralization you intend to assess in the space provided. Then use the rating scales to indicate the importance that each motive might play in the persistence of the compulsion or neutralizing response.

Neutralization/Compulsive Response: _____

_____

Determinants	Not Important	Slightly Important	Moderately Important	Very Important
1. How important is anxiety/distress reduction in the persistence of the response?	0	1	2	3
2. How important is reduction in perceived threat or achievement of harm avoidance in the persistence of the response?	0	1	2	3
3. How important is reduction in personal responsibility in the persistence of the response?	0	1	2	3
4. How important is attainment of a "just right" feeling in the persistence of the response?	0	1	2	3
5. How important is reduction in the feeling of uncertainty in the persistence of the response?	0	1	2	3

From *Cognitive-Behavioral Therapy for OCD and Its Subtypes*, Second Edition, by David A. Clark. Copyright © 2020 The Guilford Press. Permission to photocopy this material is granted to purchasers of this book for personal use or use with individual clients (see copyright page for details). Purchasers can download enlarged versions of this material (see the box at the end of the table of contents).

PART II
Theory, Research, and Practice

CHAPTER 4

Exposure and Response Prevention

THEORY AND PRACTICE

The behavioral account of OCD is particularly well suited to explain harm avoidance types of OCD, such as compulsive washing and checking. As an illustrative example, Jenna had a primary obsessional fear involving an inflated sense of responsibility for causing illness in others. She believed that she could cause this malady because they might have touched minuscule traces of bodily fluid, such as blood, urine, or salvia, which she accidentally left on objects she touched. When Jenna saw a reddish smear on the kitchen table at work, she felt intense anxiety, wondering whether the smear might be a drop of her blood. Of course, this obsessional fear precipitated an intense episode of scrubbing the table to ensure that all traces of the contaminant were eliminated.

The *anxiety reduction hypothesis* was the central concept in early behavioral theories of OCD. Compulsive rituals persisted because of their anxiety-reducing capability. The completion of a compulsive act like handwashing reduces high levels of subjective anxiety caused by the occurrence of obsessions (Carr, 1974; Teasdale, 1974). Because a reduction in anxiety or distress is reinforcing, this act ensures that the compulsive ritual will be repeated in the future. In a paradoxical manner the compulsion also preserves the fear-eliciting properties of the obsession, thereby setting up an escalating cycle of ever more frequent and intense obsessions and compulsions (e.g., Eysenck & Rachman, 1965; Rachman & Hodgson, 1980). On the other hand, obsessions are conditioned noxious stimuli that acquire anxious properties by association with a prior upsetting experience (Steketee, 1993).

The behavioral theory of OCD was based on Mowrer's (1939, 1953, 1960) two-stage theory of fear and avoidance, and it was from this formulation that the most effective psychological treatment for OCD—ERP—was born. Applications of early behavioral techniques to OCD, including systematic desensitization, modeling, operant reinforcement, aversion relief, and relaxation therapy, produced mixed results (Emmelkamp, 1982; Foa, Franklin, & Kozak, 1998; Kozak & Foa, 1997). However, in 1966 Victor Meyer introduced ERP, which substantially altered how behavioral psychologists treated obsessions and compulsions (Meyer, 1966; Meyer, Levy, & Schnurer, 1974). In the decades to follow, numerous clinical trials have shown that 60–85% of individuals with OCD who complete ERP show significant symptom improvement (for reviews and meta-analyses, see Abramowitz, 1998; McKay et al., 2015; Romanelli, Wu, Gamba, Mojtabai, & Segal, 2014; Stanley & Turner, 1995; van Balkom et al., 1994).

This chapter presents an overview of behavioral theory and treatment of OCD. Empirical support for the model is reviewed, and more recent conceptualizations of learning theory are considered (Craske, Treanor, Conway, Zborinek, & Vervliet, 2014). Step-by-step instruction on how to conduct standard ERP is provided along with guidelines and resource materials for use in treating obsessions and compulsions. As well, a more contemporary view of ERP, based on inhibitory learning theory, is presented that holds promise for enhancing treatment effectiveness. The chapter concludes by highlighting the shortcomings of ERP and a rationale for its integration with cognitive strategies.

THE BEHAVIORAL PERSPECTIVE OF OCD

Anxiety Reduction Hypothesis

Rachman (1971) argued that obsessions are *conditioned noxious stimuli* that cause pain and/or distress for vulnerable individuals and often result in the production of avoidance behaviors (or compulsions) to relieve the distress. Obsessions persist because individuals fail to habituate to the intrusive thought and show increased sensitization or responsiveness to the cognition. Several factors are responsible for this heightened sensitivity, including the presence of dysphoria, preexisting personality vulnerability (e.g., introversion, excessive conscientiousness, moral rigidity), periods of stress, heightened arousal, and perceived loss of control (Rachman, 1971, 1976, 1978; Rachman & Hodgson, 1980). In addition, the occurrence of both active (i.e., compulsive ritual) and passive (i.e., avoidance of situations that trigger the obsession) avoidance contributes to a failure of habituation and increased sensitivity to the obsession.

Compulsive rituals like cleaning, checking, and reassurance seeking persist because of avoidance learning or what Mowrer (1953) called *solution learning*. Avoidance learning occurs when a learned activity circumvents or prevents exposure to a noxious or fear stimulus (Teasdale, 1974). The avoidant activity is strengthened through a process of operant conditioning. In the case of OCD, the compulsion takes the form of active avoidance because it reduces anxiety associated with the obsession (Emmelkamp, 1982). However, anxiety reduction is often brief for individuals with severe OCD, and so the whole cycle of anxiety elicitation and relief will be repeated.

Early research provided considerable support for the anxiety reduction hypothesis. It was evident that obsessions cause a significant increase in subjective distress and heightened physiological arousal before the performance of a compulsive ritual (e.g., Boulougouris & Bassiakos, 1973; Boulougouris, Rabavilas, & Stefanis, 1977; Hodgson & Rachman, 1972; Rabavilas & Boulougouris, 1974; Roper & Rachman, 1976; Roper, Rachman, & Hodgson, 1973). Moreover, individuals with OCD rate their unwanted intrusive thoughts or obsessions as more intense, discomforting, distressing, and unacceptable than nonclinical individuals rate their unwanted thoughts (Calamari & Janeck, 1997; Rachman & de Silva, 1978). Obsessions could be provoked by external stimuli (e.g., Roper et al., 1973; Steketee et al., 1985), a finding consistent with an associative learning explanation of obsessions as conditioned noxious stimuli. Finally, experimental provocation of the obsession indicated that production of overt compulsions like washing or checking resulted in an immediate and significant decline in subjective discomfort (for reviews of this experimental literature, see Rachman & Hodgson, 1980; Rachman & Shafran, 1998). These same anxiety reduction effects were evident whether the compulsion was overt or covert (Marks et al., 2000).

As research progressed, however, there were several findings that did not support the anxiety reduction hypothesis. These are summarized in Table 4.1. The main problem for the anxiety reduction hypothesis is the persistence of some compulsions (possibly 20% or more), despite causing a significant increase in subjective anxiety (see Carr, 1974; Rachman & Hodgson, 1980). Moreover, the temporary anxiety-reducing effects of neutralization may not be specific to obsessions but may be apparent when individuals neutralize other types of thoughts, such as anxiety-provoking images (Marks et al., 2000). More recently, research on stop criteria indicate that reaching a certain level of anxiety reduction is not the primary reason for deciding when to cease a compulsive ritual (Bucarelli & Purdon, 2015; Purdon, 2017). Another major problem for the anxiety reduction theory is that most obsessions are not acquired by association with a traumatic or aversive experience, and some types of obsessions, such as those involving order or nonsensical themes (e.g., repetitive phrases or musical tunes), are not anxiety provoking (Jakes, 1996). Clearly, then, the anxiety reduction hypothesis was inadequate for explaining the pathogenesis of obsessions and compulsions.

TABLE 4.1. Problems with the Anxiety Reduction Hypothesis

- Minimal evidence that obsessions are acquired via association with a traumatic experience.
- A minority of obsessions (i.e., nonsensical tunes, phrases, exactness/symmetry) do not elicit anxiety or discomfort.
- Some compulsions persist, despite causing an increase in anxiety or discomfort.
- Many people with OCD have multiple obsessions.
- There is a nonrandom distribution to obsessional content.
- The content and form of obsessions often change over time.
- Compulsions may occur in response to other negative emotions or to reduce the likelihood of some imagined aversive consequence.
- Anxiety reduction is often not the primary stop criteria used to terminate compulsive rituals.

Emotional Processing

Early behavioral accounts had difficulty explaining the return of fear after a successful trial of exposure therapy (Jacoby & Abramowitz, 2016; Rachman, 1980). If fear or anxiety had been extinguished via repeated exposures to the obsession without intense anxiety or occurrence of the feared outcome, how can we explain the return of fear or anxiety? In 1980, Rachman introduced the concept of *emotional processing* as an alternative to the anxiety reduction hypothesis. He defined emotional processing as "a process whereby emotional disturbances are absorbed and decline to the extent that other experiences and behavior can proceed without disruption" (p. 51). Thus, any emotional disturbance, such as anxiety, will persist when emotional processing is incomplete, but will decline in strength when emotional disturbance is absorbed because of successful emotional processing.

Rachman (1980) posited several indicators of unsatisfactory emotional processing, such as the presence of obsessions, disturbing dreams, unpleasant intrusive thoughts, inappropriate expressions of emotion, return of fear, and the like. He continued to ascribe to the behavioral perspective by asserting that satisfactory emotional processing could be promoted by prolonged and repeated exposure to disturbing material, habituation training, extinction trials, and relaxation. The return of fear/anxiety or the persistence of obsessions and other forms of unwanted mental intrusions was explained in terms of incomplete emotional processing rather than a failure in anxiety reduction.

Building on Rachman's (1980) proposal, Foa and Kozak (1986) offered an elaboration and clarification of emotional processing that have become the dominant theoretical basis for contemporary ERP of OCD. Fear, the fundamental emotion in anxiety, is represented in a memory network that includes information about the fear stimulus (i.e., antecedents, triggers) and its verbal, physiological, and behavioral responses, as well as interpretive information that gives meaning to the stimulus and response elements of the structure. To achieve fear reduction, therapeutic interventions must activate the fear structure and then provide information that is incompatible with fear memory, which, when integrated into the fear structure, causes emotional change such as fear reduction. Foa and Kozak state that a change in the fear structure is the mechanism that achieves emotional processing.

Foa and Kozak (1986) posit three indicators of emotional processing: (1) an elevated initial fear response, which indicates successful activation of the fear memory structure; (2) within-session habituation (i.e., fear response decrement); and (3) across-session habituation. Table 4.2 presents various treatment elements thought to influence modification of the fear structure.

Foa and Kozak (1986) believed that fear habituation was most likely when treatment exposed the client to information that was incompatible with the fear memory structure. If we consider Jenna's fear of contaminating others, habituation of her obsessive fear and compulsive washing would be most likely when the therapist assigned prolonged *in vivo* exposure sessions that involved contact with reddish specks of dirt and smudges that were mistaken for human blood. Emotional processing of the obsessive fear would be less likely if the dirt or stains were easily identifiable as innocuous and minimal fear or anxiety occurred in the exposure session. Moreover, without evidence of within-session habituation, it is expected that

TABLE 4.2. **Treatment Ingredients That Influence the Extent of Emotional Processing**

Treatment parameters	Failed emotional processing	Successful emotional processing
Therapy information (content)	Informational elements of the treatment (exposure) fail to match informational elements in the fear memory structure.	Information encountered during treatment is coherent with key aspects of fear memory, thereby activating the fear structure.
Therapy modality (e.g., *in vivo* exposure, verbal descriptions, films, role plays, etc.)	The therapeutic process fails to represent critical elements of the fear structure and/or does not elicit sufficient recall of the fear experience.	Therapeutic process depicts the core elements of the fear memory structure.
Exposure duration	Exposure too brief to allow habituation.	Prolonged exposure is associated with habituation.
Degree of attention	Reduced attention to fear stimuli impedes encoding of incompatible information.	Heightened attention to fear stimuli facilitates encoding of incompatible information.

individuals would not show long-term habituation or successful emotional processing.

In their critical review of ERP for OCD, Jacoby and Abramowitz (2016) note that the emotional processing view of habituation means that therapists using ERP must (1) explain that repeated and prolonged exposure is necessary for fear reduction, (2) continue within-session exposure until habituation occurs, and (3) begin ERP with moderately fearful stimuli and then progress upward in a gradual manner. However, the authors conclude that empirical evidence that habituation predicts ERP treatment outcome is mixed, and within-session response decrement may not be necessary for between-session habituation. They note that the emphasis on habituation in emotional processing theory could perpetuate "fear of fear" as clients and their therapists seek to achieve an anxiety-free state rather than learning to tolerate anxiety. In addition, emotional processing does not provide a completely satisfactory explanation of the return of fear. And so, we turn to the most recent development in the behavioral conceptualization of ERP: *inhibitory learning theory*.

Inhibitory Learning Theory

According to inhibitory learning theory (ILT), the original threat association learned during fear acquisition (e.g., that a particular unwanted thought is threatening) does not disappear with extinction but rather is left intact and competes with new nonthreatening inhibitory associations (Craske et al., 2014; Jacoby & Abramowitz, 2016). In our case illustration, Jenna would never completely lose her fear of spreading contamination no matter how successful her exposure treatment. Instead her original contamination memory remains intact but weakened as it competes with new knowledge gained about personal responsibility for harming others. The new understanding gained through extinction trials involves secondary inhibitory learning in which the obsession (the conditioned stimulus) does not predict personal threat (the unconditioned stimulus) (Craske et al., 2014). For Jenna, inhibitory learning would mean discovering from exposure therapy that one can safely ignore thoughts of personal responsibility for causing inadvertent contamination of others.

Cognitive-behavioral therapists who practice *conventional ERP* are espousing an emotional processing perspective on learning whether they realize it or not. They explain to clients that effective treatment requires that one begin with moderately anxious situations in which avoidance and safety seeking are eliminated and that each exposure must continue until within-session anxiety declines to baseline levels. As well, exposures must be repeated frequently, if not daily, with clients gradually progressing to more anxiety-provoking situations in a hierarchical fashion. Emotional processing theory assumes that ERP must be offered in this manner to achieve the within-session and between-session habituation that are essential for treatment success.

However, ILT takes a very different perspective on the ERP learning process. It is not the level of fear or anxiety expressed during exposure trials that is critical but whether inhibitory learning acquired during exposure modifies fear expression at posttreatment (Craske et al., 2008). As well, ILT emphasizes the importance of fear tolerance rather than fear habituation and the introduction of "desirable difficulty" during exposure sessions to promote greater self-efficacy and fear tolerance even though fear level may remain high throughout the exposure session (Craske et al., 2008; Jacoby & Abramowitz, 2016). In sum, ILT contends that exposure therapy should increase the strength, durability, and generalization of learning so that nonthreatening associations override or inhibit accessibility and retrieval of threat-based associations (Arch & Abramowtiz, 2015).

To achieve the goals of ILT, conventional ERP for OCD requires some refinement. Craske and colleagues (2014) proposed several therapeutic strategies that would enhance inhibitory learning during exposure, with other researchers offering specific application to ERP for OCD (Arch & Abramowitz, 2015; Jacoby & Abramowitz, 2016). Table 4.3 summarizes these modifications and describes how they can be applied to OCD.

As can be seen, the ILT perspective suggests a different approach to ERP from what is normally practiced by behaviorally oriented clinicians. The overarching goal of these changes is to maximize the discrepancy between the anxiety-based associations learned during the acquisition phase and the new nondistressing associations learned during exposure. The greater the discrepancy between the old and new information, the more likely that the new inhibitory associations acquired during exposure will override existing fear (anxiety) memory structures (Craske et al., 2014). It should be noted that empirical evidence for many of the tenets of ILT are mixed, at best (for reviews, see Craske et al., 2014; Jacoby & Abraomwitz, 2016). Nevertheless, the core elements of ILT are compatible with CBT. For this reason the next section explains how to implement standard ERP for OCD and then proposes changes that improve treatment outcome by incorporating modifications based on ILT.

EXPOSURE AND RESPONSE PREVENTION FOR OCD

Origins and Overview

Beginnings

Victor Meyer (1966) published the first case report on ERP for OCD. He reasoned that if individuals with OCD could be persuaded to remain in a fear situation and were prevented from carrying out the compulsion, then they would learn that the feared consequences of ritual nonperformance

TABLE 4.3. **Inhibitory Learning Strategies for Enhanced ERP for OCD**

Strategy	Explanation	Application to OCD
Expectancy violation	Set up discrepancies between what the client expects will happen in exposure and what really happens (i.e., create "surprise").	Client articulates what she expects to experience before ERP exercise, rates the probability that expected experience will occur, and rates her ability to tolerate the experience. After ERP, the client records and rates the actual experience. The therapist helps the client reflect on the expected–actual discrepancy as a basis of new learning.
Deepened extinction	Combine multiple fear cues during exposure, or pair a novel fear cue with a previously extinguished cue.	Exposure sessions should involve complex naturalistic distressing scenarios that contain multiple obsession cues.
Occasional reinforced extinction	Occasionally include the client's most feared outcome in the exposure trial.	In some of the *in vivo* exposures, clients imagine that their actions are responsible for some dreaded outcome because of failure to neutralize.
Removal of safety signals	All forms of safety seeking, neutralization, and reassurance seeking are prevented during and after exposure trials.	Encourage prevention of overt and covert neutralization responses, avoidance, and efforts to exert mental control over the obsession.
Stimulus variability	Incorporate varied stimulus cues into the exposure so that to-be-learned information is paired with more retrieval cues.	Vary the order, duration, and intensity level of the exposures, even though this may be associated with increased subjective discomfort.
Planned retrieval cues	Embed exposure scenarios with retrieval cues that will be present in daily living after exposure treatment ceases.	Ensure that ERP is practiced in the client's daily routine settings so that certain aspects of the setting will act as retrieval cues for the learned inhibitory associations.
Multiple contexts	Conduct exposure across multiple settings to offset *context renewal*, which is the return of fear (anxiety) due to a change in context.	ERP exercises should cover a range of diverse conditions, with clients encouraged to evaluate and synthesize what they learned from their exposure assignments.
Reconsolidation	To engage in pre-exposure recall of fear memories prior to sustained trials of exposure therapy.	Have clients recall in detail memories of past OCD experiences prior to engaging in a planned exposure assignment.

Note. Based on Arch and Abramowitz (2015); Craske et al. (2014); and Jacoby and Abramowitz (2016).

would not materialize (i.e., the conditioned fear stimulus is not associated with the unconditioned fear stimulus). This would result in modification of the obsessive–compulsive goal expectation, which in turn would lead to complete cessation of the compulsion. Meyer reported some success in using ERP to treat a patient with compulsive washing and another with blasphemous sexual obsessions who neutralized with repeating and redoing rituals. Both individuals were treated by Meyer on an inpatient basis with 20–25 hours of situational ERP. In a later ERP treatment study of 15 individuals with OCD, 10 were either "much improved" or totally asymptomatic, with treatment gains maintained in two-thirds of the sample over a varying follow-up period (Meyer et al., 1974).

Exposure

Treatment begins by providing clients with a rationale for the two main components of the intervention: exposure and response prevention. A fear hierarchy is constructed that lists a variety of situations, objects, mental intrusions, or other experiences that the client finds distressing and/or avoids or that elicit obsessive–compulsive symptoms. Table 4.4 presents a hypothetical exposure hierarchy for compulsive cleaning. Clients are asked to rate the anticipated level of discomfort associated with each hierarchy item if they were prevented from carrying out the compulsive ritual. The intensity of the compulsive urge is rated in terms of subjective urge to neutralize as well as estimated ability to resist engaging in the compulsion.

Three elements of exposure must be present for treatment success. First, a high level of anxiety must be elicited and maintained during each exposure session. Treatment effectiveness depends on dosage level. Thus, the client with OCD must be exposed repeatedly to highly distressing situations and must remain in those situations until he or she experiences a significant reduction in subjective distress (de Silva & Rachman, 1992; Steketee, 1999).

Second, the therapist should provide considerable support and encouragement as individuals attempt to endure their distressing situations. Individuals with OCD are often reluctant to expose themselves to situations that cause elevated distress. In providing support, the therapist must ensure that the encouragement does not acquire neutralizing properties. The therapist can remind the client that anxiety will naturally dissipate if left alone, but the therapist must also refrain from reassuring the client that the obsessional concern will not occur (e.g., that the client will not become deathly sick by touching a doorknob). This is the core fear that must be targeted by the exposure session. Finally, the therapist should model the most appropriate response by performing each exposure task before the client is assigned between-session homework (Rachman, Hodgson, & Marks, 1971; Rachman, Marks, & Hodgson, 1973; Roper, Rachman, & Marks,

TABLE 4.4. **Illustrative Exposure Hierarchy for Compulsive Cleaning**

Hierarchy items	Discomfort level[a]	Level of compulsive urge[b]
Sitting in a friend's apartment	10	0
Wearing the same clothes on 2 consecutive days	15	5
Seeing dirt while vacuuming	25	5
Noticing dust on furniture at work	30	40
Handling books that other people probably used	30	60
Touching doorknobs in public buildings	50	75
Sitting on a park bench	55	45
Having one's pajamas touch the floor	65	60
Wearing clothes that fell on the floor	65	80
Washing clothes in a public laundromat	75	20
Pushing a supermarket shopping cart with bare hands	90	85
Shaking the hand of an unfamiliar person	90	95
Using a public toilet	100	100

[a]0 = no discomfort to 100 = maximum/peak discomfort.
[b]0 = no urge to neutralize, 50 = strong urge to neutralize but resisted for several minutes, 100 = intense urge and neutralized immediately.

1975). By modeling the appropriate behavioral response, the client is shown that despite some discomfort, contact with the provoking stimulus can be made without engaging in a neutralizing response.

Response Prevention

Response prevention involves the suppression of any compulsive ritual or other response that alleviates discomfort caused by the obsession. Exposure sessions are usually 30–60 minutes, followed by instructions to refrain from carrying out a neutralizing response. Response prevention can last up to 2 hours, with the therapist present during this entire interval. Behavioral therapists do not physically restrain clients from carrying out their compulsions, but they do use distraction, feedback, conversation, and encouragement to help clients resist their compulsive rituals (de Silva & Rachman, 1992). In addition, every effort is made to refrain from providing reassurance. For example, if asked "Are you sure nothing bad will happen if I don't check?", the therapist takes an investigative perspective, encouraging the client to wait and see what happens. The therapist must also be vigilant of substitute rituals or mental neutralizing that may be used to alleviate distress during exposure.

Practice Guidelines for (Standard) ERP

Most CBT therapists who utilize ERP assume that habituation is the core process responsible for treatment effectiveness. For this reason, the standard form of ERP described in this section is based on the emotional processing theory of learning. What is presented is a practical, step-by-step explanation of standard ERP along with clinical resource materials that therapists can use to improve ERP efficiency and effectiveness. The following are the basic components that must be included when implementing ERP: (1) treatment readiness, (2) pretreatment assessment, (3) psychoeducation, (4) hierarchy construction, (5) within-session and between-session ERP, and (6) relapse prevention. Many excellent treatment manuals provide a more detailed discussion of the many issues involved in ERP treatment for OCD (e.g., Abramowitz, 2018; Abramowitz, Deacon, & Whiteside, 2011; Rego, 2016; Steketee, 1999).

Treatment Readiness

Before offering ERP, it is important to determine the client's readiness to undertake a treatment that is quite demanding. The treatment requires a strong dose of client collaboration, commitment, and effort as individuals face their greatest fears, experience heightened levels of distress, abandon cherished safety practices, and confront situations or experiences that may have avoided for years.

There are several aspects to determining treatment readiness for ERP. These include (1) client goals and expectations, (2) past experiences and knowledge of ERP, (3) faulty ERP beliefs, (4) cost–benefit analysis of ERP, (5) practical obstacles to commitment, and (6) the collaborative contract.

Client Goals and Expectations

Assessment of client readiness begins by determining how ERP fits with the client's treatment goals and expectations. You can expect considerable variability from clients who are able to express what they want to change with therapy to others who respond with "I don't know; I just want to get better." Client-centered ERP begins with determining how the intervention can be presented in a way that helps the client achieve valued goals and avoids clashing with treatment expectations that lead to noncompliance or outright rejection of the intervention.

It is important to assess client goals and expectations during the assessment phase (see also Chapter 8) before presenting any psychoeducation on OCD and its treatment. Form 4.1 can be given as part of the assessment package at the initial contact. As indicated in the instructions, clients should formulate their treatment goals in terms of changes in their OCD symptoms that would lead to significant improvement in their daily functioning and QOL. Often individuals write general responses like "Do less washing," "Have more self-confidence," or "Be less obsessive." These entries will need further elaboration and goals/expectations highlighted that are compatible, or not, with ERP. For example, the therapist can incorporate a client goal like "Want to stop repeatedly checking doors and windows when leaving the house" into the psychoeducational phase of ERP since this is a treatment-congruent goal. However, a goal like "Be anxiety-free when leaving the house" would be incompatible with an intervention that involves confronting anxious thoughts and feelings. Expect a mixture of ERP-consistent and -inconsistent goals/expectations that will need to be taken into consideration when introducing ERP.

Past Experiences and Knowledge of ERP

Some individuals with OCD may report that they have had ERP from another therapist and that it was not helpful. When this happens, try to obtain more specific information about the therapy.

- What types of exposures did they do, how often, and for how long?
- How well did they resist the compulsive urge?
- Was an exposure hierarchy developed?
- Was exposure homework assigned and, if so, how often was it done?
- How distressing were the exposures and did the distress ever decline?
- Was exposure first done in the therapy session or were other forms of therapist-assisted exposure utilized?
- Did the therapist introduce other treatment strategies such as cognitive therapy, mindfulness, or acceptance and commitment therapy (ACT)?

If the client is vague or unsure about his or her previous treatment, the therapist can ask to see any information sheets or homework assignments associated with the previous therapy. Rego (2016) suggests that in certain cases, written consent can be obtained from the client to contact the previous therapist for further treatment information.

The Internet is a rich source of information on ERP. Clients may have visited relevant websites, read several self-help books, or may know someone treated with ERP. The therapist should inquire about the client's knowledge of ERP, being especially mindful of false information or misconceptions about the treatment. Two key points should be emphasized when discussing past ERP treatment.

1. *Therapist differences.* Like any psychological treatment, each therapist brings to ERP his or her therapy style, knowledge, and experience. This means that ERP delivered by one therapist might be quite different from another therapist. For the client, ERP delivered by a new therapist could feel like a whole new therapy.
2. *Dose–response sensitivity.* The effectiveness of ERP depends on the amount of exposure and the client's ability to resist his or her compulsions. It is possible that past exposures were too infrequent or not sufficiently challenging to be effective. One can't expect treatment to be effective if it's done only occasionally.

Faulty ERP Beliefs

Client knowledge and experience of ERP can give rise to personally held beliefs about the treatment and its impact. Some of these beliefs could be misconceptions that will undermine the client's engagement in the treatment process. It is important to address these faulty beliefs before engaging in exposure therapy. The therapist uses Socratic questioning and guided discovery to identify these beliefs, and then cognitive restructuring strategies to help the client adopt a healthier perspective on ERP. The following is a sample of faulty ERP beliefs:

- *"ERP requires that I endure more anxiety or discomfort than I can bear."* The response to this belief is that exposures occur in a graded fashion that most often involves moderate anxiety/discomfort with the goal of helping individuals learn to strengthen their ability to deal with (tolerate) anxiety/discomfort in obsessive–compulsive situations.

- *"I can't let myself get too anxious because it could be dangerous; it could harm my health."* The type of anxiety/discomfort associated with ERP is acute, but it is not harmful. It will feel uncomfortable, but this type of anxiety has a built-in thermostat that causes a person to eventually calm down. It operates a lot like the physical exertion involved in exercise (see Abramowitz, 2018).

- *"ERP forces people to do things against their will."* ERP is always done in a collaborative manner with the client highly involved in setting exposure assignments. The pace of ERP is always determined by how quickly the individual wants to progress up the exposure hierarchy.

- *"Once an OCD situation has been conquered with ERP, I should never struggle with obsessive–compulsive symptoms in that situation again.*" Like most treatments, ERP does not progress in a smooth and steady manner. On some days an exposure assignment can be accomplished with less discomfort or obsessiveness, whereas on other days the same assignment may cause a surprising amount of discomfort and urge to neutralize. The important point is that overall tolerance of obsessive concerns has improved, and obsessive–compulsive symptoms are on the decline.

Cost–Benefit Analysis

Rego (2016) suggests that the therapist engage the client in a discussion of the pros and cons of treatment to enhance client motivation and commitment to treatment. In the present context a cost–benefit analysis could focus on whether to engage in ERP versus continue with "treatment as usual." Depending on the client's experience, treatment as usual might be (1) manage OCD on his or her own, (2) rely solely on medication, (3) accept only supportive psychotherapy, or (4) engage in cognitive therapy, mindfulness, or ACT without ERP. Figure 4.1 presents an illustrative cost–benefit analysis of ERP, and a blank worksheet for client use can be found in Form 4.2.

The therapist should introduce the ERP Cost–Benefit Worksheet early in treatment as a within-session task. Clients may have difficulty listing the advantages and disadvantages of exposure therapy, so this needs to be done collaboratively in therapy. Figure 4.1 can be used as a guide, but the cost–benefit points should be specific to each client. As well, individuals are encouraged to revisit this exercise after their initial experiences with ERP, in order to modify the points or add new comments. This step will ensure that the exercise continues to have relevance for each client and acts as a motivation enhancer.

Practical Obstacles to Commitment

Because between-session homework is a critical component of ERP, it is important to identity practical obstacles that may thwart the client's full commitment to do exposure exercises outside of sessions. This discussion should occur before the first ERP session. The demands of home, work, and family may limit personal time needed for exposure. Other issues might be whether to do exposures when (1) traveling for work or leisure; (2) feeling slightly unwell, having pain, or feeling tired; (3) others are present, like family or guests; (4) the day was stressful or upsetting; (5) feeling down or generally anxious; (6) spouse or family member undermines exposure; (7) unexpected life events occur; and the like. By exploring these issues, the therapist is confronting problems that could undermine ERP effectiveness before it happens. Naturally it is important to problem-solve *with the client* any anticipated obstacles to exposure.

	Benefits, Advantages	**Costs, Disadvantages**
Treatment with ERP	1. Most effective psychological treatment for OCD 2. Treatment gains are more durable 3. Deals directly with obsessive–compulsive situations that interfere in daily living 4. Therapeutic benefits extend beyond the therapy session 5. Able to involve a spouse or family member for support and encouragement 6. Opportunity to practice skills learned in therapy	1. Requires considerable effort and personal commitment 2. Will feel moderate to high anxiety or discomfort 3. Will provoke feelings of uncertainty about dreaded outcomes 4. Will feel heightened sense of responsibility for bad outcomes to self or others. 5. Momentarily may feel worse about myself. 6. Takes time and so there is some interference in daily routine.
Treatment without ERP (i.e., treatment as usual)	1. Don't have to face my obsessional fears 2. Requires less effort, especially between sessions 3. No increase in anxiety or discomfort 4. Won't have to face the possibility of failure 5. Might achieve some symptom improvement with minimal effort	1. Greater chance of obsessive–compulsive relapse and recurrence 2. More sessions may be required, which increases therapy costs 3. Therapy may have less impact on daily living 4. Less opportunity to practice therapy skills and make meaningful change 5. Less likely to feel a sense of personal mastery over the OCD 6. OCD may continue to interfere in daily living due to avoidance

FIGURE 4.1. Sample ERP cost–benefit worksheet.

The Collaborative Contract

For some clients, a written agreement specifying the roles and responsibilities the client and therapist will adopt while working on ERP might boost treatment commitment. The agreement should list only a few general points that would apply to a broad range of exposure experiences. For example, therapist responsibilities might be to (1) provide the best evidence-based advice on ERP, (2) develop an individualized treatment plan, (3) emphasize collaboration in developing the exposure program, (4) encourage but not coerce progression through the hierarchy, and (5) teach coping skills that improve management and tolerance of distress. Client responsibilities could include (1) devoting time to do between-session exposure-based homework, (2) working on tolerating anxiety and letting it decline naturally, (3) maintaining therapy focus on ERP for several sessions, (4) collaborating on developing exposure exercises, (5) taking a problem-solving approach to difficulties encountered with an exposure, and (6) not giving up at the first signs of distress or uncertainty. The collaborative contract should be reviewed periodically throughout treatment to ensure continued relevance to the client's exposure experiences.

Pretreatment Assessment

Before introducing ERP, it is important to do a functional analysis of the obsessions and compulsions. In addition to identifying the primary obsessions and compulsions, the pretreatment assessment should include information on triggers, feared consequences, avoidance, and safety-seeking behaviors (Abramowitz, 2018). The assessment tools found in Chapter 7 are helpful in providing information needed to develop an ERP intervention, but they also assess other aspects of OCD that are critical to the cognitive therapy strategies. Form 4.3 is a worksheet that is especially useful for providing the specific information needed to construct an exposure hierarchy. It is based on the example of an exposure hierarchy for compulsive cleaning found in Table 4.4.

Psychoeducation

Psychoeducation is an important ingredient in CBT for OCD. At the outset of treatment, the therapist will provide psychoeducation on OCD and its treatment. Chapter 8 provides an extensive discussion on educating the client about the CBT model, the normalcy of unwanted intrusive thoughts, and how cognitive change can contribute to treatment effectiveness. This section focuses on psychoeducation that is specific to ERP. It can be incorporated into the general CBT psychoeducation at the beginning of therapy, or the therapist can wait and present it separately when introducing the client to ERP. The following are some of the key features of ERP that should be discussed with clients.

- *Definition of ERP.* Introduce ERP as an intervention strategy that involves intentionally focusing one's attention on obsessional thoughts or images and purposefully exposing oneself to the situations or stimuli that trigger obsessive–compulsive symptoms. It is intended that clients maintain their engagement with the obsession and its trigger for as long as it takes for distress to subside. At the same time, the person is not to engage in any behavioral or mental compulsion throughout the exposure session and for a couple of hours after the exposure ends.

• *Exposure hierarchy.* ERP is a highly systematic, structured intervention that starts with constructing an exposure hierarchy. A list of 15–20 obsessive–compulsive-relevant situations or scenarios is generated, ranging from the mildly difficult to the most difficult situations imaginable.

• *Exposure sessions.* The exposure exercises start with a moderately difficult obsessive–compulsive scenario. Clients are asked to expose themselves repeatedly to the obsession and its trigger daily for 30–60 minutes over a 1- to 2-week period. During each session, attention is maintained on the obsession, and distress can decline naturally without the use of anxiety management strategies.

• *Treatment goal.* ERP is one of the most powerful interventions for strengthening inhibitory responses to anxiety, disconfirming belief in the most feared consequence associated with obsessive–compulsive symptoms, learning tolerance of anxiety/discomfort, normalizing risk taking and uncertainty, and improving self-confidence.

• *Treatment progression.* When a client can engage in an obsessive–compulsive task with minimal distress, a more difficult obsessive–compulsive scenario is selected from the hierarchy. With each new scenario, the first exposure is done with the therapist in session before it is assigned as homework.

• *Collaboration.* The client's pace through the exposure hierarchy is set collaboratively. The therapist never cajoles the client to do an exposure against his or her will. The therapy is intended to give clients "hands-on" experience in dealing with OCD and reducing its negative impact on daily living.

• *Evidence-based treatment.* Numerous clinical trials over the last 45 years have demonstrated that ERP is the most effective treatment for OCD. It produces the most enduring effects, but it is most effective when individuals do the exposure homework assignments and complete a course of treatment. However, its effectiveness rate for treatment completers is 60–70%, and only 20–25% attain symptom-free status. Moreover, many people who complete ERP require occasional booster sessions to maintain their treatment gains.

• *Grit and commitment.* ERP requires more effort, determination, and patience than many other forms of psychological treatment for OCD. It involves facing the worst fears, exposure to high levels of anxiety or discomfort, and considerable effort at preventing compulsive responses.

Although involving some "short-term pain," the benefits of ERP are substantial for those who complete treatment.

The rationale for ERP must be individualized so that the misconceptions and faulty beliefs unique to each client are addressed in the psychoeducational phase. Clients are invited to raise questions and concerns about the treatment. For further discussion on how to address client concerns about ERP, see Abramowitz (2018) and Rego (2016).

The Exposure Hierarchy

Development of an exposure hierarchy is a core therapeutic ingredient of ERP. It is constructed in a collaborative manner, drawing on various assessment and self-monitoring worksheets (e.g., Forms 4.1 and 4.3). Figure 4.2 presents an exposure hierarchy based on Jenna's contamination and harm obsessions.

There are various indicators, such as level of anxiety or ratings on the subjective units of distress scale (SUDS), which can be used to organize the hierarchy items or scenarios. Form 4.4 uses the term *level of difficulty* because the critical determinant is the ease or difficulty of engaging in ERP when confronted with the scenario. Also, *difficulty* is a broad concept that includes level of distress, tendency to avoid, urge to neutralize, and the like.

There are several characteristics that go into creating an effective exposure hierarchy. Select 15–20 scenarios that capture the primary obsessive–compulsive concerns of the client and that range from mild to extreme difficulty. It is best to work on obsessive–compulsive-relevant situations, thoughts, or experiences that are highly impactful on daily functioning and are consistent with the client's treatment goals and expectations. Also, the best hierarchy scenarios are specific situations that are encountered daily. More items in the moderate to high difficulty range are needed, since most of the ERP work is done with these scenarios. Most clients will need considerable input from their therapist when constructing the hierarchy, and it will likely need frequent revision as treatment progresses. A copy of the exposure hierarchy should be provided so that clients can follow their treatment progress.

ERP Sessions and Homework

The first exposure session begins with a moderately difficult scenario (i.e., > 25). The Exposure Worksheet in Form 4.5 can be used to monitor ERP progress. Part I should be completed collaboratively within session, so the client has detailed instructions for engaging in the between-session ERP. It is important to specify how, when, where, and length of the exposure session. Normally, exposures last at least 30 minutes or longer to allow anxiety or distress to dissipate and for the client to consider the situation less difficult. In addition, all overt and covert compulsive rituals, reassurance seeking, safety seeking, and other neutralization strategies must be specified so the client is clear on which responses should be prevented. In Part II clients record their experience with homework exposure, and Part III provides opportunity for individuals to comment on their success or disappointment with the weekly ERP sessions.

OCD Scenarios (i.e., obsessive–compulsive-relevant situations, thoughts, or experiences)	Difficulty Level
1. People touching me, like in a crowded elevator	10
2. Shaking hands with people	12
3. Using washroom at work	20
4. See brown, reddish smear on sidewalk and wonder if it's blood	25
5. Taking a new route to work	30
6. Going through intersection and wondering if traffic light was red	40
7. Using public toilet	45
8. Changing lanes while driving alone	50
9. Merging onto a busy highway	60
10. Driving on a city street crowded with pedestrians on the sidewalks	65
11. Driving past cyclists	70
12. Seeing a reddish speck on office kitchen counter	75
13. Sitting on bus and notice a reddish smudge on another seat	75
14. Preparing a meal for guests	75
15. Using exercise equipment at gym	77
16. Sitting on a chair in doctor's office and notice a smear	80
17. Having a small bandaged cut on hand	85
18. Having a small clotted cut on hand, not bandaged	95
19. Person starts to walk toward car while I'm driving through a pedestrian crosswalk	97
20. Picking up a tissue spotted with a stranger's blood	100

FIGURE 4.2. Jenna's exposure hierarchy.

The therapist begins within-session exposure by collaborating with the client in selecting a moderately difficult scenario from the hierarchy. Modeling the exposure is a good way to introduce clients to ERP exercises. The client then imitates the therapist's demonstration and should continue with the exposure until he or she experiences a significant decline in distress. Introduce exposure early in the session to allow enough time for anxiety reduction and discussion of the homework exposure.

When an exposure scenario elicits only minimal anxiety or discomfort after several attempts, the client can engage in variations of the exposure or tackle another hierarchy scenario at the same or higher difficulty level. However, it's important that clients not start too low in the hierarchy, get stuck at an exposure level, or run ahead too quickly. Pace the exposures so they are always moderately challenging to maximize the learning experience.

Daily exposure sessions lasting about 90 minutes are recommended for moderate to severe OCD (Kozak & Foa, 1997; Steketee, 1993, 1999). Weekly exposure sessions may suffice for milder OCD. Abramowitz, Foa, and Franklin (2003) reported that twice-weekly sessions of ERP can be as effective as intensive daily treatment, especially in the long term. It is unknown whether weekly ERP therapy sessions, which are the likely modus operandi of many practitioners, are enough to produce clinically significant treatment effects.

In vivo exposure to actual feared situations is preferred over imaginal exposure, although the latter can be used initially to prepare the patient for naturalistic exposure (de Silva & Rachman, 1992). Also, imaginal exposure is useful for (1) obsessions based on fateful catastrophes such as disasters, (2) accidents happening to loved ones, and (3) imagined or remote outcomes like being punished in hell or experiencing the end of the world (de Silva & Rachman, 1992; Foa & Kozak, 1997). Self-directed exposure can be as effective as therapist-assisted exposure (Emmelkamp & Kraanen, 1977; Emmelkamp et al., 1989), and family members or spouses can act as co-therapists or coaches (Emmelkamp & De Lange, 1983; see also Emmelkamp, 1982). Coaches should only encourage and support the client in doing exposure and ritual prevention and avoid giving reassurance, using physical restraint, making threats, or using persuasion or rationalization to dissuade the client about his or her obsessive–compulsive symptomatology (Rego, 2016). Finally, various therapeutic strategies such as cognitive restructuring, mindfulness, and ACT can be incorporated into ERP to strengthen the client's commitment to the exposure sessions.

Relapse Prevention

In the final sessions of ERP, it is important to discuss relapse prevention and prepare the client for treatment termination. There are several issues that should be addressed when focusing on relapse prevention.

1. *Expect setbacks and symptom recurrence.* Few individuals are completely symptom-free after a trial of ERP. Therefore, clients should expect that their obsessive–compulsive concerns will linger but in a greatly diminished manner. As well, obsessive–compulsive symptoms can gain strength during times of stress, depressed mood, health problems, and the like. In addition, the individual could encounter a novel situation or have an experience that approximates his or her most feared consequence. It is important to discuss the many ways in which individuals can experience a resurgence of obsessive–compulsive symptoms so that they are prepared to deal with these perceived setbacks.

2. *Adopt an ERP lifestyle.* Abramowitz and colleagues (2011) consider it important that clients adopt a lifestyle approach to ERP that involves "making choices to take advantage of additional opportunities to practice confronting, rather than avoiding, fear cues" (p. 119). Take time to review with clients their daily living routine and how they could build in more naturalistic exposure opportunities to ensure the continuation of ERP long after treatment termination. Encourage clients to be vigilant for any obsessive intrusions, avoidance of obsessive–compulsive triggers, or the emergence of compulsive rituals. When this happens, intentionally engage in ERP. Identify any barriers to confronting daily situations that still make the client uncomfortable. For someone with physical contamination OCD, "lifestyle exposure" might mean repeatedly using the airport washrooms when traveling, being the first person to open doors with bare hands, or offering to push the luggage cart without gloves or use of hand sanitizer. It is important that clients view ERP as a "new way of living" rather than as a time-limited treatment strategy.

3. *Confront "mini-rituals."* Abramowitz (2018) describes mini-rituals as brief, subtle, and discreet responses that are driven by obsessive–compulsive symptoms but possibly unrecognized by the individual. These actions are taken to feel a sense of comfort or safety. Examples include continually looking in the rearview mirror while driving, having hand sanitizer available at all times, saying "God willing" whenever talking about the future, wearing a lucky bracelet or other clothing, never varying the route to work, always having the same morning routine, etc. Often these mini-rituals involve an avoidance of the unfamiliar. It is important to help the client identify these obsessive–compulsive-related habits of living and to practice countering with exposure to novelty, uncertainty, and ambiguity.

4. *Follow-up sessions.* Consider whether to schedule booster sessions to preserve treatment gains and reduce risk of relapse. The first booster session is normally scheduled 4–6 weeks after the final session, with subsequent sessions scheduled at increasing time intervals. Booster sessions provide an opportunity to evaluate the client's progress, encourage daily

ERP, and problem-solve difficulties that might represent early signs of relapse (Rego, 2016). At the very least, therapists should encourage clients to schedule a follow-up session as soon as possible if they are concerned about the return of obsessive–compulsive symptoms.

Boosting ERP with Inhibitory Learning

Conventional ERP emerged from the two-factor conditioning model of fear and anxiety and later became rooted in emotional processing theory. Contemporary CBT still utilizes standard ERP as a key therapy ingredient, although exposure exercises are often framed as behavioral experiments designed to provide disconfirming evidence of faulty OCD appraisals and beliefs (e.g., Abramowitz, 2018; Clark, 2004; Rachman, 2004; Salkovskis, 1999).

As discussed previously, ILT proposes that the effectiveness of ERP depends on learning nonthreatening secondary associations and tolerance of fear and anxiety rather than a process of habituation (Craske et al., 2008, 2014). This reformulation of the ERP learning process has treatment implications. The most critical modifications that might enhance ERP effectiveness are summarized in the following sections (Abramowitz, 2018; Arch & Abramowitz, 2015; Jacoby & Abramowitz, 2016).

Expectancy Violation

In ILT, exposure sessions should be developed so that the person experiences a violation or disconfirmation of his or her expectations about the feared consequences associated with the obsession and failure to neutralize. Craske and colleagues (2014) state that "a mismatch between expectancy and outcome is critical for new learning" (p. 4). The greater the discrepancy between expectation and outcome, the stronger the inhibitory learning. For expectancy violation to occur in treatment of OCD, it is necessary that compulsive rituals and other forms of neutralizing are prevented. To boost expectancy violation, the client should make expectancy ratings before a new exposure session, record actual exposure experiences, and then work on understanding the discrepancy at the next therapy session. Form 4.6 (Expectancy Exposure Worksheet) can be used along with the Exposure Worksheet (Form 4.5) to highlight expectancy violations.

It is important to spend time in the subsequent session reviewing Forms 4.5 and 4.6 to highlight the discrepancy between what was expected and the actual outcome of the exposure homework. As well, the cognitive therapist will want to use this discrepancy as disconfirmation of the individual's faulty appraisals and beliefs (see Chapter 9). The therapist and client should collaborate on writing a summary statement in the client's own words that expresses what he or she has learned from the exposure. In subsequent exposures this could be used as a coping statement to help the client succeed with even harder ERP exercises.

Variability and Surprise

To increase inhibitory learning, the length of exposure sessions, their timing, intensity, and stimulus properties are varied. Rather than do the same exposure over and over and then progress in a linear fashion to the next scenario in the hierarchy, ILT recommends that individuals jump back and forth between higher- and lower-intensity exposures. As well, the time of day that exposure homework is done and the length of the exposure are varied from day to day. In addition, the client should vary the exposure situation, in order to experience exposure to multiple contexts. For Jenna, this might mean driving past cyclists and imagining that one of them swerved toward the car; on another day, she might use the washroom at the mall; and on a third day, she would visit the doctor's office and sit close to sullied furniture in the waiting room. Abramowitz (2018) noted that exposure variability enhances learning when the client is surprised by what happened in the exposure session. Jenna might be surprised that her fear of harm and contaminating others subsided much faster than she expected.

Exaggerated Exposure

Craske and colleagues (2014) state that occasional reinforced learning during extinction can facilitate inhibitory learning. This would involve building the client's feared outcome into an intense exposure session. In the case of Jenna, this might mean leaving a used tissue on the counter in the office kitchen for a day and then observing any untoward health effects on coworkers. The other possibility is to intentionally make oneself more anxious or hyperaroused in the exposure situation by breathing excessively, ingesting caffeine, engaging in intense physical exercise, or the like. Of course, the therapist must ensure that the exposures match the client's obsessive–compulsive concerns and are done in an ethical and compassionate manner.

Complete Cessation of Neutralization (Safety Seeking)

There is considerable debate on whether safety seeking undermines exposure or whether it could facilitate inhibitory learning by enabling the individual to tolerate greater distress or anxiety (Blakey & Abramowitz, 2016). Rachman, Radomsky, and Shafran (2008) argued that judicious use of safety behaviors in the early stages of treatment can facilitate treatment effectiveness because individuals still are able to experience disconfirmation of their faulty threat-related beliefs. Of course, the argument for retaining safety-seeking behaviors is more difficult to support in OCD when this behavior takes the form of compulsive rituals. Craske and colleagues (2014) concluded that the general consensus is to fade out safety-seeking behavior over the course of exposure, and Abramowitz (2018) recommended that clients should do their best to resist performing safety-seeking rituals. With this in mind, the therapist should help the client develop reasonable, normalized responses to his or her obsessive–compulsive concerns that do not become safety-seeking behaviors. For example, a person with a fear of contamination would need to develop a set of guidelines for cooking with raw meat that would not constitute compulsive washing or safety seeking.

Promote Anxiety/Distress Tolerance

Jacoby and Abramowitz (2016) suggest that rather than teach clients to reduce or control their anxiety/discomfort, the ILT perspective is that ERP is an intervention that teaches anxiety/distress *tolerance*; that is, that the obsessive–compulsive concerns of the client are common, inevitable, and nonthreatening. To achieve this goal, ILT introduces *desirable difficulties* into the exposure by the modifications described previously. Throughout treatment, the therapist continues to emphasize distress tolerance. In fact, physical exercise is an accurate analogy for ERP. Just as exercise is intended to build physical strength, so ERP is designed to build anxiety/distress tolerance of the client's obsessive–compulsive concerns.

CONCLUSION

After 50 years of research and clinical application, ERP remains the single most potent treatment ingredient for OCD (e.g., McKay et al., 2015; Öst, Havnen, Hansen, & Kvale, 2015). Probably most clinicians who use ERP believe that its underlying mechanism is the habituation of fear or anxiety, and this is the rationale that is communicated to clients. And yet, early conditioning and emotional processing theories of ERP have been found lacking. Instead, the inhibitory learning perspective offers a radically different understanding of ERP that moves it much closer to the cognitive theory of OCD. However, the empirical support for inhibitory learning is mixed, and there is no research on whether the modifications to ERP outlined previously are more or less effective than standard ERP (see Jacoby & Abramowitz, 2016, for a critical review). In their more extensive review of exposure augmentation techniques based on ILT, Weisman and Rodebaugh (2018) concluded that empirical support has fallen short of theoretical expectation. However, they note that elimination of safety behaviors, maximizing of expectancy violation, introducing variability into the exposures, and using multiple exposure contexts have some credence for

TABLE 4.5. **Shortcomings of ERP**

- A significant minority of individuals with OCD (20–30%) refuse ERP.
- Approximately 25% of ERP completers fail to improve.
- ERP is less suited for obsessions, especially when overt compulsions are absent.
- Certain subtypes of OCD, such as those with repugnant obsession, overvalued ideation, and possibly order and symmetry compulsions, may show less effective response.
- Residual symptoms persist in treated patients.
- Comorbid conditions, such as depression, may reduce treatment effectiveness.
- Other negative emotions associated with OCD, such as guilt, may be unresponsive to ERP.
- Residual social and occupational impairment is evident at posttreatment.
- Treatment factors like low motivation, homework noncompliance, and pessimistic attitude toward treatment can reduce effectiveness.
- Cognitive dysfunctions and biases are prominent in OCD.

augmenting exposure. From a cognitive therapy perspective, the ILT modifications look very similar to the exposure-based behavioral experiments proposed in CBT (see Chapter 9).

Despite the success of ERP, several prominent OCD researchers have questioned whether this treatment is necessary, given the emergence of cognitive approaches and the high rate of client unacceptability associated with ERP (Shafran, Radomsky, Coughtrey, & Rachman, 2013). Table 4.5 summarizes major limitations in ERP that are still applicable today.

The theoretical and clinical limitations of a strictly learning theory approach to OCD resulted in a paradigmatic shift toward the cognitive features of the disorder (Rachman & Hodgson, 1980; Salkovskis, 1985). Salkovskis (1985, 1989a, 1999) can be credited as pioneering this more cognitive-behavioral perspective in theory and treatment of OCD, which emerged from an amalgamation of Beck's cognitive therapy for depression and Rachman's exposure-based approach to the disorder. In the past three decades this cognitive-behavioral perspective has emerged as the dominant psychological treatment for OCD.

FORM 4.1. OCD Treatment Goals and Expectations Worksheet

Instructions: Most people with OCD know how the condition affects their life. There are things they would like to do, but the OCD stops them, or there are things they'd like to stop doing but they can't because of their OCD. Using the form below, write down what changes you would like to make in your behavior, your emotions, and your thoughts that would represent a significant reduction in your OCD. In other words, what would need to change for you to "feel normal" again? Try to be specific. Think about all the ways in which OCD interferes in your daily life.

Domains	Want to Reduce or Eliminate from My Life	Want to Increase or Improve in My Life
Behaviors (i.e., what I want to do or won't do, how I act, how I respond, what I avoid, my compulsions, my strategies to feel safe or comfortable, etc.)		
Feelings (i.e., my daily moods, momentary feelings, positive emotions, negative emotions, etc.)		
Thoughts (i.e., desirable and undesirable thoughts, spontaneous intrusive thoughts, intentional thinking, images, memories, etc.)		

From *Cognitive-Behavioral Therapy for OCD and Its Subtypes, Second Edition*, by David A. Clark. Copyright © 2020 The Guilford Press. Permission to photocopy this material is granted to purchasers of this book for personal use or use with individual clients (see copyright page for details). Purchasers can download enlarged versions of this material (see the box at the end of the table of contents).

FORM 4.2. ERP Cost–Benefit Worksheet

Instructions: This worksheet is designed to help you decide whether to make a commitment to include exposure and response prevention (ERP). Your therapist has already explained to you that *ERP involves daily, systematic, and repeated exposure to your obsessive fears and concerns while not allowing yourself to engage in a compulsive response.* Before deciding to include ERP in your treatment, consider both the short-term and long-term advantages and disadvantages of the treatment. Compare ERP with your usual or current treatment, which might be medication alone, supportive therapy or counseling, or some other form of psychological treatment but without exposure.

	Benefits, Advantages	Costs, Disadvantages
Treatment with ERP		
Treatment without ERP (i.e., treatment as usual)		

From *Cognitive-Behavioral Therapy for OCD and Its Subtypes, Second Edition*, by David A. Clark. Copyright © 2020 The Guilford Press. Permission to photocopy this material is granted to purchasers of this book for personal use or use with individual clients (see copyright page for details). Purchasers can download enlarged versions of this material (see the box at the end of the table of contents).

FORM 4.3. Pre-Exposure Worksheet

Instructions: For several days record your most common experiences of obsessions and/or compulsions on this worksheet. In the second column rate the intensity of distress (i.e., anxiety, fear, guilt, frustration) associated with that episode on a 100-point scale, with 100 indicating the most distress. Likewise, in the third column rate the intensity of your urge to neutralize the obsession or alleviate the distress by performing a compulsive ritual, leaving the situation, seeking reassurance, etc.

Note. 0 = no associated distress, 50 = moderate distress, 100 = worst distress ever felt; 0 = no urge to neutralize, 50 = moderate urge, 100 = immediate, irresistible urge.

OCD Episode	Distress/ Discomfort (0–100 rating)	Urge to Neutralize (0–100 rating)
1.		
2.		
3.		
4.		
5.		
6.		
7.		
8.		
9.		
10.		

From *Cognitive-Behavioral Therapy for OCD and Its Subtypes, Second Edition*, by David A. Clark. Copyright © 2020 The Guilford Press. Permission to photocopy this material is granted to purchasers of this book for personal use or use with individual clients (see copyright page for details). Purchasers can download enlarged versions of this material (see the box at the end of the table of contents).

FORM 4.4. Exposure Hierarchy Worksheet

Instructions: Use the form below to construct your exposure hierarchy. In the first column, list a variety of situations, thoughts, or experiences that trigger your obsessions and compulsions. It is important to have 15–20 OCD scenarios listed in your hierarchy that range from mild to moderate to intense difficulty. They should be arranged in a stepwise fashion, starting with the easier experiences first, followed by the moderately difficult, and then progressing to the most difficult scenarios. Use the second column to rate each scenario on a 1–100 difficulty scale, with 100 indicating the most difficult.

Note. Difficulty refers to the extent that a scenario would be hard to do without neutralizing (doing a compulsion), avoiding, seeking reassurance, and the like. Use a rating of 1–25 to represent fairly easy scenarios, 26–60 for moderately difficult, and 61–100 for the most difficult scenarios.

OCD Scenarios (i.e., obsessive–compulsive-relevant situations, thoughts, or experiences)	Difficulty Level
1.	
2.	
3.	
4.	
5.	
6.	
7.	
8.	
9.	
10.	
11.	
12.	
13.	
14.	
15.	
16.	
17.	
18.	
19.	
20.	

From *Cognitive-Behavioral Therapy for OCD and Its Subtypes, Second Edition*, by David A. Clark. Copyright © 2020 The Guilford Press. Permission to photocopy this material is granted to purchasers of this book for personal use or use with individual clients (see copyright page for details). Purchasers can download enlarged versions of this material (see the box at the end of the table of contents).

FORM 4.5. Exposure Worksheet

Instructions: This form is designed so that clients know how to do their homework exposure exercise and have an accurate record and evaluation of their exposure experiences. Part I should be completed collaboratively while assigning the exposure homework. Next, individuals rate each exposure session in Part II and write down their general impression of the exposure homework in Part III prior to the next therapy session. The form should be thoroughly reviewed at the subsequent therapy session and any necessary changes made to the exposure assignment.

Name: _____ Date of Therapy Session: _____

I. Description of Exposure Assignment

1. What I need to do (exposure activity): _____
   _____

2. What I need *not* to do (response prevention): _____
   _____

II. Exposure Homework Record

Date	Initial Discomfort (0–100)	Final Discomfort (0–100)	Exposure Duration (minutes)
1.			
2.			
3.			
4.			
5.			
6.			
7.			

III. Observations

Were your exposure sessions successful or not? If you are disappointed with your progress, what changes are needed? _____
_____

From *Cognitive-Behavioral Therapy for OCD and Its Subtypes, Second Edition*, by David A. Clark. Copyright © 2020 The Guilford Press. Permission to photocopy this material is granted to purchasers of this book for personal use or use with individual clients (see copyright page for details). Purchasers can download enlarged versions of this material (see the box at the end of the table of contents).

FORM 4.6. Expectancy Exposure Worksheet

Instructions: This form is designed to encourage inhibitory learning from exposure assignments. Part I, on exposure prediction, should be completed collaboratively with the client when assigning the exposure exercise. In Part II individuals briefly describe their exposure experience in response to the questions posed in this section. Part III asks the client to state what was learned from the exposure exercise. The client's responses should be thoroughly reviewed at the subsequent therapy session, with the therapist elaborating on responses that strengthen inhibitory learning.

Name: _____ Date of Therapy Session: _____

I. Exposure Prediction

1. What are you worried will happen if you expose yourself to this obsessive–compulsive situation and resist doing a compulsion or other form of neutralizing?
   _____
   _____

2. What is the likelihood that your worries will come true (0 = not at all; 100 = certain to happen)? _____%

3. Do you think you can do this exposure, prevent the compulsion, and tolerate the anxiety, discomfort, risk, and uncertainty? If not, why? _____
   _____
   _____

II. Actual Exposure Outcome

Briefly summarize what happened in your exposure sessions. Consult your exposure worksheet to generate this summary. What was the worst that you experienced with the exposures? What was the most difficult? Did your worries come true? What went better than you expected? How well did you cope with the anxiety, discomfort, and uncertainty?
_____
_____
_____

III. Learning

What did you learn about your OCD and how you can manage it from your exposure sessions? Did you expect worse than what actually happened? Discuss what you've learned with your therapist and together write a summary in the space below.
_____
_____
_____

Note. Based on Arch and Abramowitz (2015).

From *Cognitive-Behavioral Therapy for OCD and Its Subtypes*, Second Edition, by David A. Clark. Copyright © 2020 The Guilford Press. Permission to photocopy this material is granted to purchasers of this book for personal use or use with individual clients (see copyright page for details). Purchasers can download enlarged versions of this material (see the box at the end of the table of contents).

CHAPTER 5

The Cognitive-Behavioral Model

THEORY AND RESEARCH

If intrusive thinking is normal, why does it become obsessive for people vulnerable to OCD? This is the central question addressed by cognitive-behavioral theories of OCD. Not only is this question critical for understanding the etiology and maintenance of OCD, but it also informs treatment of the disorder.

The cognitive approach to OCD is an appraisal-based theory, which posits that a core aspect of all emotional states is "a person's subjective evaluation or appraisal of the personal significance of a situation, object, or event on a number of dimensions or criteria" (Scherer, 1999, p. 637). In clinical psychology appraisal theories focus on the content and product of a biased information-processing system to understand the etiology and persistence of psychopathology. Although criticisms have been raised against this perspective (MacLeod, 1993), a vigorous defense of its validity has been offered, citing various factors, not the least being its significant contribution to improved treatment of clinical disorders (McNally, 2001).

This chapter presents the generic CBT model of OCD. It begins with a brief discussion of the historical roots of cognitive theory and treatment of OCD. Next the generic cognitive appraisal model of OCD is presented, drawing heavily on the contributions of Salkovskis, Rachman, Freeston, and the Obsessive Compulsive Cognitions Working Group (OCCWG). This is followed by a critical review of empirical support for the model. The chapter concludes by delineating the main tenets of the CBT approach and their implications for the treatment of OCD.

HISTORICAL ROOTS OF THE COGNITIVE APPROACH TO OCD

The cognitive revolution in clinical psychology did not include OCD until publication of Salkovskis's (1985) article on the cognitive-behavioral analysis of obsessions and compulsions. Beck's (1967, 1976) early writings on his cognitive formulation of emotional disorders made scant reference to obsessional states. The first cognitive therapy treatment manual for anxiety disorders excluded OCD (Beck & Emery, 1985). Furthermore, Hollon and Beck (1986) concluded that the most effective treatment for OCD was ERP and that "it also remains possible that explicit cognitive interventions have little to offer this disorder" (p. 467).

Carr (1974) proposed one of the first cognitive theories of OCD in response to limitations with the anxiety reduction hypothesis. The core tenet of his model is that obsessional states are characterized by an abnormally high subjective estimate of the probability that unfavorable outcomes will occur. In OCD, any situation that involves potential harm (i.e., high subjective cost) will result in heightened threat or anxiety, because the individual generates an elevated estimate of the probability of occurrence of the undesired outcome. Compulsive rituals develop as threat-reducing activities that function to lower the subjective probability of an undesired outcome. The occurrence of obsessive–compulsive symptoms in a specific situation depends on the person perceiving high subjective cost (i.e., harm) and probability of the undesirable outcome. Cognitive compulsions will occur when an appropriate threat-reducing behavior is not available. Cognitive or behavioral compulsions become ritualistic because the person perceives that they are the most efficient way to reduce the probability of an unfavorable outcome. Carr admitted that the threat appraisal model does not explain what causes people initially to make high subjective probability estimates. Moreover, it may be that overestimated threat appraisals are more important in the pathogenesis of phobias and other anxiety disorders than they are in OCD (e.g., see Volans, 1976).

McFall and Wollersheim (1979) began with Carr's (1974) notion that individuals with OCD make a faulty primary threat appraisal. However, they also proposed an erroneous secondary appraisal process in which individuals underestimate their ability to cope with the threat. Both primary threat and secondary vulnerability appraisals are based on certain maladaptive preconscious beliefs such as (1) it is necessary to be perfect, (2) mistakes should be punished, (3) one has the power to prevent terrible outcomes by magical rituals or ruminative thinking, (4) certain thoughts are highly unacceptable because they can cause a catastrophic outcome, (5) it is easier and more effective to engage in neutralizing activity than to confront one's feelings, and (6) feelings of uncertainty and loss of control are intolerable. The faulty primary and secondary appraisals give rise to feelings of uncertainty, loss of control, and anxiety. Because obsessional individuals perceive that they cannot deal with this distress in a realistic or adaptive manner, they resort to magical rituals and compulsive strategies as the best option for reducing distress. Based on this model, McFall and Wollersheim (1979) recommended that behavioral exercises and cognitive restructuring, based on rational–emotive therapy, be used to directly modify faulty appraisals.

Salkovskis (1985) was critical of the McFall and Wollersheim formulation because of (1) their attempt to bridge the gap between behavioral and psychoanalytic theory, (2) their emphasis on preconscious and unconscious cognitions without elaborating on the direct cognitive and behavioral expression of these concepts, and (3) a failure to specify how the primary threat appraisals in OCD differ uniquely from the threat appraisals seen in other anxiety disorders. Although Salkovskis's critique is warranted, it is interesting that contemporary cognitive models include several constructs like those of McFall and Wollersheim (1979) (e.g., inflated responsibility, thought–action fusion [TAF], and excessive concern with thought control).

One of the most important contributions to the development of the CBT approach to OCD can be found in the seminal text published in 1980 by Rachman and Hodgson and simply titled *Obsessions and Compulsions*. Many of the central tenets of the CBT perspective were first proposed by Rachman and Hodgson in this thoughtful and visionary explanation of the psychology of OCD. We see in this text recognition that healthy individuals can have unwanted intrusive thoughts involving obsessive–compulsive content and that the problem in OCD is the individual's distorted meaning and intolerance of certain types of mental intrusions. Rachman and Hodgson considered neutralization and avoidance critical processes in the persistence of obsessions. They also noted that obsessions are characterized by poor mental control, and that efforts should be made to teach individuals more efficient and effective methods of controlling unwanted intrusions. Their theoretical insights were a major catalyst in bringing the "cognitive revolution" to OCD.

FOUNDATIONAL MODELS OF CBT

Salkovskis: Inflated Responsibility

A significant development in the cognitive-behavioral approach to OCD occurred with the publication of Paul Salkovskis's (1985) influential paper titled "Obsessional–Compulsive Problems: A Cognitive-Behavioural Analysis." Salkovskis asserted that obsessional thinking has its origins in normal intrusive thoughts. If an individual evaluates the intrusive thought as meaningful in terms of being responsible for harm or its prevention to self or others, then the intrusion will cause discomfort. Salkovskis (1999) viewed *inflated responsibility* as encompassing both enduring beliefs and immediate appraisals to specific intrusive thoughts, and defined the construct as "the belief that one has power which is pivotal to bring about or prevent subjectively crucial negative outcomes. These outcomes are perceived as essential to prevent. They may be actual, that is, having consequences in the real world, and/or at a moral level" (p. S32).

The inflated responsibility appraisals focus either on the occurrence or on the content of the intrusive thought (Salkovskis & Wahl, 2003). For example, an individual with multiple obsessions might misinterpret his failure to dismiss intrusive thoughts as a sign that he is losing control and could be responsible for committing some horrendous act of violence. In this case the responsibility appraisal is associated with the occurrence of any unwanted cognitive intrusion. However, if the content of an intrusive thought suggests a specific reaction, then neutralization will occur to limit the person's experience of the obsession. An individual with the obsession "I might get sick and vomit" interpreted this thought as a sign that she must take responsibility for her health and ensure that she does not get sick. Here we see a neutralization response that is associated with the content of the intrusion, rather than to its mere occurrence.

Salkovskis (1989a, 1998) argues that appraisals of responsibility for harm are specific to obsessional thinking. What distinguishes obsessions from other forms of anxious and depressive thinking is their association with appraisals of responsibility. If a thought results only in harm or danger appraisals, then the emotional response will be anxiety, whereas appraisals of loss will be associated with depression (Salkovskis, 1999). It is further argued that the inflated responsibility misinterpretation is necessary for an intrusion to become pathological; "without appraisal of responsibility, an obsessional episode would not result" (Salkovskis, 1989a, p. 678). The adverse mood (e.g., discomfort, guilt, anxiety) associated with an obsession arises from misinterpretations of responsibility (Salkovskis, 1999).

To terminate the intrusive thought and discharge perceived responsibility for harm, the individual adopts behavioral and cognitive neutralizing strategies that include compulsive rituals, avoidance, reassurance seeking, thought suppression, and the like (Salkovskis 1985, 1989b, 1999). However, the neutralizing responses are inadequate because the obsession-prone individual has unrealistic criteria for completion of the response and tries too hard to exert control over the unwanted thought (Salkovskis, 1999; Salkovskis et al., 1995). In the end neutralization strengthens the individual's preexisting beliefs related to the misinterpretation of unwanted thoughts as indicating personal responsibility and increases the person's preoccupation with such thinking (Salkovskis, 1999; Salkovskis et al., 1998). What then develops is a vicious spiral of ever more frequent cognitive misinterpretations and counterproductive neutralizations. Later, Salkovskis and colleagues noted that compulsions also persist because individuals with OCD use multiple, subjective, internally based criteria when deciding to "stop," such as striving to attain a "just right feeling" (Wahl et al., 2008). These criteria elevate the evidence required to terminate a neutralization response, thereby ensuring its persistence and significant contribution to the vicious cycle of obsessive thinking.

Clinical Implications

In the Salkovskis formulation, treatment focuses on changing the client's faulty beliefs and misinterpretations of responsibility for harm through exposure-based experiences that disconfirm the individual's assumptions about threat and danger. The case conceptualization is based on the responsibility model, and cognitive restructuring is employed to help clients normalize the experience of intrusions and develop alternative, nonthreatening interpretations of the obsession (Salkovskis, 1999). Exposure-based behavioral experiments are designed to disconfirm erroneous threat-related responsibility beliefs about the obsession and curtail deleterious neutralization responses. The goal of treatment is normalization of the obsession; that is, the client learns to evaluate the obsession as an unwanted mental intrusion that signifies no personal responsibility for harm and that requires no effortful response, despite its distressing quality.

Rachman: Misinterpretation of Personal Significance

Drawing from D. M. Clark's (1986) cognitive theory of panic and Salkovskis's (1985) cognitive-behavioral formulation of obsessions, Rachman (1997, 2004) asserts that certain types of unwanted intrusive thoughts escalate into obsessions when a person misinterprets the intrusion as a personally significant and threatening phenomenon. Like the inflated responsibility model, Rachman starts with the premise that unwanted intrusive thoughts, images, or impulses are universally experienced—but unlike Salkovskis's conceptualization, he proposes that only thoughts with particular content (e.g., sex, aggression, blasphemy, contamination) can escalate into obsessions (Rachman, 1998; Rachman, Coughtrey, Shafran, & Radomsky, 2015). This type of thought content becomes obsessional when individuals misinterpret their mental intrusions in a personally significant and threatening manner (Rachman, 2003). Misinterpretations of significance involve the erroneous view that an intrusive thought is an indication of something meaningful about one's character that could result in serious negative consequences. Thus, Rachman (1998) asserts that mental intrusions turn into obsessions only if they are misinterpreted as *personally significant* and as *signifying a threat*. Furthermore, which intrusive thought becomes obsessional depends on whether it is "important in the patient's system of values" (Rachman, 1998, p. 390). Once an intrusive thought is misinterpreted, the obsession persists if the misinterpretations of significance continue but decreases when the misinterpretation is weakened or eliminated (Rachman, 1997, 2003).

Rachman proposed several cognitive biases that contribute to the escalation of "normal" unwanted intrusive thoughts into highly persistent clinical obsessions.

- *Misinterpretation of anxiety.* The physical sensations of anxiety or discomfort (e.g., trembling, sweating) can be misinterpreted as a loss of control. This line of thinking will reinforce the individual's conviction of the importance of the obsession and its negative consequences (Rachman, 1998). Avoidance and the consequent reduction in anxiety will further reinforce the individual's belief that a negative consequence has been averted and prevent disconfirmation that there is no catastrophic consequence to the obsession (Rachman, 1998, 2003).

- *TAF bias.* This is the tendency to equate thoughts with actions, in which occurrence of the obsession is believed to increase the likelihood of a feared outcome (TAF–Likelihood) or that having the obsession is morally equivalent to engaging in the forbidden action (TAF–Moral) (Rachman & Shafran, 1998). The presence of TAF is thought to contribute to the catastrophic misinterpretation of certain unwanted intrusive thoughts.

- *Inflated responsibility.* Rachman (1997, 2003) acknowledged that responsibility appraisals and beliefs can contribute to the catastrophic misinterpretations of significance, but their presence is neither necessary nor sufficient to ensure the pathogenesis of obsessions. In this way inflated responsibility plays a less prominent role in Rachman's theory of obsessions than it does in Salkovskis's formulation.

- *Threat overestimation.* A tendency to overestimate the probability and severity of harm, threat, or danger is another cognitive bias that can contribute to misinterpretations of significance (Rachman, 2003). This cognitive bias is not unique to OCD, as it is readily evident in all the anxiety disorders (Clark & Beck, 2010).

In addition to misinterpretations of significance, Rachman (1997, 2003) also considered neutralization a major contributor to the persistence of obsessions. "Successful" neutralization reinforces the individual's belief that the neutralization response was responsible for preventing a feared event from occurring, or that the discomfort caused by the obsession would persist without having engaged in the designated neutralization process (Rachman, 1998). Temporary relief resulting from neutralization confirms the client's erroneous belief that the upsetting obsession is dangerous and that neutralization is a necessary and effective way to deal with it (Rachman, 2003). Neutralization, then, prevents opportunities to experience confirmation that the obsession is actually much less significant and inconsequential than assumed.

Rachman (1998) also recognized that *excessive thought control* is a consequence of catastrophic misinterpretations of significance. As the perceived significance of an intrusion increases, the individual engages in ever more vigorous attempts to suppress or control such thoughts. However, these control efforts are bound to fail, which then contributes to an increase in the frequency of the intrusion, which in turn will strengthen the significance of that intrusion (Rachman, 2003).

Clinical Implications

There are several clinical implications that can be drawn from Rachman's formulation. Assessment and case formulation must focus on the personal meaning and significance of the obsession. Once the client's misinterpretations of significance are fully understood, experientially based cognitive interventions are needed that disconfirm the client's faulty obsessional fears. The therapist then helps the individual discover healthier, more realistic interpretations that recognize a more benign meaning and inconsequential outcome associated with the obsession. In addition, other cognitive biases will need to be addressed, including TAF and overestimated threat. The response prevention component of treatment needs to be expanded to include all forms of neutralization, avoidance, and thought control. More recently, Rachman has offered more specific cognitive formulations and treatment protocols for OCD subtypes such as physical and mental contamination, obsessions, and checking. These are discussed more fully in Part IV.

OCCWG: Schema Vulnerability

At the World Congress of Behavioral and Cognitive Therapies in Denmark (July 1995), a group of OCD researchers agreed to collaborate in the development of self-report measures and experimental procedures to investigate the cognitive basis of OCD. Called the Obsessive Compulsive Cognitions Working Group (OCCWG), the group consisted of 46 OCD researchers from nine countries. Under the leadership of Gail Steketee and Randy Frost, the group sponsored several research meetings, developed self-report measures, conducted multisite collaborative research, and published their findings in a series of articles that appears in *Behaviour Research and Therapy*.

One of the most important accomplishments of the OCCWG was the identification of six belief domains that were thought to characterize OCD and constitute a cognitive vulnerability for the disorder (OCCWG, 1997). Individuals who endorsed these beliefs were thought to have a greater propensity to misinterpret unwanted intrusive thoughts and adopt maladaptive neutralization strategies (see also Freeston, Rhéaume, & Ladouceur, 1996). Table 5.1 presents definitions of the six belief domains developed by the OCCWG (1997).

One noteworthy contribution was the OCCWG's delineation of beliefs about the overimportance of mental control. The group proposed that this belief domain consisted of several facets: (1) the importance of monitoring and staying hypervigilant for certain types of mental events, (2) the moral consequences of not controlling thoughts, (3) the psychological and behavioral consequences of failure to control thoughts, and (4) the efficiency of mental control. The first five belief domains were thought to be specific to OCD, whereas the sixth domain, perfectionism, was considered important but not exclusive to OCD (see also Taylor, 2002).

Clinical Implications

The most important clinical contribution of the OCCWG was to suggest that cognitive therapy for OCD must target additional dysfunctional beliefs and appraisals, such as importance and control of thoughts, perfectionism,

TABLE 5.1. The Six Belief Domains of OCD Proposed by the OCCWG

Belief domain	Definition
Inflated responsibility	"the belief that one has power which is pivotal to bring about or prevent subjectively crucial negative outcomes" (OCCWG, 1997, p. 677)
Overimportance of thoughts	"beliefs that the mere presence of a thought indicates that it is important" (p. 678)
Overestimation of threat	"an exaggeration of the probability or severity of harm" (p. 678)
Importance of controlling thoughts	"the overvaluation of the importance of exerting complete control over intrusive thoughts, images and impulses, and the belief that this is both possible and desirable" (p. 678)
Intolerance of uncertainty	Beliefs about the necessity of being certain, the personal inability to cope with unpredictable change, and difficulty in functioning in ambiguous situations
Perfectionism	"the tendency to believe there is a perfect solution to every problem, that doing something perfectly (i.e., mistake free) is not only possible but also necessary, and that even minor mistakes will have serious consequences" (p. 678)

and intolerance of uncertainty. As vulnerability constructs, CBT therapists should focus on these beliefs to ensure maintenance of treatment gains and reduce risk of relapse.

Clark and Purdon: Mental Control

Clark and Purdon (1993) argue that dysfunctional beliefs about thought control are a significant contributor to the pathogenesis of obsessions. The individual vulnerable to OCD may hold unrealistic beliefs about unwanted intrusive thoughts and the need to exert control over these thoughts. If complete control over the intrusion is not attained, vulnerable individuals may envision catastrophic consequences to their perceived loss of mental control. To gain control, the person's initial response might be the more usual thought control strategies such as distraction, thought replacement, avoidance of triggers, thought suppression, and the like. However, failure to obtain an adequate level of control causes the person to escalate neutralization efforts to more extreme strategies, such as overt or covert compulsive rituals. Purdon and Clark (1999) suggested that ego-dystonic intrusive thoughts are especially salient threats that the person will feel most compelled to control. In sum, the obsession-prone person tries too hard to control his or her obsessive intrusive thoughts, increasing the likelihood of failed control, mounting distress, and a need to resort to more extreme responses, such as compulsive rituals.

In a further elaboration of mental control, Clark (2004) proposed that individuals with OCD generate negative appraisals of their failure to control the obsession. Obsessive–compulsive prone individuals may consider their inability to attain satisfactory control of the obsession a highly significant threat. They believe that they should be able to control their unwanted thoughts and so their loss of control portends an even more serious state of affairs, such as the possibility that they will lose control of their actions. Here we see a type of TAF bias in which loss of mental control is equated with loss of behavioral control, or even worse, loss of sanity. In this case the person believes, "If I can't control the obsession, this means I'm mentally weak and capable of losing all control." The result is that individuals who consider their incomplete mental control unacceptable and problematic will be motivated to exert even greater control over the intrusion. However, this increased exertion only increases the chances that they will succumb to the *paradox of mental control,* which is the harder one tries to suppress an unwanted thought, the more one is drawn to the thought (Clark, 2018).

Criticisms have been raised about the inclusion of failed mental control in the CBT formulation of obsessions. Cougle and Lee (2014) argued that greater use of mental control strategies could be a consequence rather than cause of frequent obsessional intrusions. Salkovskis and Millar (2016) reasoned that beliefs about control are subsumed under the construct of responsibility and that thought control strategies are just another form of safety-seeking behavior. Salkovskis and Millar are also critical of Clark and Purdon's (1993) comments on neutralization, claiming that the authors downplay its role in the pathogenesis of obsessions. In their reply, Clark and Purdon (2016) noted that differentiating mental control beliefs and responsibility has heuristic value and contributes to a more precise formulation of the cognitive basis of OCD. As well, empirical evidence supports the validity and likely clinical utility of including appraisals of mental control failure in the CBT model of obsessions.

Clinical Implications

According to this perspective, CBT case formulation and therapy should include an emphasis on mental control. This would consist of an assessment of the mental control strategies that clients use in response to their obsessions, their appraisals of control failure, and their beliefs about mental control. Cognitive restructuring and behavioral experiments could focus on evaluating whether the client has succumbed to the paradox of mental control and whether letting go of mental control efforts is a more effective way to deal with the obsession (see Clark, 2018, for further discussion). The goal of treatment is to guide the individual toward discovering more effective responses to the obsession, such as focused distraction, learning that failed mental control is inevitable and acceptable, and that giving up on excessive control effort is the most effective way to diminish the salience of the obsession. It should be noted that these goals are very similar to those of mindfulness and ACT of OCD.

THE GENERIC CBT MODEL

Figure 5.1 presents a diagram of the generic model of CBT. This theoretical account integrates the various cognitive constructs discussed in the previous chapters. The cognitive case conceptualization found in Chapter 7 is derived from the generic model, which is also the basis for the specific subtype formulations found in later chapters. There are several processes delineated in the CBT model that form its main tenets and guide CBT treatment protocols.

Most often, the involuntary and unwanted intrusions that characterize obsessive thinking are elicited by certain stimuli or environmental contexts. For example, the person who has obsessive doubts such as "Did I express myself clearly and honestly?" may only experience such thoughts when in conversation with a valued individual. Rachman (1981) commented that unwanted intrusions may be more likely when an individual is alone and bored, thereby occurring as spontaneous, unintended thought without external precipitants. Julien and colleagues (2009) found that only 33% of the intrusions in their OCD sample had a direct link with the context, and 16% had no relationship with their context. This finding would suggest that obsessive-like intrusive thoughts are not always triggered by external or internal cues but instead can arise independently, without elicitation by contextual determinants.

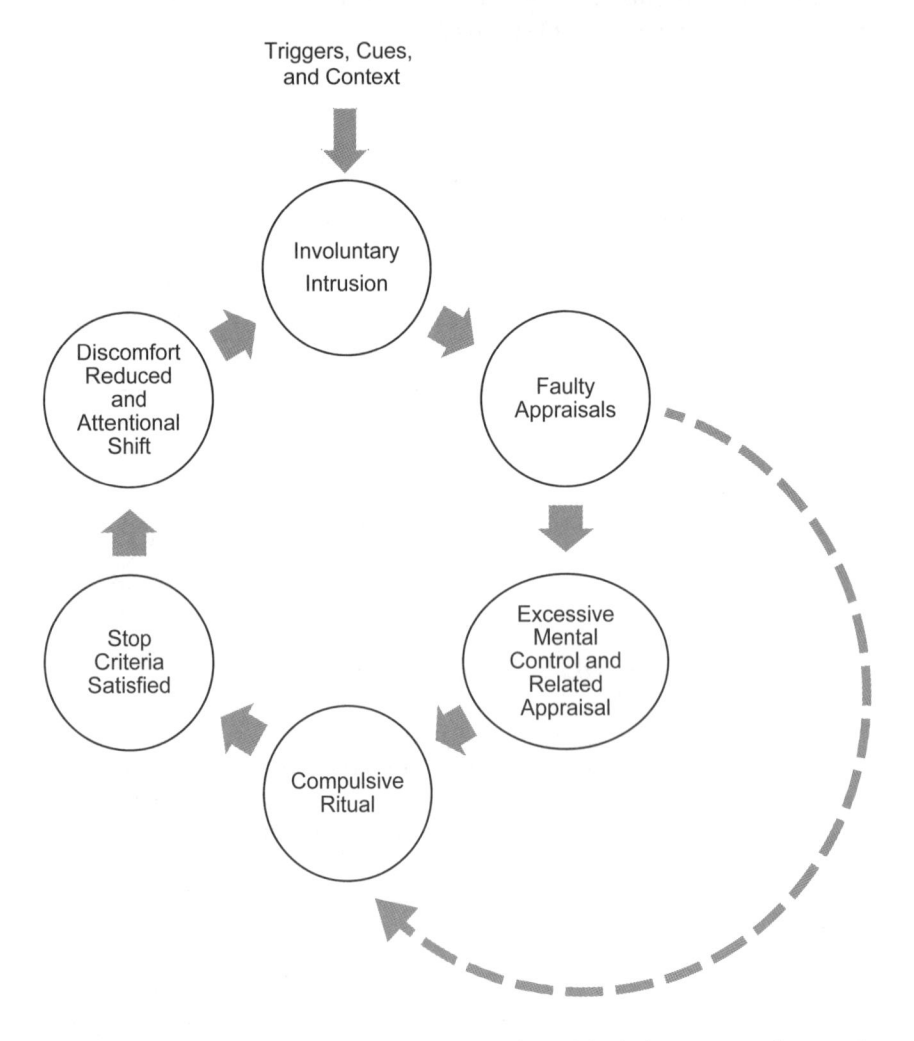

FIGURE 5.1. The generic cognitive-behavioral model of obsessions and compulsions.

The generic model recognizes two possible pathways in the progression to obsessional thinking after faulty appraisals endow the intrusion with greater personal significance and threat. In the early phase of the disorder, individuals will try to exert direct mental control of the intrusion via common control strategies. The failure of these efforts is appraised as a highly threatening outcome, and so the individual migrates to more extreme forms of neutralization, such as compulsive rituals. However, with chronic OCD, individuals are more likely to skip over mental control and go directly to a compulsive ritual. Sometimes the production of a compulsion is so automatic that the individual has difficulty even identifying the obsession.

The overt or covert compulsion will continue until a person's termination criteria has been met. As discussed in Chapter 3, the stop criteria in OCD tend to be vague, internally based standards such as attaining a "just right feeling." As well, the vulnerable person requires a higher evidentiary standard for deciding when to stop his or her compulsions. As a result, compulsive rituals and other forms of neutralizing persist much longer in OCD.

The final goal state of the person with OCD is a significant reduction in negative emotion or discomfort and an attentional shift away from the obsession. Although both states can be achieved temporarily, the more enduring effect is a strengthening of the frequency and salience of the obsession-relevant intrusive thought.

EMPIRICAL STATUS

The cognitive-behavioral explanation for the etiology and maintenance of obsessions and compulsions has spawned considerable research on both clinical and nonclinical samples. Empirical support for the main tenets of the model is mixed, although more substantial than for other theoretical explanations. In this section we consider the empirical evidence for several key hypotheses of the generic CBT model. A more focused review of the literature can be found in each of the subtype chapters.

Universality of Unwanted Intrusions

The generic model assumes that unwanted intrusive thoughts are a normal feature of cognitive functioning and so will be found universally in all individuals regardless of their clinical status. Moreover, clinical obsessions have their origin in these spontaneous mental intrusions, and so it is expected that individuals with emotional disturbance will have a higher frequency of unwanted intrusive thoughts, images, and impulses.

Cognitive neuroscience research indicates that 25–50% of our waking hours is spent in spontaneous, stimulus-independent thought such as daydreaming, mind wandering, unwanted mental intrusions, and the like (Christoff, 2012; Kane et al., 2007). In fact, this type of thinking is so common that it has been called the brain's "default mode of operation" (Killingsworth & Gilbert, 2010). Stimulus-independent thought or mind wandering increases when there is a reduction in processing demands, although individual differences exist in the amount of stimulus-independent thought generated (Mason et al., 2007). Individuals with lower working memory capacity may experience more mind wandering during tasks requiring concentration than individuals with high working memory (Kane et al., 2007). Moreover, a cortical network has been identified that is activated when individuals are engaged in spontaneous thought. It involves the medial prefrontal cortex, posterior cingulate–precuneus region and the temporal–parietal junction, which all have functional connections to the dorsolateral prefrontal cortex and anterior cingulate cortex (Dixon, Fox, & Christoff, 2014; Smallwood & Schooler, 2015). Clearly, spontaneous thought appears to be a baseline condition to which the brain returns when cognitive resources are not required for some novel or demanding external task. Unintended intrusive thought, then, is a prominent feature of human consciousness that is a universal cognitive process of *Homo sapiens'* neocortex.

The effects of unintended, stimulus-independent thought depend on its content and context (Smallwood & Schooler, 2015). Spontaneous thought or mind wandering that tends to be negative, past-oriented, and repetitive is associated with unhappiness, low mood, and poor performance on demanding tasks (Killingsworth & Gilbert, 2010; Poerio, Totterdell, & Miles, 2013; Smallwood & Schooler, 2015). Moreover, spontaneous mind wandering was found to have a significant relationship to obsessive–compulsive symptoms in a large nonclinical sample (Seli, Risko, Purdon, & Smilek, 2017). Nevertheless, there are also benefits to mind wandering, such as improved planning and goal directedness, heightened creativity, increased self-reflection and understanding, and restorative mental breaks from boring or monotonous activities (Smallwood & Schooler, 2015).

Unwanted intrusive thinking, then, is a type of unintended, self-generated thought that occurs regularly in the daily life of individuals. Clinical researchers have investigated whether healthy, nonclinical individuals experience the same types of negative intrusions that are found in OCD. There is a robust research literature showing that nonclinical individuals experience negative mental intrusions with obsessive–compulsive-relevant content but with less frequency, intensity, distress, and uncontrollability as seen in OCD samples (see Chapter 3 for review). In the largest cross-cultural study of obsessive intrusive thoughts in nonclinical individuals, Radomsky, Alcolado, and colleagues (2014) found that over 90% of individuals in 13 countries reported at least one obsessive-like intrusion in the last 3 months. Moreover, intrusions involving dirt/contamination, doubt, and miscellaneous content were unique, significant predictors of obsessive–compulsive symptoms in this international sample (Clark et al., 2014). Other correlational studies also found a significant relationship between frequency of unwanted intrusions and obsessive–compulsive symptoms (e.g., Barrera & Norton, 2011; Clark, 1992; Freeston, Ladouceur, Thibodeau, & Gagnon, 1992; Purdon & Clark, 1993).

Research comparing individuals with OCD and non-OCD clinical and healthy controls find that the OCD samples have more frequent and distressing unwanted mental intrusions than other clinical and nonclinical groups (e.g., Bouvard et al., 2017; García-Soriano & Belloch, 2013; García-Soriano, Belloch, Morillo, & Clark, 2011; Morillo et al., 2007; Rachman & de Silva, 1978). In their meta-analysis of thought suppression, Magee and colleagues (2012) concluded that unwanted mental intrusions are significantly more frequent in psychopathology. Moreover, negative involuntary thoughts may be more highly associated with psychopathology (Krans, de Bree, & Moulds, 2015), and the thought content of intrusions in OCD samples is more bizarre, autogenous, or independent of their context, and more irrational or lacking real-life evidence (Audet et al., 2016; Julien et al., 2009; Rassin & Muris, 2006; Rassin et al., 2007). Critics of the CBT model have argued that these differences indicate that intrusive thoughts with obsessive content may not be universal but instead unique to individuals vulnerable to OCD (Cougle & Lee, 2014; Julien, O'Connor, & Aardema, 2007).

The most compelling evidence for the importance of unwanted intrusions is experimental data showing a causal relationship between the experience of intrusions and the development of obsessive–compulsive symptoms. There is evidence that the production of unwanted, negative intrusive thoughts causes heightened distress and discomfort (e.g., Forrester et al., 2002; Ólafsson et al., 2014; Purdon & Clark, 2001; Reynolds & Salkovskis, 1992), although negative results also have been reported (Purdon, Gifford, McCabe, & Antony, 2011; Purdon, Rowa, & Antony, 2007). Unfortunately, there is scant experimental research demonstrating that unwanted intrusions cause obsessive–compulsive symptoms, and there is no longitudinal data supporting the etiological significance of unwanted intrusions in OCD. A retrospective OCD study found that greater attention to one's thoughts was a significant factor in the escalation of participants' obsessive–compulsive symptoms (Coles et al., 2012).

Research to date supports the cognitive-behavioral contention of continuity between normal, obsessive-like intrusive thought content and the clinical obsessions in OCD. Individuals with OCD generally report more frequent and distressing negative unwanted intrusions than nonclinical healthy controls, and possibly non-OCD clinical groups. Mental intrusions have a significant association with obsessive–compulsive symptoms, although research is lacking on the causal relationship between intrusions and symptoms.

Faulty Appraisals and Beliefs

According to CBT the main factor in the pathogenesis of obsessions is the faulty interpretation of unwanted intrusions as significant personal threats that must be controlled or eliminated to reduce threat and/or prevent a dreaded consequence to self or others. A tendency to generate misinterpretations of significance is thought to arise from preexisting beliefs about unwanted, spontaneous thought and their control. Thus, the review in this section considers both appraisals and beliefs associated with the six types of metacognitive appraisal: inflated responsibility, TAF or overimportance of thought, threat overestimation, importance of thought control, intolerance of uncertainty, and perfectionism.

Are Faulty Appraisals and Beliefs Elevated in OCD?

If dysfunctional appraisals and beliefs are important cognitive constructs in the pathogenesis of obsessions, they should be significantly more prominent in OCD samples than in healthy controls or even in non-OCD clinical groups. Several studies have used self-report measures of appraisal and found that OCD samples score significantly higher on negative appraisal ratings than healthy controls (e.g., Calamari & Janeck, 1997; García-Soriano & Belloch, 2013; Morillo et al., 2007), although Bouvard and colleagues (2017) found that individuals with OCD were significantly higher than nonclinical individuals on measures of the importance of thought, intolerance of anxiety, need to control, and intolerance of uncertainty, but not on measures of threat, responsibility, perfectionism, TAF, and unacceptability/ego dystonicity. Differences in appraisals comparing OCD and non-OCD clinical groups have been more mixed, with OCD groups significantly higher only on select appraisals such as responsibility, importance of control, overestimated threat, and unacceptability (see García-Soriano et al., 2014; Morillo et al., 2007; Romero-Sanchiz, Nogueira-Arjona, Godoy-Ávila, Gavino-Lázaro, & Freeston, 2017).

One of the best-researched constructs in the CBT model is TAF, with the 19-item TAF Scale (Shafran, Thordarson, & Rachman, 1996) the measure of choice. Unfortunately, it is unclear whether the TAF Scale items assess appraisals or beliefs (Berle & Starcevic, 2005). Most, but not all, of the items appear to take an appraisal orientation because they refer to a specific thought or situation. Thus, most researchers consider the TAF Scale a self-report appraisal measure. Research comparing OCD samples with nonclinical controls find significant differences mainly on the TAF–Likelihood subscales and not on the TAF–Moral subscale (Abramowitz, Whiteside, Lynam, & Kalsy, 2003; Shafran et al., 1996), although contrary results have been reported (Bailey, Wu, Valentiner, & McGrath, 2014). The most parsimonious conclusion is that TAF appraisals are elevated in OCD, especially interpretations that one's thoughts can influence the probability of harm to others, although evidence of disorder-specificity is lacking (for further discussion, see Berle & Starcevic, 2005; Hezel & McNally, 2016; Shafran & Rachman, 2004).

Most research on the belief structure in OCD has utilized the 44-item Obsessive Beliefs Questionnaire (OBQ-44) developed by the OCCWG (2003, 2005). Three factors emerged in the original factor analysis: Responsibility/Threat Estimation, Perfectionism/Intolerance of Uncertainty, and Importance/Control of Thoughts. The OCD sample scored significantly higher than non-OCD-anxious controls on OBQ Responsibility/Threat Estimation and Importance/Control of Thoughts but not on Perfectionism/Intolerance of Uncertainty (OCCWG, 2005). Others found that individuals with OCD were significantly higher than non-OCD-anxious controls on Importance/Control of Thoughts and, to a lesser extent, Perfectionism/Intolerance of Uncertainty but not on Responsibility/Threat Estimation (Fergus & Wu, 2010; Tolin et al., 2006). Using the original six subscales of the 87-item OBQ, Sica and colleagues (2004) found that only intolerance of uncertainty, control of thoughts, and perfectionism were elevated in OCD when compared to those with generalized anxiety. Still others reported findings that question whether OBQ scores are uniquely elevated in some or even all individuals with OCD, especially when compared with non-OCD clinical groups (Baptista, Magna, McKay, & Del-Porto, 2011; Taylor et al., 2006; Viar, Bilsky, Armstrong, & Olatunji, 2011). In a meta-analysis, Pozza and Dèttore (2014) found that responsibility beliefs were significantly higher in OCD samples than in non-OCD-anxious and non-clinical controls.

Overall, the group comparison studies indicate that faulty appraisals and beliefs are significantly elevated in OCD relative to healthy, nonclinical controls. Differences tend to be more variable when compared with non-OCD-anxious or other clinical groups, and it is likely that only certain appraisals and beliefs, such as Importance/Control of Thoughts, are distinctly elevated in OCD.

Do Faulty Appraisals and Beliefs Have a Specific Association with Obsessive–Compulsive Symptoms?

Numerous studies have examined cognitive-symptom specificity in clinical and nonclinical samples. The CBT model predicts that faulty appraisals and beliefs should have significant, and possibly unique, associations with the frequency and distress of unwanted intrusive thoughts as well as with obsessive–compulsive symptoms. Various correlational studies have shown that frequent and/or distressing unwanted intrusive thoughts are characterized by increased faulty appraisals (e.g., Clark & Claybourn, 1997;

Corcoran & Woody, 2008; Freeston et al., 1991; Freeston & Ladouceur, 1993; García-Soriano et al., 2014; Parkinson & Rachman, 1981a; Purdon & Clark, 1994a, 1994b; Rachman & de Silva, 1978; Romero-Sanchiz et al., 2017; Whitaker et al., 2009). In a sample of 28 individuals with OCD, Rowa and colleagues (2005) found that individuals' most upsetting obsession was evaluated as significantly more meaningful and more likely contradicted valued aspects of the self than the least upsetting obsessions. Likewise, self-reported faulty appraisals of unwanted intrusions or obsessions, including TAF, are significantly associated with obsessive–compulsive symptoms (e.g., Corcoran & Woody, 2008; Freeston et al., 1992; García-Soriano & Belloch, 2013; García-Soriano et al., 2014), although negative findings have also been reported (Barrera & Norton, 2011). However, it is evident that most types of frequent and distressing intrusive thoughts are associated with faulty appraisals of significance, but it is unclear whether some appraisals are more characteristic of obsessive–compulsive symptoms than others. TAF appraisals, especially likelihood–self, are significantly associated with obsessive–compulsive symptoms, but again evidence for appraisal-symptom specificity has been questionable (Abramowitz, Whiteside, Lynam, et al., 2003; Bailey et al., 2014; see Berle & Starcevic, 2005).

Obsessive–compulsive symptom specificity has been investigated at the belief level. Numerous studies have shown that dysfunctional beliefs about responsibility, importance and control of thoughts, threat overestimation, perfectionism and intolerance of uncertainty are significantly associated with obsessive–compulsive symptom severity (e.g., Fergus & Carmin, 2014; Julien et al., 2006; Myers, Fisher, & Wells, 2008; OCCWG, 2003, 2005; Sica et al., 2004; Tolin et al., 2008; Viar et al., 2011; Wheaton, Abramowitz, Berman, Riemann, & Hale, 2010; Woods, Tolin, & Abramowitz, 2004), although negative findings also have been reported (Myers et al., 2017). However, not all belief domains have the same degree of obsessive–compulsive symptom specificity. Beliefs about the importance and control of thoughts, and possibly perfectionism, have greater specificity with at least certain obsessive–compulsive symptom subtypes. Responsibility beliefs also show obsessive–compulsive symptom specificity in many studies, although this finding has been challenged by Pozza and Dèttore's (2014) meta-analysis. Finally, the association between beliefs and obsessive–compulsive symptoms may be influenced by symptom severity, with beliefs about responsibility relevant at less severe obsessive–compulsive symptom levels and beliefs about the importance/control of thoughts evident at all levels of severity (Kim et al., 2016).

In sum, faulty appraisals and beliefs are significantly related to the frequency and distress of unwanted intrusive thoughts and obsessive–compulsive symptoms. However, the specificity of this relationship is less clear, although importance/control of thoughts may be one of the more specific appraisal and belief domains. As well, certain types of appraisals and beliefs may be more relevant to some OCD symptom subtypes than others, and mediating factors such as negative affect, anxiety, or depression may account for significant variance in appraisal–symptom specificity (Abramowitz, Whiteside, Lynam, et al., 2003; Tolin et al., 2006).

What Is the Causal Status of Faulty Appraisals and Beliefs?

There is evidence that thoughts perceived as spontaneous are more likely to be interpreted as revealing something meaningful about oneself than deliberately generated cognition (Morewedge, Giblin, & Norton, 2014). This finding is consistent with the CBT model, which predicts a reciprocal causal relationship between unwanted mental intrusions and their appraisal. Thus, when unwanted spontaneous thoughts are experienced, they are more likely to activate faulty appraisals of significance, and production of faulty appraisals will increase the frequency and distress of unwanted intrusions. Likewise, production of faulty appraisals in reaction to intrusive thoughts will contribute to the production of obsessive–compulsive symptoms.

Experimental studies are needed to determine the causal relationship between faulty appraisals and unwanted intrusions. Much of this research has focused on responsibility appraisals. Lopatka and Rachman (1995) first reported that individuals assigned to a low-perceived-responsibility manipulation evidenced significant decreases in perceived discomfort, urge to check, and estimates of harm and criticism, whereas those in the high-responsibility condition showed a nonsignificant trend for increased perceived discomfort, urge to check, and severity of anticipated criticism. Shafran (1997) found that a high-responsibility ERP treatment condition was associated with increased ratings of urge to neutralize, subjective discomfort/anxiety, and estimates of threat probability. Arntz, Voncken, and Goosen (2007) compared OCD, non-OCD-anxious, and nonclinical controls on a high- and low-responsibility manipulation. Only the individuals with OCD in the high-responsibility condition showed a significant increase in OCD-like subjective experiences and checking behavior. A more recent systematic review of 16 experimental studies that manipulated responsibility concluded that the negative effects of heightened responsibility were variable, although there was more consistent evidence that heightened responsibility had a negative impact on threat appraisals and anxiety/distress, to a lesser extent (Mantz & Abbott, 2017). The effects of responsibility were no greater in OCD than in other comparison samples. Thus, the causal status of responsibility appraisals has not been established. Its effects do not appear to be specific to OCD, and whether heightened responsibility has a distinct influence beyond threat appraisals remains to be determined.

In a study that compared an OCD and a nonclinical group, ambiguous scenarios that included a negative intrusive thought were rated by the

OCD group as more anxiety-provoking and distressing than scenarios that included a neutral intrusion (Forrester et al., 2002). Gentes and Ruscio (2015) provided nonclinical students with negative, normalizing, or no feedback in response to self-generated worry, rumination, and obsessive thoughts. They found that individuals with higher scores on a metacognitive beliefs measure that were assigned to the negative appraisal group reported more negative and less positive affect. Newby and Moulds (2011) reported that negative appraisals of intrusive memories predicted depressive symptoms at 6 months. In another study, provision of educational information on the nature of intrusive thoughts resulted in a significant reduction in maladaptive appraisals. Finally, two treatment process studies found that reduction in maladaptive obsessive–compulsive beliefs mediated symptom improvement (Diedrich et al., 2016; Wilhelm, Berman, Keshaviah, & Schwartz, 2015). A more complicated picture emerges from a CBT trial for obsessions in which importance/control beliefs and appraisals of personal significance accounted for treatment effects on the YBOCS Obsessions subscale, but analysis of temporal precedence indicated that prior symptom severity determined subsequent changes in appraisals (Woody, Whittal, & McLean, 2011).

More experimental research on specific faulty appraisal and belief constructs is needed before firm conclusions can be made about their causal role. There is preliminary empirical evidence that negative appraisals and beliefs can influence individuals' experience of unwanted intrusive thoughts and the presence of obsessive–compulsive symptoms. Various review studies have concluded that empirical evidence of an association between faulty appraisals, beliefs, and obsessive–compulsive symptoms is strong, but the causal pathway predicted by the CBT model has only weak empirical support (Cougle & Lee, 2014; Hezel & McNally, 2016; see also Julien et al., 2007).

Excessive Mental Control and Its Appraisal

As indicated in Figure 5.1, exaggerated appraisals of personal significance will lead to excessive effort to control the unwanted intrusive thought or obsession. When these initial mental control efforts fail to produce the desired outcome, vulnerable individuals interpret this failure as a highly threatening, even catastrophic, state of affairs. Several predictions arise from this aspect of the generic model.

Does Excessive Mental Control Characterize Vulnerability to OCD?

Since the seminal white bear thought suppression study by Wegner, Schneider, Carter, and White (1987), hundreds of studies have investigated the effects of intentional thought control on unwanted cognitions. At first it was found that thought suppression produced a paradoxical effect on thought frequency, with suppression causing a rebound effect when suppression efforts ceased, or an immediate enhancement of the unwanted thought during the suppression period. To explain this phenomenon, Wegner (1994a) proposed the ironic process theory of mental control. However, there have been many failures to replicate the thought suppression enhancement and rebound effects (for reviews, see Abramowitz, Tolin, & Street, 2001; Magee et al., 2012; Purdon, 1999; Purdon & Clark, 2000; Rassin, 2005). This has led others to suggest that thought suppression might have a negative impact on (1) distress but not on frequency of the intrusion (Najmi, Riemann, & Wegner, 2009), (2) the natural habituation of repeated unwanted and unintended thought occurrences (Hooper & McHugh, 2013), (3) metacognitive evaluations of the intrusion, (4) appraisals of mental control failure, or (5) mood state (see Purdon, 1999, 2004b). Despite inconsistent findings, this research has relevance for understanding the effects of mental control effort. As expected, individuals assigned to a suppression condition expend greater mental effort to "not think," whereas those assigned to "monitor only" let their thoughts come and go with less effortful control (e.g., Najmi & Wegner, 2008; Purdon & Clark, 2001; Purdon et al., 2005). At the very least, it is evident that efforts to suppress unwanted thoughts are counterproductive responses (Najmi et al., 2009).

Although most thought suppression experiments involve nonclinical participants, a few have examined thought suppression in OCD samples. In their quantitative review, Magee and colleagues (2012) concluded that individuals with OCD symptoms who suppressed intrusive thoughts had less initial enhancement and rebound effects than nonclinical controls. Thus, individuals with OCD are as capable as non-OCD-anxious and nonclinical groups in short-term control of unwanted thoughts (see similar results for thought dismissibility by Purdon et al., 2011). However, the thought suppression findings indicate that individuals with OCD are highly motivated to suppress their unwanted intrusive thoughts, and in fact, will show natural active resistance to unwanted thoughts (Purdon et al., 2005). Likewise, a 3-day diary study of 37 individuals with OCD found that individuals engaged in frequent, strenuous, and time-consuming attempts to control their unwanted thoughts (Purdon, Rowa, et al., 2007). Moreover, some individuals with OCD will continue to suppress even when assigned to the "do not suppress" control group (Purdon et al., 2005; for contrary results, see Najmi et al., 2009), and in other studies suppression has a more negative effect on unwanted intrusions for at least some people with OCD (Janeck & Calamari, 1999; Tolin, Abramowitz, Przeworski, & Foa, 2002; for contrary results, see Najmi et al., 2009; Purdon et al., 2005). Individuals with OCD also rate the importance of controlling their most disturbing intrusive thought significantly higher than non-OCD-anxious and nonclinical groups (Morillo et al., 2007).

Studies based on clinical or analogue groups found that thought suppression was characterized by more intrusions, greater distress, and more negative appraisals than the "do not suppress" or "monitor only" conditions (Marcks & Woods, 2007; Morillo et al., 2007). Likewise, Corcoran and Woody (2009) found that appraisals of personal significance and greater thought control effort together predicted increased posttask negative affect in a nonclinical thought suppression experiment. Based on an undergraduate sample, Grisham and Williams (2009) found that less perceived thought controllability during thought suppression was associated with obsessive–compulsive symptoms, which in turn was associated with greater spontaneous suppression efforts. The deleterious effects of suppression have been attributed to heightened accessibility of the target thought (Najmi & Wegner, 2008) or to deficits in cognitive inhibitory processes (Tolin, Abramowitz, Przeworski, et al., 2002). Both processes have been implicated in OCD.

It is expected that individuals with elevated scores on trait measures of thought suppression would be characterized by high mental control effort. The White Bear Suppression Inventory (WBSI; Wegner & Zanakos, 1994) was developed to assess the tendency to engage in thought suppression. There is some evidence that individuals with OCD score significantly higher on the WBSI than non-OCD-anxious and nonclinical controls (Yorulmaz, Karanci, Bastug, Kisa, & Goka, 2008), although others have failed to find group differences (Belloch, Morillo, & García-Soriano, 2009). Correlational studies have reported significant associations between the WBSI and obsessive–compulsive symptom measures (Rafnsson & Smári, 2001; Wegner & Zanakos, 1994; Yorulmaz et al., 2008), although Höping and de Jong-Meyer (2003) found that it was the unwanted intrusive thoughts dimension rather than the suppression items that accounted for this relationship (see also van Schie, Wanmaker, Yocarini, & Bouwmeester, 2016).

As predicted by the generic model, the most consistent finding from the thought suppression research is that obsessionality is characterized by heightened effort to control unwanted thoughts. Even though individuals with OCD are capable "thought suppressors," at least in the short term, there is clear evidence that thought suppression is a counterproductive coping strategy. It has a negative impact on the experience of unwanted intrusions and increases the likelihood of faulty appraisals of significance (Corcoran & Woody, 2009; Marcks & Woods, 2007). Moreover, individuals who believe that it is important to control unwanted mental intrusions may exhibit more effort to control their unwanted thoughts (Purdon, 2004b), although research is needed on whether the beliefs included in the OBQ determine the level of suppression effort in thought control studies.

Is Maladaptive Thought Control More Evident in OCD?

It is possible that the mental control problem in OCD is not simply excessive control effort, but also reliance on less effective mental control strategies. As noted previously, thought suppression is considered a maladaptive control strategy, along with self-punishment or criticism, reassurance seeking, worry, thought stopping, and rationalization or analysis (Freeston et al., 1991; Freeston, Ladouceur, Provencher, & Blais, 1995; Wells & Davies, 1994). To varying degrees, these maladaptive strategies are associated with increased frequency and distress of unwanted intrusive thoughts, although not to the same degree as negative appraisals (Belloch, Morillo, Lucero, Cabedo, & Carrió, 2004; Freeston et al., 1991, 1992; Purdon & Clark, 1994b). Levine and Warman (2016) found that individuals were more likely to recommend maladaptive response strategies with more distressing intrusive thoughts.

Freeston and Ladouceur (1997b) found that only a third of the cognitive strategies and one-quarter of the behavioral strategies used by individuals with OCD to control obsessions could be considered cognitive rituals or neutralization. They concluded that individuals with OCD use a variety of thought control strategies in a similar proportion to nonclinical individuals. However, other researchers have investigated this question more directly. Abramowitz, Whiteside, Kalsy, and colleagues (2003) found that individuals with OCD reported more use of self-punishment and worry in response to unpleasant thoughts than non-OCD-anxious and nonclinical controls. Morillo and colleagues (2007) found their OCD sample scored significantly higher than nonclinical groups on a variety of maladaptive control strategies, although other studies found fewer differences (Bouvard et al., 2017; Calamari & Janeck, 1997; García-Soriano & Belloch, 2013; see also García-Soriano et al., 2014).

To date, the research is inconsistent on whether individuals with OCD rely on more maladaptive mental control than nonclinical individuals. Obviously, overt and covert compulsions are more common in OCD, which is true by definition. Maladaptive control strategies do contribute to the frequency and distress of unwanted intrusions and obsessions, but significantly less than negative appraisals. Finally, little is known about the use of adaptive mental control strategies in OCD because self-report measures of control are overly weighted on maladaptive strategies.

Are Faulty Appraisals of Thought Control Failure More Prominent in OCD?

The generic model (see Figure 5.1) predicts that vulnerable individuals will consider their unsuccessful mental control efforts to be a significant personal threat. This appraisal will contribute to an increased focus on the unwanted intrusion, greater mental control effort, and adoption of even more extreme control or neutralization strategies. Others have also suggested that vulnerable individuals might interpret thought control failures in a catastrophic manner (Abramowitz et al., 2001; Magee et al., 2012; Purdon, 2004b). A few studies have investigated this question using the thought suppression paradigm.

In a nonclinical thought suppression experiment, Purdon (2001) found that regardless of thought suppression conditions, negative mood state was predicted by greater concern that thought recurrences indicated an undesirable personality characteristic (i.e., ego dystonicity), poor mental functioning, and negative future events. Tolin, Abramowitz, Hamlin, and colleagues (2002) found that individuals with OCD endorsed more internal, negative attributions for their suppression failures than nonclinical controls. Magee and Teachman (2007) also found that internal, self-blaming attributions for suppression failure and ascribing importance to unwanted thoughts predicted greater distress and frequency of unwanted thought recurrence. Purdon and colleagues (2005) conducted a thought suppression experiment on 50 participants with OCD and found that negative appraisals over failures in thought control predicted suppression effort, discomfort associated with thought recurrences, and negative mood state. A subsequent dismissability experiment found that an OCD group had higher scores on concerns over thought recurrence than a panic disorder group, but the appraisals of thought control failure were equally related to dismissability in both groups (Purdon et al., 2011). Finally, Najmi and colleagues (2010) showed that beliefs about the futility of thought suppression could be altered by a brief psychoeducational intervention in nonclinical but not in OCD samples.

Unfortunately, too few studies have investigated the role of thought failure beliefs and appraisals to determine their influence on the persistence of unwanted intrusive thoughts and obsessions. However, the positive findings that have been reported suggest this is a fruitful area for future research. From this review, it is evident that individuals with OCD do exhibit a problem in mental control, as predicted by the generic model. It is most likely that excessive mental control effort and faulty appraisals of control failures are key features of the mental control problems associated with OCD.

Compulsive Rituals

Chapter 3 presented an extensive discussion of compulsive rituals and other forms of neutralization. Two issues are germane to the CBT model: (1) Are neutralization responses to unwanted intrusions more characteristic of OCD? (2) Does neutralization increase the recurrence and distress of unwanted mental intrusions or obsessions?

Practically all individuals with OCD exhibit overt or covert compulsions in response to unwanted, obsessive thoughts, images, or impulses (Foa et al., 1995; Leonard & Riemann, 2012; Williams, Farris, et al., 2011). Moreover, individuals with OCD are more likely to act to prevent harm in response to intrusive thoughts of harm than are nonclinical controls (Wroe, Salkovskis, & Richards, 2000; for similar results, see Morillo et al., 2007), and overt compulsions are related to obsessive–compulsive symptom severity (Belloch et al., 2015). When examining mental control strategies, OCD groups are more often distinguished by their greater use of compulsive rituals (Bouvard et al., 2017; García-Soriano et al., 2014; Romero-Sanchiz et al., 2017). Generally, there is considerable evidence that neutralization is more prominent in obsessional states.

In the generic CBT model, compulsions arise from certain unwanted intrusions, their faulty appraisal, and initial efforts at thought control. Thus, neutralization should influence the experience of unwanted intrusions. In an early nonclinical investigation, Rachman and colleagues (1996) found that neutralization immediately led to significant declines in anxiety, guilt, threat estimates, responsibility, and urge to neutralize. A second nonclinical study found that neutralization, but not distraction, resulted in more discomfort and an urge to neutralize even after a 30-minute delay (Salkovskis et al., 1997). Similar results were obtained with an OCD sample and a 15-minute delay before a second presentation of the unwanted intrusion. However, van den Hout and colleagues (2001) found that 2 minutes of neutralizing had the same effect on anxiety reduction and urge to neutralize as 20 minutes of spontaneous decay. In a second study, no difference in anxiety reduction was evident between a neutralization and no-neutralization group, but this was due to spontaneous self-generated neutralization in the "no-instruction" control group (van den Hout et al., 2002).

Overall, the results of these studies indicate that production of a compulsive response or neutralization can quickly reduce distress associated with an intrusive thought, and then cause an increase in distress with subsequent recurrence of the intrusion. What is not known is the extent to which neutralization boosts distress with thought recurrences relative to conditions in which spontaneous neutralization is prevented. Also, the effects of neutralization on negative appraisals of intrusion recurrences have not been adequately explored.

The generic CBT model posits that obsessions and their faulty appraisals elicit neutralization (i.e., compulsive rituals) in obsession-prone individuals. However, others have challenged this assumption, arguing that compulsions give rise to obsessions (Gillan & Sahakian, 2015). According to Gillan and colleagues (2011) the habit learning hypothesis proposes that OCD involves a general impairment in goal-directed action control, in which repetitive behavior results in the dominance of the automatic habitual system. Overreliance on habits may appear more efficient, but it is also characterized by loss of behavioral flexibility and possibly by the development of compulsivity. Gillan and colleagues suggest that the goal-directed impairment in OCD is associated with a neurobiological dysfunction in the cortical–striatal pathway. Gillan and Sahakian (2015) argue that obsessions may reflect an agitated mental urgency or a cognitive representation of "abstract feelings of anxiety and compulsive urges" (p. 248) that arise from compulsions.

The habit learning hypothesis of OCD is entirely contrary to the CBT understanding of the functional relationship between obsessions and compulsions, which harks back to the early behavioral view that compulsions arise from obsessions in most OCD cases (Rachman & Hodgson, 1980). Furthermore, phenomenological research indicates that certain aspects of the obsessional experience, such as the presence of sensory–perceptual experiences, can influence the frequency and impairment associated with compulsive behavior (Moritz, Purdon, Jelinek, Chiang, & Hauschildt, 2017), and obsessions and compulsions often load on the same dimensions on self-report measures (see Chapter 3). At present, there is considerable empirical evidence of a functional relationship between obsessions and compulsions that is consistent with the generic model. Like other constructs in the model, the direction of causality between neutralization and frequency of unwanted intrusions has not been established (Cougle & Lee, 2014).

Stop Criteria

The generic model posits that compulsive rituals will be repeated until the vulnerable person's stop criteria are satisfied. Chapter 3 introduced the concept of stop rules and the heightened evidence requirement used by individuals with OCD to decide when a compulsion has been satisfied. A few studies have investigated this topic and found that individuals with OCD use more subjective and multiple criteria when deciding when to cease a compulsive action (Bucarelli & Purdon, 2015; Salkovskis et al., 2017; Wahl et al., 2008). However, many questions remain, such as whether certain stop criteria are more efficient than others, whether elevated compulsion repetition degrades stop rule effectiveness, and the role of evaluations and sensory perceptions in signaling whether to terminate a compulsion. Given the positive findings in these preliminary studies, it is evident that stop criteria are an important component in the CBT model of obsessions and compulsions.

CONCLUSION

The CBT perspective on OCD emerged from the conceptual and therapeutic limitations of the behavioral approach and its exclusive focus on exposure and response prevention (see Chapter 4). A more cognitive approach to OCD was advanced by Salkovskis, Rachman, Freeston, and others who proposed new constructs such as inflated responsibility, TAF, misinterpretations of personal significance, neutralization, and the like to explain the etiology and treatment of obsessions and compulsions. From this work, a generic CBT model can be formulated, as depicted in Figure 5.1.

In the last 25 years, an extraordinary amount of empirical research has investigated various aspects of the CBT model. Research has spanned clinical, analogue, and nonclinical samples with both correlational and experimental methodologies employed. Empirical support for the basic tenets of the generic model is significant. Individuals with OCD:

- Experience more frequent and distressing unwanted mental intrusions.
- Tend to generate more faulty appraisals of these intrusions because of underlying maladaptive beliefs about mental control.
- Expend more effort in mental control (i.e., suppression) and may interpret their control failures more negatively.
- Resort to more extreme neutralization responses such as compulsive rituals and reassurance seeking.
- Employ more subjective criteria to determine when to stop a compulsion.

In addition, the cognitive constructs in the generic model, such as faulty appraisals, maladaptive beliefs, mental control effort, and neutralization, have a causal connection with the experience of unwanted intrusive thoughts or obsessions, although the direction of causality is still debated.

There are several criticisms and limitations of the model that must be recognized. First, there is the problem of specificity. Many of the cognitive appraisals and beliefs proposed in the model, such as inflated responsibility, TAF, threat overestimation, intolerance of uncertainty, reassurance seeking, and the like, are found in other forms of psychopathology (Julien et al., 2007). Second, the causal elements of the generic model have not been demonstrated. For example, it could be that greater mental control effort could be a consequence rather than cause of frequent obsessional intrusions (Cougle & Lee, 2014). Likewise, faulty appraisals of significance could be the consequence of obsessive–compulsive symptom exacerbation rather than its cause. Contextualism is a third issue for CBT models. There is evidence that the presence of obsessive–compulsive-relevant cognitive disturbance and maladaptive responses may depend on the situational elements of the intrusion experience rather than representing a generalized approach to any occurrence of an unwanted negative intrusion (Audet et al., 2016; Freeston et al., 1995; Julien et al., 2009). Fourth, it is likely that some cognitive constructs are more important in the pathogenesis of obsessions than others, but the research is too inconsistent at this time to suggest which belief or appraisal construct is most critical. And finally, the CBT model assumes that OCD develops from a cognitive vulnerability to the disorder. However, little progress has been made on determining the etiological role of cognitive constructs (see Coles et al., 2012, for an exception).

Despite these outstanding issues, there is enough empirical support for the CBT model to justify the cognitive treatment modifications and OCD subtype adaptions described in Part IV. However, before delving into the subtype models and treatment protocols, the chapters in Part III present the major treatment components of the CBT approach, based on the generic model presented in this chapter. We begin with the therapeutic relationship: a necessary but not sufficient precondition for effective CBT of OCD.

PART III
Fundamentals of CBT for OCD

CHAPTER 6

The Therapeutic Relationship

Like all forms of psychotherapy, CBT occurs within an interpersonal context with client and therapist entering into a professional relationship in which various therapeutic processes and interventions occur for the sole benefit of the client. Although conceptualization and intervention are the major concerns in CBT research and practice, there is little doubt that the therapeutic relationship plays an integral role in its treatment effectiveness (Kazantzis, Dattilio, & Dobson, 2017). From its inception, cognitive therapy has emphasized the importance of the therapeutic relationship (Beck, Rush, Shaw, & Emery, 1979). However, when treating clients with OCD, there are many factors that can undermine the quality of the therapeutic relationship, as evident in the following case example.

Since childhood Benjamin had struggled with obsessive–compulsive concerns about contamination, harming others, correctness, balance, and symmetry. He had many compulsions that included washing, redoing, counting, and checking, as well as extensive avoidance of anything that might trigger his obsessive–compulsive symptoms. As a result, he isolated himself at home, unable to work, travel, or socialize. His treatment history was extensive; he had tried many medications and seen several mental health professionals. Nothing had helped, and now he was referred to another psychologist, a supposed "expert in OCD." Benjamin stated, "My entire existence is a trigger, so I am having obsessions every moment of the day." He ended our first session by stating, "I don't think therapy can help me, but you're my last resort."

It was evident from that first contact that establishing an effective therapeutic relationship would be a critical factor in determining treatment outcome. A hint of delight could be detected as he told about past failed treatment and his prediction that I too would likely fail. Benjamin dominated the session with detailed and yet rambling descriptions of his OCD. He spoke of many things that he could not do and seemed resigned to a life of isolation and dependency on others. Attempts to bring organization and focus to the interview were met with generalities and digressions. There were inconsistencies in his self-report, as indicated, for example, by his comment that he felt "at that moment" his usual obsessive–compulsive concern about correctness (e.g., "Am I sitting correctly in the chair?"), and yet there were no observable compulsions or signs of distress. From that initial session it was possible that several issues might thwart efforts to engage Benjamin in the therapeutic enterprise:

- Was he capable of collaboration and considering alternative perspectives, or was he overly invested in his OCD worldview?
- Did he have sufficient trust, respect, and confidence in the therapist to commit to the therapy process?
- Would his negative treatment expectations and history of past failures or "defeats" weaken his motivation to invest in therapy once again?
- Could his domineering style be subdued enough to allow collaboration?
- Did he possess enough intrinsic motivation for change?
- Would avoidance, intolerance of uncertainty, and perfectionism sabotage openness to new learning?

From this case example, one can deduce several features of OCD that could threaten the quality of the therapeutic relationship. And yet, a strong therapeutic alliance is as critical for effective CBT for OCD as it is for treatment of any anxiety disorder or depression. This chapter discusses how the therapeutic relationship can be strengthened to improve treatment effectiveness. It begins by considering the conceptual distinction between the therapeutic relationship and a working alliance, and the empirical evidence that the latter is a significant factor in symptom improvement. The importance of collaboration, empiricism, Socratic questioning, and guided discovery are discussed—all CBT-specific elements of the therapeutic relationship. Finally, the chapter concludes by delineating prominent features of OCD that can undermine the therapeutic relationship and how the therapist can address these threats in order to strengthen the working alliance. (This chapter draws heavily on a highly informative clinical handbook on the therapeutic relationship by Kazantzis et al., called *The Therapeutic Relationship in Cognitive-Behavioral Therapy: A Clinician's Guide* [2017]. I strongly recommend this resource to all clinicians who want to sharpen their clinical skills and effectiveness.)

BROAD FACTORS

Until recently, CBT research focused exclusively on outcome or process issues such as the relative contribution of behavioral versus cognitive interventions, treatment integrity, cognitive restructuring, therapist competence, homework compliance, and other active treatment ingredients. The quality of the therapeutic relationship was recognized but only as the context needed for treatment effectiveness. In the original cognitive therapy manual for depression, Beck and colleagues (1979) stated, "This chapter describes the general nature of the therapeutic collaboration in cognitive therapy and the characteristics of the therapist which we believe facilitate the application of specific techniques for cognitive therapy" (p. 45). Later, J. S. Beck (2011) recognized that the quality of the therapeutic relationship has a more direct impact on treatment outcome. And so, CBT clinicians have become much more interested in the therapeutic relationship, offering a more thoughtful analysis of its constituent elements and investigating how these various elements affect treatment outcome (i.e., Kazantzis et al., 2017). Before considering the relevance of this research for CBT of OCD, it's imperative to understand the cognitive-behavioral perspective on the therapeutic relationship and its empirical status.

The Therapeutic Relationship: Concepts and Research

The *therapeutic relationship* is a broad term that refers to an exchange between therapist and client in which highly personal thoughts, beliefs, and emotions are shared to facilitate a client-focused change process (Kazantzis et al., 2017). An effective therapeutic relationship is characterized by empathy, understanding, positive regard, respect, honesty, collaboration, and feedback (Beck et al., 1979; Kazantzis et al., 2017). Although the therapist takes responsibility in setting the tone of the therapeutic relationship, its quality will be determined by client and therapist characteristics. A positive relationship is accomplished not only by the therapist's interactional style, but how the therapy itself is structured and delivered. Dobson and Dobson (2013) discuss how session structure that includes setting the agenda, reviewing homework, and soliciting client feedback can promote collaboration and a positive therapeutic context. When there is a collaborative client–therapist relationship, an individual will feel trust, mutual respect, a sense of safety, and a connection with the therapist that will promote engagement in the therapeutic enterprise (Kazantzis et al., 2017).

The American Psychological Association Task Force on Evidence-Based Therapy Relationships concluded from their review of a dozen meta-analyses that the therapeutic relationship plays a significant role in determining who improves or fails to improve with treatment (Norcross

& Wampold, 2011). Based on their conclusions and recommendations, the working alliance, empathy, and eliciting client feedback have the strongest empirical evidence for promoting symptom improvement, whereas positive regard, collaboration, and goal consensus are probably effective but not yet empirically substantiated. Table 6.1 lists various treatment processes that can strengthen the critical elements of the therapeutic relationship.

There is little empirical research on the contribution of these more generic therapeutic relationship elements to symptom improvement

TABLE 6.1. Strengthening the Critical Elements of the Therapeutic Relationship

Elements	Methods for enhancing the therapeutic relationship
Working alliance	Collaborate in treatment goal setting; have client prioritize goals; practice joint session agenda setting; develop homework assignments together; have clients write therapy summaries (e.g., coping statements) in their own words.
Empathy	Communicate a deep understanding of the client's OCD; acknowledge and validate the client's personal distress and suffering; recognize the idiosyncratic aspects of the client's OCD; express genuine concern about the negative impact of OCD on the client's daily living.
Client feedback	Elicit client feedback when presenting the case conceptualization; always obtain end-of-session feedback; elicit client reactions to homework assignment and review; explicitly ask for client understanding of therapist summaries and "interpretations."
Positive regard	Do a review of the pros and cons of the client's OCD; recognize the client's readiness for change; express understanding and compassion for obsessive–compulsive fears and concerns; discuss client's OCD as occurring along a continuum of normality; validate the client's struggle with self-disclosure; present the case conceptualization in a compassionate, respectful manner; make frequent encouraging, affirming, and positive statements about the client.
Collaboration	Ensure client participation in session agenda setting and homework assignments; do within-session cognitive and behavioral interventions before between-session assignments; practice Socratic questioning and guided discovery; engage clients in setting the pace of therapy; be flexible in dealing with immediate client issues and crises.
Goal consensus	Collaborate on treatment goal setting and session agenda setting; client prioritizes goals; periodically review progress toward treatment goals; collaboratively revise treatment goals throughout treatment course; mutually agree on treatment termination.

(Kazantzis et al., 2017). However, it would be hard to argue that positive regard, empathy, collaboration, and the like play little role in treatment effectiveness. At the very least, CBT therapists need to be cognizant of the importance of a high-quality therapeutic relationship when treating clients with OCD and to periodically conduct an audit of its quality and function in the therapy. It is common for strain and even ruptures to appear in the relationship between client and therapist when both are engaged in a very intense and demanding treatment like CBT for OCD.

The Working Alliance

The therapeutic *working alliance* refers to collaboration between client and therapist that consists of (1) agreement on therapeutic goals, (2) consensus on the tasks or activities that comprise the therapy, and (3) the bond between client and therapist (Bordin, 1979; Horvath, Del Re, Flückiger, & Symonds, 2011). Most of the empirical research on the therapeutic relationship and its impact on symptom improvement has focused on the working alliance. In these studies, self-report questionnaires such as the Working Alliance Inventory (WAI; Horvath & Greenberg, 1989) are administered to clients, therapists, and/or observers to measure the quality of the therapeutic relationship. CBT is well represented in most of these process studies, with depression and anxiety the most common clinical problems. In a large meta-analytic review of over 200 studies covering a broad range of psychotherapies, Horvath and colleagues (2011) concluded that the working alliance had an effect size of $r = .275$, which indicates a modest but significant contribution to treatment outcome. A subsequent multilevel longitudinal analysis again found a modest but robust relationship between working alliance and treatment outcome across all treatment modalities, including CBT (Flückiger, Del Re, Wampold, Symonds, & Horvath, 2012). Treatment allegiance had a moderating influence on the early alliance–outcome relationship.

It may be that the relationship between the working alliance and treatment outcome is more nuisance than first thought. Strunk, Brotman, and DeRubeis (2010) found that adherence to cognitive therapy methods was a better predictor of symptom improvement in cognitive therapy for depression than the therapeutic alliance. Based on an observer-rated version of the WAI, Lorenzo-Luaces, DeRubeis, and Webb (2014) found that the alliance–outcome relationship was significant only for individuals with fewer than three depressive episodes. However, correlations between alliance and depression scores were mostly nonsignificant in a treatment process study of interpersonal psychotherapy and cognitive therapy for depression (Lemmens et al., 2017). A large CBT treatment study of outpatients that included individuals with OCD found that a positive therapeutic alliance, problem coping skills, and emotional involvement within sessions were significant predictors of next-session symptom improvement (Rubel, Rosenbaum, & Lutz, 2017).

A few studies have examined therapeutic alliance effects on treatment outcome in OCD. The therapeutic alliance was a significant predictor of posttreatment outcome in exposure-based CBT for OCD (Vogel, Hansen, Stiles, & Götetam, 2006), although this effect may be mediated by patient adherence to ERP homework assignments (Simpson et al., 2011). Wheaton, Huppert, Foa, and Simpson (2016) found that patient adherence and engagement in therapy tasks but not the therapeutic alliance predicted treatment outcome. In the most recent study, Strauss, Huppert, Simpson, and Foa (2018) assessed common and specific treatment effects in 111 individuals with OCD, randomly assigned to ERP or stress management. Only 32% of symptom improvement was due to common factors, with early therapeutic alliance and treatment expectancy weak predictors of symptom improvement. Moreover, cross-lag analysis indicated that the therapeutic alliance was a consequence rather than cause of symptom improvement. At the very least, these findings indicate that the specific treatment ingredients of ERP are far more important to symptom improvement than nonspecific factors like the quality of the therapeutic relationship.

Nevertheless, there can be little doubt that the quality of the therapeutic relationship plays some role in treatment effectiveness. This conclusion appears to be applicable to a broad range of psychotherapies, including CBT. However, the therapeutic alliance accounts for approximately 7.5% of treatment outcome variance (Horvath et al., 2011), and so other treatment variables, such as treatment fidelity, probably play an even more important role. Likewise, the therapeutic relationship may be more important earlier in treatment or for individuals with more acute forms of disorder.

It is worth noting that the alliance–outcome relationship is largely due to therapist characteristics, with some therapists consistently better at forming alliances and achieving better treatment outcomes than others (i.e., Del Re, Flückiger, Horvath, Symonds, & Wampold, 2012). Several studies have investigated which therapist characteristics have either a positive or a negative impact on the therapeutic alliance (e.g., Heinonen et al., 2014; Hersoug, Høglend, Havik, von der KIppe, & Monsen, 2009). Table 6.2 lists potentially positive and negative characteristics.

Kazantzis and colleagues (2017) noted four essential skills needed to become a competent CBT therapist. It is likely that these competencies also contribute to a positive therapeutic relationship and are prerequisite clinical skills for effective CBT for OCD.

- *Interpersonal effectiveness:* the ability to communicate effectively to a range of people in a manner that conveys knowledge of the cognitive approach and its relevance to the client's condition.
- *Cognitive case conceptualization:* the ability to formulate a broad

perspective on the client that goes beyond session-by-session issues. This is analogous to being able to "see the forest instead of the trees."
- *Encourage client experimentation:* the ability to encourage and promote client commitment to engage in between-session interventions.
- *Knowledge of cognitive theory:* possesses and is able to convey a full understanding of the cognitive model and its interventions in treatment of OCD.

A positive therapeutic relationship and healthy working alliance are critical for effective CBT for OCD. The cognitive-behavioral approach requires a high level of client involvement, which some individuals may find overwhelming. A positive working alliance will be necessary to promote client engagement in the therapy process. In other words, individuals with OCD need to "like their therapists." If the therapist or therapy style grates against the client, then it is unlikely he or she will respond to CBT interventions. It is incumbent on each therapist to evaluate the quality of the therapeutic relationship periodically throughout treatment. Table 6.3 is a self-reflective exercise that can be used to pinpoint potential problems in the therapeutic relationship.

TABLE 6.2. Positive and Negative Therapist Characteristics That Impact the Therapeutic Alliance

Positive characteristics	Negative characteristics
Demonstrates good relational skills (i.e., composed, responsive to others, empathy for wide range of human experience, ability to feel and communicate authentic concern)	Perceives self as possessing advanced skills in therapy (i.e., conveys arrogance, detachment)
Demonstrates an engaging and encouraging quality	Conveys hostility, empathic deficiency, and frustration with client
Demonstrates high therapeutic skillfulness and efficacy (i.e., competence)	Conveys boredom, anxiety, and/or uncertainty
Demonstrates enjoyment in therapy work	Is distant, disconnected, and indifferent
Experiences close personal relationships	Is rigid, uncertain, critical, tense, and distracted
Is trustworthy, warm, flexible, honest, interested in and openly responsive to clients	

TABLE 6.3. **Self-Reflection on the Quality of the Therapeutic Relationship**

1. "Have I communicated understanding, relevance, and knowledge of CBT theory and treatment and how it applies to the client's OCD?"
2. "Have I expressed empathy, positive regard, and compassion toward the client?"
3. "Have I encouraged collaboration in treatment goal setting, the session agenda, and formulating homework assignments?"
4. "Do I regularly elicit client feedback on the homework assignments, within-session interventions, and end-of-session review?"
5. "Does the client have sufficient trust to engage in self-disclosure of potentially embarrassing and distressing obsessions and compulsions?"
6. "Have I been flexible and adaptable in my therapy style?"
7. "Have I been open and responsive to client needs and initiatives?"
8. "Do I convey interest and enjoyment in my therapy work?"
9. "Have I been composed, confident, and goal-directed in my therapy approach?"
10. "Do I regularly validate the client, recognizing his or her efforts and contributions to the therapeutic enterprise?"
11. "Am I honest and emotionally authentic in my interactions with the client?"
12. "Have I encouraged client independence as therapy progresses?"

CBT-SPECIFIC FACTORS

Over the years, CBT manuals have tended to emphasize therapy content over process, despite the introduction of several therapeutic processes that represent innovations in how treatment is delivered to clients (i.e., J. S. Beck, 2011; Beck et al., 1979). This section focuses on three CBT-specific relational elements: collaboration, empiricism, and Socratic questioning (Kazantzis et al., 2017). Along with the broad factors of the therapeutic relationship discussed previously, these three processes are considered critical to effective CBT for OCD.

Collaboration

In CBT, clients take an active role in treatment planning, delivery, and evaluation. The need for active participation in the therapeutic process may be foreign to many clients, so the therapist must educate each client into the collaborative nature of treatment. Early in therapy the clinician takes a more dominant role in guiding the client in adopting interventions that facilitate progress toward treatment goals. As therapy progresses, more and more responsibility for the direction of therapy is shifted to the client (Kazantzis et al., 2017). In this way the therapist encourages greater client self-determination in the therapy process.

According to Kazantzis and colleagues (2017), *collaboration* in CBT is the "active and shared work between therapist and client" (p. 51). Client motivation and engagement in therapy, which are essential for active treatments like CBT, will be enhanced when collaboration is emphasized. Kazantzis and colleagues note that collaboration is promoted when the therapist seeks client feedback, provides rationales, suggests interventions, and responds to client contributions, whereas the client contributes to decisions and choices and offers suggestions throughout treatment. Therapists who dominate the therapy session, make unilateral decisions, select treatment goals, control the session agenda, impose homework assignments, and rarely solicit client feedback or evaluation will undermine collaboration. It is easy to see how this domineering therapeutic style would lead to a rupture in the therapeutic relationship and client disengagement from the therapy process.

Tee and Kazantzis (2011) offer a conceptual basis for the importance of collaboration in CBT. Based on self-determination theory, they argue that collaboration promotes a client's sense of autonomy, which in turn strengthens motivation for behavioral change. When collaboration is present, the client is more likely to attribute change to his or her own efforts, which will increase a sense of autonomy, competence, and efficacy. This represents a form of "introjected [internalized] regulation," which is more likely to promote sustained behavioral change. On the other hand, low collaboration reduces the client's sense of self-determination so that change will be attributed to external causes, such as the therapist's clinical skill. When this happens, therapeutic change will be less stable and enduring.

Collaboration does not come naturally to the therapy process; it must be actively cultivated by the therapist from the initial contact to treatment termination. Therapy must be presented as "shared work" characterized by balanced decision making, balanced contributions to therapy sessions, and mutual respect, interest, and responsiveness (Kazantzis, Tee, Dattilio, & Dobson, 2013). However, Padesky and Greenberger (1995) remind us that collaboration alone is insufficient without visible progress in solving the client's problems.

A modified therapy excerpt illustrates a confrontational, didactic therapeutic style, followed by a more facilitative collaborative approach. The situation involves a Christian fundamentalist who suffers pathological doubt. She cannot decide to do even routine daily tasks (e.g., wash, get out of bed) because she is not sure whether she will make the right decision that pleases God.

Didactic, Confrontational Style

CLIENT: God is continually putting me to the test to see if I will make the right decision that pleases Him.

THERAPIST: It is impossible to know whether one pleases a deity.

CLIENT: Well, it is important that I try to discern whether God is pleased with me or not.

THERAPIST: Your distress is caused by trying to answer an impossible question. You would feel less anxious if you gave up trying to please God and focused more on your own personal needs.

CLIENT: But that would make me selfish. Pride is one of the most serious of sins.

THERAPIST: Your God appears harsh and judgmental. If you focused more on the loving, forgiving nature of God, you would not be so upset by thoughts of displeasing Him.

CLIENT: But the Bible tells us that God will judge our every deed and punish the sinner.

THERAPIST: You are striving to attain an impossible level of Christian obedience that is not humanly attainable. Each time you think about making a decision, you feel anxious because you search endlessly for signs that one decision or the next is the right one. Instead of this obsessive questioning, the next time you wonder if God is pleased, I want you to take an immediate course of action, and then monitor your thoughts and feelings over the next few hours.

Collaborative, Nonconfrontational Style

CLIENT: God is continually putting me to the test to see if I will make the right decision that pleases Him.

THERAPIST: How does this thought make you feel?

CLIENT: Well, I feel very upset, frightened by the thought of not pleasing God by my decisions.

THERAPIST: So, the question or doubt of whether you pleased God causes you a lot of anxiety, distress. This is obviously an important issue for you. What makes this doubting thought so important to you?

CLIENT: If I can't be certain that I've made the right decision that pleases God, then maybe I have displeased Him. If God is displeased, then I am not putting Him first, I'm not totally sold out to Him.

THERAPIST: What's so bad about that?

CLIENT: I have dishonored God; He will turn His back on me and condemn me to hell.

THERAPIST: This is obviously a terrible outcome, but especially for someone who is trying so hard to make the right decision that is honoring to God. Do you have any way of knowing when you may have made a right or wrong decision?

CLIENT: Well, when I feel at peace I think that my decision may have pleased God, but when I have doubts and turmoil, I am convinced that my decision may be displeasing to God.

THERAPIST: I see. So, you have a theological explanation for your distress. You believe that the problem (i.e., feeling distress) is due to not pleasing God, while the solution (i.e., peace of mind) is found in finding the right course of action that pleases God. Certainly, that is one way to look at your obsessional doubt. However, I wonder if we could explore to see whether there is another, possibly psychological, explanation for your distress and its remedy.

CLIENT: What might that be?

THERAPIST: Well, I was wondering whether there might be something in the way that you respond to your doubting thoughts that makes them more intense and upsetting. Would you like to look at this possibility and see what we can find?

CLIENT: *(with some reluctance)* I suppose we could look at this possibility, but I am convinced that my problem is spiritual.

Empiricism

Cognitive therapy is an empirically based therapy in which individuals' maladaptive beliefs and behaviors are tested against their experience. In CBT, *empiricism* refers to helping clients use the scientific method to bring new understanding to their experiences (Kazantzis et al., 2017). Therapist and client act as co-investigators to identify, evaluate, and test alternatives to maladaptive thoughts and beliefs. In CBT the therapist takes an empirical approach to developing the case conceptualization and then guides the client toward observing, evaluating, and learning from his or her personal experiences. For example, a client might say, "I can't touch that dirty doorknob and not wash my hands because the anxiety will be unbearable." In taking an empirical approach, the therapist might inquire about experiences in which touching the doorknob led to unbearable anxiety and then ask the client whether there were other times when he or she touched the doorknob, but the anxiety was bearable. Maybe, for example, the client was able to touch the doorknob without washing his or her hands and didn't feel overly anxious because someone was present. So rather than engage in a verbal dispute on whether touching doorknobs is associated with unbearable anxiety, a therapist who values empiricism invites the client to evaluate this belief from the perspective of the client's own experience and then draft an alternative belief. In the end the therapist seeks to teach clients to evaluate and critique their thoughts, feelings, and behavior through the lens of their own experience (Kazantzis et al., 2017). In other words, the CBT motto could be, *Don't believe everything you think*. First *evaluate the thought in terms of real-life experience and then formulate a more valid, realistic alternative.*

While the empirical approach is a fundamental element of all forms of CBT, it is especially critical in treatment of OCD. As discussed below, there are many features of OCD that can threaten the therapeutic alliance. Therapists who take an empirical approach (e.g., "Let's see what we can learn from your experience") will be able to navigate many of the challenges in working with people with OCD. Since obsessive–compulsive-related beliefs and coping responses are often held with rigid conviction, it's important to avoid verbal disputation or persuasion. Trying to reason with a client about the irrationality or improbability of an obsessive–compulsive fear will only lead to treatment failure and termination. Instead the therapist adopts an *empiricist* approach, inviting the client to test out his or her obsessive–compulsive thoughts, beliefs, and appraisals through real-life experiences. Behavioral assignments, empirical hypothesis testing, and ERP are interventions the therapist uses so that individuals can learn new ways of thinking and responding. Collaborative empiricism is the therapeutic style that most effectively addresses the maladaptive beliefs about exposure, distress tolerance, and readiness for change that characterize clients with OCD (Clark, 2013).

Socratic Questioning

The previous therapy excerpt on collaboration illustrates two other important features of the cognitive-behavioral therapeutic style: Socratic questioning and guided discovery. These concepts were introduced by Aaron T. Beck to ensure the development of a collaborative therapeutic relationship between therapist and client (Beck & Emery, 1985). Socratic questioning involves a form of inductive questioning used by therapists to guide clients into discovering their own problematic thoughts, interpretations, and beliefs. Kazantzis and colleagues (2017) defined *Socratic questioning* as "a process of communication adopted by the therapist that fosters client engagement in cognitive change strategies" (p. 72). Beck and Emery (1985) observed that good questioning expands the client's constricted thinking and helps establish structure, collaboration, and motivation.

Guided discovery is a process in which a series of Socratic questions are asked about the meaning of thoughts, so the client becomes aware of underlying dysfunctional beliefs and subsequently evaluates the validity and functionality of these beliefs (J. S. Beck, 1995). Padesky and Greenberger (1995) noted that guided discovery involves the following:

- Questions that identify information outside the client's current awareness.
- Concentrated listening and reflection

- Statements that summarize the client's responses.
- A synthesizing question that requires the client to apply newly discovered information to the dysfunctional belief.

Kazantzis and colleagues (2017) noted that guided discovery involves a style of questioning in which dialogue is the process, discovery is the outcome, and change is the goal.

There is some empirical evidence that Socratic questioning is related to symptom improvement. In one study observer ratings of the first three sessions of cognitive therapy for depression revealed that within-session Socratic questioning significantly predicted session-to-session symptom change across early treatment sessions (Braun, Strunk, Sasso, & Cooper, 2015). Similarly, Kazantzis and colleagues (2017) reported on their own study in which variations in Socratic dialogue predicted subsequent depression outcome. In both studies, Socratic questioning predicted outcome even after controlling for the therapeutic alliance. Clearly, then, Socratic questioning appears to be a therapeutic communication style that facilitates treatment effectiveness. The following is a hypothetical therapy segment that illustrates the use of Socratic questioning and guided discovery with our case example of Benjamin.

> THERAPIST: Benjamin, you've told me that you stay in bed most of the day because if you do anything, you immediately become concerned that it was not done correctly. Is that right?
>
> BENJAMIN: That's right. I'm constantly feeling anxious and distressed that I'm not thinking or doing the right thing.
>
> THERAPIST: To understand your OCD concerns better, could we focus on one specific example, let's say a moment in time when you felt overcome with anxiety and distress because of your concern about correctness. Is there an example that comes to your mind?
>
> BENJAMIN: Yesterday I was lying in bed and suddenly became concerned that I was lying on my left side too long. I kept thinking that I should roll over on my right side, but I was unsure whether I'd spent more time on my left or on my right. I could feel myself get more and more anxious.
>
> THERAPIST: Why do you think you became so upset when you had the thought "Am I lying too much on my left side?"?
>
> BENJAMIN: It's because I have OCD. I get very anxious when I think that my life is not balanced.
>
> THERAPIST: You're right; this definitely sounds like an OCD experience, but I wonder if we might try to break down this experience and identify exactly what caused the thought "Maybe I'm lying too much on my left side" to be so anxiety-provoking. If we can discover the psychological causes to the anxiety, this might lead us to a treatment strategy.

BENJAMIN: I'm not sure what you mean. Isn't the thought about lying too much on my left side the cause of my anxiety?

THERAPIST: Yes, I agree. If you didn't have the thought, then you wouldn't feel anxious. But let's assume it's perfectly normal for people who are lying down to think "I need to roll over on my other side." Do you think these people feel anxious when they have this thought?

BENJAMIN: Probably not.

THERAPIST: Exactly! So, I wonder what it is about this thought that makes you anxious, but the same thought doesn't make other people anxious. Would you like to do some work on this question and see if we can discover the differences? From this we might learn what is causing you to feel so uncomfortable with the thought and how you can normalize the thought so that it is not anxiety-provoking.

BENJAMIN: I can see how this might be helpful, but I've no idea how to do this.

THERAPIST: Great! Glad to hear that you're on board for this type of work. I have some ideas on where we can start.

Despite the importance of the Socratic dialogue for treatment effectiveness, this therapeutic style may need modification when interviewing clients with severe doubt. Individuals with obsessional doubt and indecision may find Socratic questioning particularly anxiety-provoking as they search to provide the therapist with the "perfect" or "most correct" answer to each question. In such cases the therapist may have to use more summary statements and suggestive probes to avoid overwhelming the client or paralyzing the pace of therapy.

OCD THREATS TO THE THERAPEUTIC RELATIONSHIP

Creating a positive therapeutic relationship and working alliance can be more challenging for some clients. This section discusses 10 features of OCD that can have a negative impact on the therapeutic relationship. In each case suggestions are provided to address the threat posed to the working alliance.

Ambivalence

There are many reasons why an individual with OCD might not be fully committed to the treatment process. Some may feel coerced into treatment because family and friends are more convinced of the debilitating effects of the disorder than the client. Others battling a long course of OCD may come to therapy discouraged and demoralized, believing that nothing can be effective in dislodging well-entrenched obsessive–compulsive symptoms. Or clients may have experienced a series of "treatment failures" and so can see no reason to believe that CBT will be different. Other individuals may be so convinced of the biological basis of their symptoms that it is hard for them to accept a psychological treatment. Often the OCD becomes such an important part of their self-identity that individuals find it difficult to imagine themselves without obsessive–compulsive concerns. The end result may be ambivalence toward change and diminished commitment to the therapy process.

Ambivalence occurs when clients seek treatment because of a desire for change but at the same time fear and resist it (Westra & Norouzian, 2017). Ambivalence is an important aspect of treatment resistance and when it occurs, it tends to weaken the therapeutic alliance, undermine effectiveness, and lead to premature termination (Szkodny, Newman, & Goldfried, 2014; Westra & Norouzian, 2017).

Ambivalence may be especially problematic in OCD because of perfectionism. Perfectionism has long been recognized as a major feature of OCD (Frost, Novara, & Rhéaume, 2002; OCCWG, 1997). Rigid adherence to high standards for completion of rituals, need for exactness and completeness, fear of making mistakes, importance of control, and intolerance of uncertainty are all aspects of the perfectionism evident in OCD (see Egan, Wade, Shafran, & Antony, 2014). In their treatment manual, *Cognitive-Behavioral Treatment of Perfectionism,* Egan and colleagues (2014) note that ambivalence is a common therapy issue. Individuals may misattribute advantages to their perfectionism and downplay the negative impact it is having on their daily life. This response can result in difficulty choosing between committing to and working toward change and maintaining their dysfunctional perfectionism (Egan et al., 2014).

A second source of ambivalence is rooted in the self-view of individuals with OCD. Bhar and Kyrios (2007) proposed that individuals with OCD have a fragile or ambivalent self-view in which contradictory or opposing elements are contained within the self-concept. Others proposed that the self-representation in OCD confuses possibilities with reality (Aardema & O'Connor, 2007). In this way OCD concerns about responsibility for harm, doubts about errors and omissions, immorality, and loss of control can become important parts of the individual's self-representation. If the person with OCD comes to see him- or herself in terms of cleanliness, strong moral character, conscientiousness, meticulousness, and the like, he or she may be hesitant to engage in a therapeutic process that involves fundamental changes to cherished values and self-attributes.

There are two approaches the therapist can take in response to client ambivalence. First, it is important that therapists not direct anger, criticism, and blame toward the client. As well, a confrontational, direct, and problem-solving therapeutic orientation may increase disengagement in the resistant or ambivalent client (Westra & Norouzian, 2017). Instead, therapy may need to become less directive and more supportive, with the therapist more sensitive to signs of resistance in the form of disagreeing, ignoring, interrupting, withdrawing, criticizing, and the like (Westra & Norouzian, 2017).

One of the best approaches to ambivalence is to integrate elements of motivational interviewing (MI) into the therapy program. MI stresses the development of a safe and collaborative therapeutic context, in which therapists help clients sort out their conflicting ideas about change (Miller & Rollnick, 2013; Westra & Norouzian, 2017). Egan and colleagues (2014) recommended that therapists return to a discussion of shared treatment goals and common aims. As well, certain erroneous beliefs might maintain ambivalence for change. Often individuals with OCD believe that the aim of CBT is to turn them into the opposite of their obsessive–compulsive concerns. Thus, the person with pathological doubt becomes reckless and irresponsible, or the person with contamination fear becomes dirty and infectious. With the use of Socratic questioning and guided discovery, the therapist helps the client identify these cognitive impediments to change and explores a more balanced treatment perspective in which the aim of therapy is normalization of obsessive–compulsive concerns, rather than their complete eradication.

Another MI approach to ambivalence is to encourage clients to write down the costs and benefits of change versus no change (Egan et al., 2014). Form 6.1 is a worksheet that clients can use to list the advantages and disadvantages of maintaining versus reducing their OCD symptoms in various major life domains.

The cost–benefit exercise should be used only when clients express ambivalence about change. It should be introduced early in the treatment phase and the therapist may need to begin the exercise within the session, since some individuals may find it difficult to think about the benefits of no symptom change. However, when done collaboratively, Form 6.1 can be a useful tool for fully exploring the client's ambivalence toward therapy. When introducing ERP, the therapist can return to the same exercise (see also Form 4.2) to work on the client's reluctance to engage in exposure-based homework.

Excessive Reassurance Seeking

Individuals with OCD often seek reassurance from their therapist (see Chapter 3 for further discussion of excessive reassurance seeking [ERS]). This can have a significant negative impact on the therapeutic relationship in two ways. First, therapists who inadvertently provide reassurance to their clients with OCD undermine the effectiveness of treatment by obfuscating an opportunity to learn to tolerate distress and uncertainty. And second, the therapist's response to requests for reassurance can convey a detachment and uncaring attitude toward the client's distress. When ERS is handled poorly by the therapist, a rupture can occur in the therapeutic relationship.

Cognitive-behavioral therapists must be vigilant for the emergence of ERS in the therapy session. For example, in response to an exposure-based homework assignment for harm obsessions, a client may say to the therapist, "Do you think it's possible to run over a pedestrian without knowing it?" The unwitting therapist might respond by helping the client seek out information on the probability of running over someone without knowing it. Although a standard cognitive intervention, the therapist is providing reassurance to the client. The better response would be "I understand why you are asking me this question, but do you think you're looking for reassurance? In the past, has reassurance from friends, family, or the Internet been very helpful? Don't you think the same thing will happen to my reassurance? Would you like to explore an alternative response to your concern about harming others?"

Several problems arise when therapists fall into the ERS trap. First, the therapist ends up reinforcing a maladaptive neutralization strategy that is an important maintaining factor in OCD. Second, the exposure-based exercises designed to test obsessive–compulsive beliefs and intolerance of distress will be weakened by the provision of reassurance. Third, the relief obtained from the therapist's reassurance will be temporary at best, thereby undermining the credibility of the therapist and his or her treatment. Fourth, ERS usually involves the request for a specific response (e.g., "It's impossible to run over someone without knowing it"), which undermines the more collaborative, investigative nature of CBT. And fifth, ERS can escalate in frequency and intensity so the therapy can become dominated by client requests for more and more reassurance from the therapist.

Therapists, of course, need to discuss the issue of ERS with composure, understanding, and empathy to preserve the therapeutic relationship. After all, refusing to provide reassurance is tantamount to turning your back on the client's distress—an experience that many vulnerable individuals will find very rejecting. The following are some suggestions for dealing with the ERS issue:

- Review with clients their experience with reassurance and its effectiveness, emphasizing that therapist reassurance will eventually become ineffective as well.
- Normalize reassurance seeking, noting that most people seek reassurance but ultimately find it unpersuasive.

- In a highly collaborative manner, discuss how you, as therapist, can respond to ERS in a sensitive, caring manner that still maintains the integrity of the treatment.
- Set a homework assignment in which therapist reassurance is provided about a specific exercise and monitor its effects on distress. This could be compared with an exercise in which reassurance is not provided. What was the difference in the intensity and duration of distress? Was therapist reassurance as effective and helpful as the client anticipated?

Rigidity and Inflexibility

Deviating from a routine, facing the unfamiliar, or doing something that is novel or ambiguous can be highly threatening to the individual with OCD (e.g., Kusunoki et al., 2000). In addition, cognitive and behavioral inflexibility are well-established deficits in OCD (e.g., Gruner & Pittenger, 2017; Meiran, Diamond, Toder, & Nemets, 2011). Consequently, individuals with OCD often seek order, routine, and the predictable in their daily lives. CBT, on the other hand, emphasizes seeking out new learning opportunities and disrupting well-established patterns of thinking and behaving. For the individual who finds uncertainty (or ambiguity), novelty, and flexibility difficult and distressing, therapy represents a daunting and highly threatening situation. Each challenge to think and respond differently can be met with fear and resistance, again putting great strain on the therapeutic relationship.

When clients lack psychological flexibility, therapy can feel like a "push and pull" exercise. For the reluctant client, the therapist's focus on evaluating the old and trying out a new approach can lead to resistance and even outright therapist–client conflict. To avoid this adverse effect on the therapeutic relationship, the therapist should acknowledge and validate the client's struggle with change. Dysfunctional beliefs about change can be addressed and together client and therapist can break down therapeutic tasks into less threatening steps. Above all, therapists need to remember that for many individuals with OCD, change in daily living can be a terrifying prospect.

Need for Control

The need for control is one of the most prominent cognitive features of OCD (see Chapters 3 and 5 for further discussion). Fear of losing control, especially over unwanted thoughts, has been repeatedly demonstrated in OCD (Clark, 2004; Clark & Purdon, 1993, 2016). In severe OCD, one's entire day can be reduced to excessive control of the most trivial of obsessive–

compulsive-related concerns, with family members often controlled by the client's obsessive–compulsive symptomatology. For the approximately 25% of individuals with comorbid OCPD, perfectionism along with desire for order and control will be especially prominent (see discussion in Chapter 1; Egan et al., 2014). It is little wonder, then, that issues of control can creep into the therapeutic relationship, causing conflict between client and therapist.

The collaborative nature of CBT can feel foreign to a client with OCD who is used to getting his or her own way, at least when it comes to OCD. The client may feel uncomfortable sharing the responsibility and control of his or her obsessive–compulsive concerns with the therapist. When disagreement, hostility, and criticism arise in the therapy session, the therapist needs to explore whether fear of losing control might be an issue that is threatening the therapeutic relationship. Therapy sessions may need to shift focus to maladaptive beliefs related to fear of losing control. Exploring with the client more adaptive beliefs about control and how therapist and client together might share in control of the therapy agenda should be discussed. At the very least, it is important that the therapist directly address control issues when they arise and threaten to undermine the therapeutic relationship.

Concealment

Often individuals with OCD, especially those with repugnant obsessions, can be so embarrassed and fearful when attempting to talk about their obsessions that they may refuse to verbalize the obsessional content to the therapist (Newth & Rachman, 2001). Concealment is a form of avoidance and needs to be overcome if any progress is to be possible. A good therapeutic relationship is the key to providing a therapeutic context that feels safe enough for clients to talk openly and honestly about their most frightening obsessions. If a working alliance has not been established, clients are more likely to refuse full disclosure of their obsessions. Alternatively, they may rationalize the obsession or downplay its irrationality and severity, which again threatens treatment effectiveness. Chapter 12, on repugnant obsessions, provides an extended discussion of concealment and how the CBT therapist can deal with this problem. When concealment is evident, the therapist will need to slow down the pace of treatment and focus on creating a safe therapeutic context that encourages full disclosure of obsessional fears and concerns.

Interpersonal Deficiencies and Emotional Detachment

For many individuals with severe OCD, the disorder becomes so all-encompassing that they cease to have healthy relationships with others.

They may retreat into their "OCD world," in which their entire attention is focused on obsessions and compulsions. Social withdrawal and isolation become extreme, and any contact with others is distorted by a total preoccupation with their disorder. When individuals with pathological doubt and severe repeating compulsions try to interact, their communication can be odd and incomprehensible, causing others to withdraw from the individual. In addition, comorbid social anxiety disorder is evident in 40% of individuals with OCD and approximately 10% may have avoidant personality disorder (see review in Chapter 1, pp. 21–23). Individuals with comorbid OCPD may lack emotional expressiveness, appearing cold and detached when talking about their obsessional concerns.

Difficulty with interpersonal relatedness and emotional detachment presents special challenges when attempting to form a therapeutic alliance. In order to mitigate the negative effects of poor relational skills on the therapeutic relationship, the therapist first must determine if social anxiety disorder, OCPD, or avoidant personality disorder are present. If so, therapy will need to be adjusted to take these comorbid conditions into account. However, low interpersonal functioning and emotional detachment can still be present in those who do not meet criteria for a personality disorder or social anxiety disorder. When these problems arise in the therapy session, the CBT therapist will need to dial back on the relational aspects of therapy. The early sessions of therapy may need to take a more formal, emotionally detached, and problem-focused approach to reduce the interpersonal demands on the client. Once safety and comfort have been established in later sessions, the therapist can shift to greater interpersonal familiarity, openness, and disclosure, which are better for building a working alliance.

Doubt and Indecision

Doubt and indecision are pervasive features of OCD. Their severity will vary greatly among individuals, with those presenting with checking and repeating compulsions exhibiting the most severe forms of doubt and indecision (see Chapter 11). However, both problems can put significant strain on the therapeutic relationship, especially in CBT in which Socratic questioning is the preferred *modus operandi*. Using Socratic questioning with a client who exhibits significant doubt and indecision can be frustrating. The therapist may ask a question to which the client takes an incredibly long time to respond, often qualifying and correcting his or her answers. This can slow the therapeutic process down to a crawl, causing the therapist to feel frustrated and impatient.

There are several suggestions for dealing with OCD clients who are incredibly slow and indecisive.

- Directly acknowledge and then validate the client's struggle in the therapy session with indecision, doubt, and their associated distress.
- Use moments of indecision to identify the faulty appraisals and beliefs that underlie the indecisiveness, and work on developing a healthier response to thoughts of doubt and concern about mistakes and correctness.
- Discuss how the therapist could change his or her communication style so it's less likely to prime indecision and doubt. For example, less Socratic questioning, at least in the early phase of treatment, may be preferable.
- Design specific behavioral tasks that encourage quicker and more efficient decision making. In fact, within-session decision-making tasks could be devised so that the client can practice more efficient decision making in the presence of the therapist.

Moral Inflexibility and Religiosity

OCD can be characterized by distortions in moral reasoning as indicated by overly strict, rigid, and inflexible moral codes pertaining to specific obsessional concerns. For example, individuals with OCD exhibit reduced use of utilitarian (flexible) moral judgments to impersonal moral dilemmas compared to healthy, but not non-OCD-anxious, controls (Whitton, Henry, & Grisham, 2014). The TAF–Moral subscale is significantly elevated in OCD (i.e., Abramowitz & Deacon, 2006; A. D. Williams, Lau, & Grisham, 2013), as are threats to the moral selfhood domain (Doron, Sar-El, & Mikulincer, 2012). The hypermorality in OCD is highly selective, focused only on the client's primary obsessive–compulsive concern, but its effect on the therapeutic relationship can be devastating.

Collaboration and willingness to consider alternatives are *sine qua non* to CBT, and yet these are the very attributes that the morally inflexible find intolerable. When this is combined with religiosity, the client may exhibit strong resistance to the therapist's perspective. Therapy can degenerate into verbal arguments, with the client dismissing the therapist as lacking in moral integrity or attempting to undermine his or her religious faith. When this happens, the working alliance ruptures and premature treatment termination is likely.

Chapter 12 (see Table 12.1) presents specific treatment recommendations for religious obsessions. It is important to validate and respect the client's moral and religious code, and to maintain focus on the client's treatment goals. The therapist should continue to emphasize collaboration, working with the client to formulate alternative responses to his or her obsessive–compulsive concerns that would be consistent with his or her moral values and faith. The client may respond with accusations of therapist incompetence, like "You're not a Christian, so how can you understand my problem?"; "You're trying to turn me from my faith, so I can't trust you"; or "I believe that some thoughts are sinful and from the devil, even if you think this is foolish."

Even when feeling threatened and rejected by the client, the therapist needs to maintain composure and continue to focus on the client's stated treatment goals, always framing the problem in terms of OCD rather than of morality or theology. The therapist can encourage the morally preoccupied client to consider the moral code of respected friends or family. Is it possible to alter some aspects of the client's moral code and values that would converge with those he or she most admires? Whatever the specific strategy, the CBT therapist approaches moral issues with respect, gentleness, and compromise to persevere a healthy therapeutic relationship. It is important to remember that the morally harsh and rigid individual is still vulnerable and suffering from his or her obsessive preoccupation with right and wrong.

Low Confidence in Memory

Individuals with OCD have lower confidence or trust in their memory than those without OCD (e.g., Radomsky, Rachman, & Hammond, 2001; van den Hout & Kindt, 2003b; see Chapter 11 for further discussion). It is obvious that distrust in one's memory can have a negative impact on the therapeutic relationship. Obtaining relevant information that is not immediately apparent to the client is an important part of guided discovery (Padesky & Greenberger, 1995). However, individuals with low memory confidence may have difficulty recalling the details of past experiences. The problem is not memory accuracy but rather confidence in recalling prior experiences. This means that clients with OCD might (1) claim to have poor knowledge of past experiences, (2) fail to respond to questions that probe for more specific thoughts and interpretations, or (3) qualify all their answers. This can make the therapeutic process a slow and frustrating experience. Therapy sessions could come to feel like an interrogation exercise. Once this happens, the therapeutic relationship is disrupted, and the client might consider terminating because the therapy feels cold and pedantic.

To deal with this problem, the therapist should acknowledge the client's problem with low memory confidence, accept tentative and partial answers to questions, and seek further clarification later. The therapist should encourage the client to answer questions even when unsure, noting that these are the types of experiences that can be considered "acting against the OCD." As well, therapists should return to experiences in later sessions, asking clients if they remember anything more about the experience. This approach demonstrates to clients that any recall can be elaborated or corrected later, which in turn reduces their fear that their poor memory recall may have permanent negative effects on therapy.

Ego Dystonicity

Often the obsessions evident in OCD are inconsistent or in conflict with the person's core values, ideals, or moral tenets—a self-evaluative process known as *ego dystonicity* (Clark, 2004; Purdon, 2004a). For example, a highly moralistic, conscientious individual might have repugnant obsessions of harming others or committing disgusting and illegal sexual acts. As well, the obsessions might represent aspects of a feared self (Aardema et al., 2013). The implication for the therapeutic relationship is that clients may become anxious, defensive, and resistant to focusing on such issues in their therapy sessions.

Chapter 12 provides an extensive discussion of ego dystonicity and various intervention strategies for dealing with this feature of OCD. Once again, it is important that therapists acknowledge individuals' struggle with these uncharacteristic mental intrusions and discuss how to talk about such disturbing material in the therapy session. It may be that certain dysfunctional beliefs, such as "The more we talk about these disgusting thoughts, the more likely I'll act on the obsessions" (TAF–Likelihood), must be addressed in the therapy session. As well, it may be necessary to do cognitive work on the feared self; that is, the client's belief that having such repugnant thoughts has some meaning about his or her true self. In the end, the ego-dystonic nature of obsessions will have less negative impact on the therapeutic relationship if the therapist utilizes collaborative empiricism to take a measured, knowledgeable, and focused approach to the repulsive intrusive thoughts driving the individual's obsessional fears.

CONCLUSION

A healthy therapeutic relationship is critical in providing effective CBT for OCD. A strong working alliance, therapist empathy and positive regard, client collaboration, and shared goal setting are important processes for building a positive therapist–client relationship. Collaborative empiricism is the "trademark" of CBT. Collaboration between client and therapist as well as taking an empirical approach to changing maladaptive thoughts and behaviors do not occur automatically in the therapy process. Therapists must be intentional in creating collaborative empiricism in the therapy session. Achieving collaborative empiricism is more likely when the therapist uses Socratic questioning and guided discovery, and ensures client participation in goal setting, case formulation, session agenda setting, and homework assignments. However, the importance of the therapeutic relationship should not be overstated. The treatment process research indicates that the specific treatment ingredients of CBT are far more important to symptom change than common factors. Moreover, the treatment effects of the therapeutic alliance may be mediated by extent of client engagement in within- and between-session therapy tasks.

There are many threats to the therapeutic relationship that are specific to OCD. Ambivalence, reassurance seeking, rigidity and cognitive inflexibility, need for control, concealment, interpersonal deficiencies and emotional detachment, pathological doubt and indecision, moral inflexibility and high religiosity, and ego dystonicity are issues that can put a strain on the therapeutic relationship. In many respects, these correlates of the disorder can elicit negative therapist reactions, such as frustration, criticalness, and uncertainty that undermine the therapeutic relationship. When treating OCD, it is incumbent on the therapist to periodically audit the therapeutic relationship and to immediately address ruptures in the therapy process.

FORM 6.1. OCD Cost–Benefit Worksheet

Instructions: Making changes in your OCD requires a significant investment of your time and effort. Like any investment, it is important to consider the advantages and disadvantages of working on your OCD versus maintaining the status quo. The following worksheet asks that you reflect on the effects of change versus no change in various areas of life. Write down all the pros and cons of change versus no change in each of the life domains. If you need more space, use additional sheets of paper.

		Costs/Disadvantages	Benefits/Advantages
Maintain OCD	Family relations:		
	Work:		
	Intimate relationship:		
	Finances:		
	Social life:		
	Leisure/recreation:		
	Spirituality:		
	Health:		
	Community:		
Reduce OCD	Family relations:		
	Work:		
	Intimate relationship:		
	Finances:		
	Social life:		
	Leisure/recreation:		
	Spirituality:		
	Health:		
	Community:		

From *Cognitive-Behavioral Therapy for OCD and Its Subtypes, Second Edition*, by David A. Clark. Copyright © 2020 The Guilford Press. Permission to photocopy this material is granted to purchasers of this book for personal use or use with individual clients (see copyright page for details). Purchasers can download enlarged versions of this material (see the box at the end of the table of contents).

CHAPTER 7

Assessment and Case Formulation

Clinical assessment and case formulation have been the bedrock of cognitive behavior therapy since its inception. Beck and colleagues (1979, p. 104) asserted that cognitive therapy begins with "developing a common conceptualization," which in subsequent years was refined and elaborated in further iterations of CBT (e.g., J. S. Beck, 2011; Clark & Beck, 2010; Greenberger & Padesky, 2016; Persons, 2008). Moreover, cognitive–clinical assessment has been the special topic of numerous research papers and published volumes (see Clark & Brown, 2015, for review). Thus, most CBT treatment manuals for obsessions and compulsions emphasize assessment and case formulation as critical treatment components (e.g., Clark, 2004, 2018; Rachman et al., 2015; Rego, 2016; Wilhelm & Steketee, 2006), although more behavioral treatment places less emphasis on case conceptualization (e.g., Abramowitz, 2018).

This chapter takes a distinctively cognitive approach toward assessment and case conceptualization. Assessment instruments, procedures, and protocols are presented that emphasize measurement of frequency, intensity, and salience of the cognitive and behavioral constructs that comprise the generic CBT model of OCD (see Figure 5.1). It is assumed that delivery of effective treatment depends on determining how unwanted mental intrusions, misinterpretations of significance, mental control efforts, neutralization efforts, and stop criteria are uniquely responsible for the persistence of obsessions and compulsions in each individual. The chapter begins by considering special challenges that face clinicians when assessing individuals with OCD. Next, normative measures of OCD symptoms and disorder-specific cognitive processes are reviewed, with special attention to their psychometric properties and clinical utility. As well, idiographic forms of self-monitoring and ratings are presented for use in treatment management and evaluation. The chapter concludes with a presentation of a generic cognitive case formulation for OCD and a discussion of the issues related to its implementation.

SPECIAL ASSESSMENT PROBLEMS IN OCD

Obsessional features such as intolerance of uncertainty, exactness, concern about making mistakes, pathological doubt, and indecision can undermine the assessment process. For example, individuals with obsessional checking may show such extreme doubt and concern about making mistakes that responding to a questionnaire with numerous items and multiple response options becomes a daunting prospect. Filling out a questionnaire or even answering questions in a clinical interview will likely provoke heightened anxiety. Under these circumstances, the client experiences the very pathology that defines the disorder (i.e., repeated checking), resorts to excessive reassurance seeking, or refuses to complete the assessment (i.e., escape and avoidance).

Summerfeldt (2001) discusses several issues that arise in the assessment of obsessive–compulsive symptoms. Taylor, Thordarson, and Söchting (2002) also highlight various difficulties in the assessment of OCD, such as the client's reluctance to talk about obsessive–compulsive symptoms, the presence of contamination fears, a minimization of symptoms, and slowness. In addition, the clinician may have difficulty distinguishing obsessions and compulsions from related clinical phenomena. Table 7.1 provides a summary of (1) pertinent issues in the assessment of OCD, which are categorized as problems intrinsic to the clinical disorder, and (2) difficulties arising from the response style or test-taking behavior of individuals with OCD.

Disorder-Related Problems

Shared Symptoms

At times obsessions are difficult to distinguish from other negative forms of cognition like rumination, worry, traumatic intrusions, pathological jealousy, or sexual fantasy (Taylor, Thordarson, et al., 2002). Chapter 2 provides an extended discussion of the distinct features of clinical obsessions that can be used to distinguish obsessions from other forms of repetitive thought (see Tables 2.2–2.4). Compulsive rituals and other types of neutralization can be difficult to distinguish from certain pathological behaviors like tics, impulse-control disorders, sexual compulsions, or intentional

TABLE 7.1. Potential Difficulties Encountered in OCD Assessment

Disorder-related problems

- Overlapping or common symptom features
- Heterogeneity of symptom content and expression
- Concealment of symptoms
- High comorbidity rate
- Symptom instability and shift
- Symptom multiplicity

Response style problems

- High anxiety during assessment
- Heightened concern about exactness, correctness, and intolerance of uncertainty
- Pathological doubt and indecision
- Slow response rate
- Compulsive rituals (i.e., repeating, checking, redoing)
- Lack of insight; high fixity of belief
- Activation of faulty appraisals and beliefs
- Noncompliance and avoidance

---

mental control (Summerfeldt, 2001). The distinctive features of clinical compulsions, discussed in Chapter 3, can be consulted when conducting an assessment.

Symptom Heterogeneity

Since any unwanted intrusive thought can become obsessional, thought content can be diverse with individuals reporting obsessions and neutralization responses that are unique to their life experiences and circumstances. A flexible and comprehensive assessment approach is needed to cover the varied symptom presentation in OCD. As discussed later, cognitive-behavioral therapists treating OCD rely heavily on idiographic measures that can be easily modified to capture the unique symptom features of each client.

Concealment

Often individuals with OCD minimize their symptoms to conceal highly upsetting, embarrassing, or immoral obsessions or compulsions (Newth & Rachman, 2001). When clients are reluctant to talk about their obsessions during assessment, therapists should not insist on full disclosure but instead proceed with other aspects of the assessment. Chapters 6 and 12 discuss the importance of building a collaborative therapeutic relationship, which includes waiting until the client is ready to provide full disclosure.

A tentative clinical assessment and case formulation can be developed in the early phase of treatment without full disclosure of obsessional content.

High Comorbidity

The co-occurrence of other disorders such as depression, social phobia, and GAD will increase the multiplicity of symptoms and make it more difficult to determine the disorder specificity of clinical phenomena. Including a structured diagnostic interview in the assessment is useful in clarifying the temporal and functional relations between OCD and other past and current psychopathology. It can also help with treatment planning when it may be difficult to know whether to start with treatment of OCD or a coexisting condition like major depression.

Temporal Instability

Obsessive–compulsive symptoms often shift over time, as few individuals maintain the same constellation of symptoms throughout the course of the condition (Skoog & Skoog, 1999). It is also common for obsessional content to change, so that individuals will report a new obsession after weeks or months of preoccupation with a previous theme. It is important to obtain a rough chronology of client's past obsessions and compulsions as well as their principal current obsessive–compulsive concerns, and to determine whether any life experiences may have contributed to the shift in their symptom presentation. For example, a client may have started with a physical contamination fear and washing compulsion, but later transitioned to harm obsessions and checking rituals. During assessment, the clinician might ask, "It's interesting that you conquered your fear of contamination; do you know what happened or how you overcame this fear?"; "Did something happen, or did you change how you thought about or responded to the possibility of harm and injury that led to your current obsession?" Notice that this line of questioning could be helpful in developing the case formulation and supporting the CBT treatment rationale.

Multiplicity

Although some individuals with OCD report a single obsession, many others experience multiple obsessions. This can make it difficult to know which symptoms to target in treatment. In the extreme case, some individuals with severe OCD will claim that practically all their thoughts are obsessive and so they experience no reprieve from their mental agony. In such cases, the clinician should look for dominant themes in the thought content, and then collaborate with the client on choosing one of these obsessional concerns.

Response Style Problems

High Assessment Anxiety

Individuals with OCD can become more anxious about completing questionnaire items or providing answers to structured interview questions than individuals with depression or anxiety disorders. This is because the assessment elicits the very pathology for which they seek treatment. Measurement items may trigger unwanted obsessions and repetitive neutralization responses. Clinicians should warn clients that they might find the assessment process anxiety-provoking and suggest strategies for handling the anxiety. Some cognitive restructuring may be needed to deal with maladaptive beliefs about the assessment. For example, an obsessive client might be thinking, "I can't possibly answer all these questions; it's too much for me"; or "I don't really know what I think or feel"; or "I need to be completely honest with my answers." Notice that in each of these situations, the clinician is introducing a challenging therapy task at the very first session. For individuals with doubt and indecision, exposure-based treatment begins before the assessment is completed.

Elevated Exactness and Correctness

Perfectionism and fear of making mistakes are common in OCD. Individuals with these concerns strive to provide the perfectly correct answer to each question. Because most assessment items are highly subjective, relying on personal opinion and judgment, this subjectivity increases the ambiguity and vagueness for the person with OCD who is earnestly trying to give the best possible answer. To deal with this problem, the clinician could explain that a person doesn't need to provide "absolutely correct answers" and that the questionnaires were designed to take into account measurement error. If the client's answers were perfectly accurate, the test responses would be difficult to interpret because they would differ from the response style adopted by most people.

Pathological Doubt and Indecision

For highly perfectionistic clients, the assessment process can be associated with continual doubt over the accuracy and honesty of their responses. Often individuals with OCD find dichotomous response options (e.g., true/false) especially difficult because they may interpret the item in terms of being "absolutely true" or "absolutely false." To the obsessive-prone person, this type of item might feel like it demands a higher level of certainty that makes decision making more difficult. Alternatively, some individuals will write copious qualifications or explanations for their answers in the margins of the questionnaire. Clinicians can help clients with their doubt by emphasizing that they, the clinicians, expect clients' responses to change over time and so will give clients the opportunity to complete the measures several times over the course of treatment. Clinicians could inform individuals who write in the margins that questionnaire scoring instructions require that written explanations of answers must be ignored. However, clinicians could review the written explanations in a subsequent therapy session.

Extreme Slowness

Individuals with OCD may take an inordinate amount of time to complete questionnaires or answer interview questions. Patience and extra time should be given to complete assessment measures. The clinician may need to address the client's slow response time and identify its determinants. Slowness could be due to checking rituals or severe perfectionism. In rare cases, the client may be suffering from primary obsessional slowness, which is a particularly difficult type of OCD to treat (Clark, Sugrim, & Bolton, 1982; Rachman, 1974). In these cases, treatment may have to proceed with some leniency toward normative testing guidelines.

Ritualizing

Assessment may trigger compulsive rituals that involve checking and rechecking answers, repeating statements just made in an interview, or other forms of redoing. When this happens, the therapist may need to instruct the client to select questionnaire items that can be done on their own with minimal ritualizing, and then deal with the skipped items that provoke more urge to neutralize in the therapy session. Clearly, it is counterproductive if the assessment elicits so much compulsive activity that it pushes the client toward terminating therapy before it even begins.

Lack of Insight

Individuals who lack insight into their obsessions or have high fixity of belief in their obsessional fears may believe that their concerns about the assessment process are reasonable. For instance, some clients may believe that participating in the assessment is making their OCD worse, or they may be afraid of not answering the questions correctly and so will provide misleading information to the therapist. In some cases, individuals are fearful that they are being dishonest, or they become confused and uncertain when asked about subjective states. As before, the clinician may need to deal with these matters directly before continuing with the assessment.

Faulty Appraisals and Beliefs

Faulty appraisals and beliefs may be underlying factors in the obsessive person's struggle with the assessment. For example, some individuals have expressed concern that giving a wrong answer could undermine treatment effectiveness. Several faulty appraisals are evident in this type of thinking, including an overestimation of threat ("Treatment will fail because of my incorrect answers"), inflated personal responsibility ("It is my responsibility to make sure my therapy is successful, and it starts by providing the most accurate answers possible"), and personal significance ("I've failed again if I can't provide the most accurate information to my therapist"). If these cognitive determinants are evident but not too disabling, the therapist should make note of them and proceed with the assessment. However, if the client is struggling, cognitive restructuring may need to be applied to the interfering beliefs before continuing the assessment.

Noncompliance and Avoidance

Most individuals with OCD can participate in an assessment process and manage their obsessional tendencies, although sometimes with considerable effort. In severe OCD, though, the doubt, indecision, and compulsive checking may be so incapacitating that the client gives up and refuses to continue with the assessment. In their meta-analysis of 37 randomized controlled trials (RCTs) of CBT for OCD, a median of 11% failed to show up for the first treatment session (Öst et al., 2015). OCD researchers have noted that refusal and attrition rates for CBT of OCD are unacceptably high (Shafran et al., 2013). Although reasons for refusal have not been sufficiently researched, it is likely that some of these treatment refusals begin at the assessment phase when clients are confronted with an array of self-report measures.

Therapeutic Strategies for Assessment of Noncompliance

The CBT therapist may need to modify the assessment protocol to address the special needs of individuals with OCD. Table 7.2 lists several therapeutic strategies that may be needed during assessment (see also Clark & Beck, 2002; Taylor, Thordarson, et al., 2002).

Validation

It is important that the therapist acknowledge the respondent's anxiety with the assessment process. (See Leahy, 2001, for extensive discussion of validation in response to resistance in cognitive therapy.) The clini-

TABLE 7.2. **Strategies to Improve Assessment Compliance**

1. Acknowledge and validate the respondent's anxiety about assessment.
2. Provide an explanation for assessment.
3. Explain the therapeutic value of assessment.
4. Provide limited reassurance and vicarious responsibility to improve compliance rates.
5. Offer a concise, focused assessment protocol.
6. Allow additional time for assessment.
7. Identify faulty appraisals and beliefs triggered by the assessment.
8. Present assessment as a dynamic, continuous, and collaborative process that extends over the course of treatment.

cian should adopt an empathic, supportive, and collaborative style, like the orientation used during treatment. It should be explained that many people with OCD find answering questions and completing questionnaire items anxiety-provoking, because the assessment format often activates obsessive–compulsive symptoms such as doubts, indecision, and fear of making mistakes. Support and encouragement should be provided to the client who finds the assessment stressful. The therapist should collaborate with the client on ways to reduce distress without jeopardizing the validity of the assessment process. For example, the therapist can review each questionnaire before it is assigned to ensure that clients understand how to interpret questionnaire items. Creating a positive therapeutic relationship begins with the therapist showing empathy and understanding of the distress experienced by clients struggling with the demands of an assessment.

Psychoeducation

When introducing the assessment phase, information should be provided that includes a description of the various assessment instruments and their purpose. It should be explained that questionnaires, interviews, and rating scales provide the therapist with (1) a better understanding of the client's experience with OCD, (2) guidance in formulating a treatment plan, and (3) a means to evaluate treatment effectiveness. In addition, therapists can explain the therapeutic benefits of the assessment in terms of providing structured tasks that involve decision making and response generation. For individuals with compulsive checking, pathological doubt, and indecisiveness, questionnaires and rating scales are exposure exercises that require confronting their obsessional fears and preventing a neutralization response (i.e., rechecking answers). For these individuals, participation in the assessment may have some early therapeutic benefits. The provision of a full rationale for assessment is intended to reduce anxiety and improve motivation to comply with the assessment process.

Vicarious Reassurance and Responsibility

At times, the person with OCD may become so anxious that a more drastic intervention is required. Although it is normally not advisable to offer reassurance, the therapist could provide the following instruction:

> "The assessment instruments I'm giving you were designed to be completed in a specific manner. People are asked to provide the first answer that pops into their mind without thinking too hard about the question or changing their answer. I want you to go with the first answer that pops into your mind. That's the one we're looking for. If you start to analyze the question, think hard about the answer or change your answers, then you are less likely to provide the best answer. Do you think you could do this?"

If the client has doubts that he or she could respond quickly and without undue reflection, the therapist needs to spend time dealing with the client's reluctance. It may be necessary to coach the person in item endorsement by helping the client respond to a few items in the therapy session.

The therapist may need to assume some degree of responsibility for client responses in order to obtain complete assessment data. Rachman (2003) noted that individuals with OCD will sometimes agree to a temporary *transfer of responsibility* to the therapist for a specific, well-defined purpose. In the manual for the Clark–Beck Obsessive–Compulsive Inventory (CBOCI; Clark & Beck, 2002, p. 12), we suggested the following intervention to encourage questionnaire completion.

> "I understand you are finding it difficult to answer these questionnaire items. [validation statement] Why don't you complete the questionnaire on your own, based on your first impression? [instructions to counter obsessive–compulsive symptoms] I will then look over your questionnaire responses and if I think that any of your answers seem different or inaccurate given what you have already told me about your OCD, I will discuss them with you and we can make the appropriate changes. [transfer of responsibility] In this way it will be my responsibility to make sure you completed the questionnaire correctly."

Naturally, this form of vicarious responsibility is only temporary and should be withdrawn as soon as the assessment process is completed.

Focused Assessment

Because of the difficulty individuals with OCD may experience with assessment, the entire process should be kept as brief as possible. Select measures that directly target the individual's core symptomatology and critical disorder-specific cognitive and behavioral processes. The choice of assessment measures should be guided by the CBT model and the information needed to develop a case conceptualization. The instruments recommended in the following sections were selected with these criteria in mind.

Extended Time

Most individuals with OCD take longer to complete assessment measures. Therefore, the therapist must be flexible and allow extra time. Although most therapists prefer to complete an assessment within the first two or three sessions before starting treatment, this sharp demarcation between assessment and treatment may not be possible in cases involving OCD. Instead, the therapist may need to integrate assessment and therapy sessions, possibly extending self-monitoring exercises well into the initial treatment sessions.

Faulty Appraisals and Beliefs

When obsessive–compulsive appraisals and beliefs are activated by the assessment process, it may be possible to simply note which faulty appraisals and beliefs are prominent and refer back to these experiences during treatment. However, when this cognitive disturbance impedes the client's ability to participate in the assessment, it will be necessary to introduce cognitive restructuring strategies to deal with the faulty beliefs before continuing with assessment.

Let's assume that a client is extremely slow working on an obsessive–compulsive questionnaire. The therapist discovers that the person is thinking, "There are so many questionnaire items that it's going to take forever to finish this; the anxiety is going to build until it becomes intolerable"; "This whole process is making me worse, not better." The therapist could take the following cognitive restructuring approach to this belief and ask, "Were there other times when this happened to you?"; "Were there any times when you completed a form and the anxiety was less than you expected?"; "Are there things that increase or decrease the anxiety?"; "I wonder if we could try a few different approaches and see if your anxiety could be reduced to a tolerable level." The therapist could then assign a behavioral task to test the client's level of anxiety. The individual could be asked to complete just 10 questions at a time and hand these to the therapist. Then a second set of 10 items could be completed, and so on until full completion of the instrument. Not only would this strategy result in the eventual collection of complete questionnaire data, but it would be a direct behavioral test of the faulty belief that "I can't stand the anxiety associated with this questionnaire; it's only making me worse."

Assessment as Continuous

Many individuals with OCD are concerned that they will provide information that will lead the therapist astray, so they end up a treatment failure. In this case the therapist can explain that assessment is an ongoing process that continues as long as the person is in therapy. Consequently, new information is being discovered in each session, which requires that the case formulation and treatment strategy be refined, elaborated, and corrected. Thus, there is nothing the client can provide in the assessment that cannot be qualified or changed later in therapy. It is important that therapists correct clients' erroneous beliefs that their answers are static, immutable, and irreconcilable facts about their experiences. The goal is to help individuals with OCD view assessment as a flexible, dynamic, exploratory, and collaborative process of self-discovery.

DIAGNOSTIC AND SYMPTOM MEASURES

Assessment for OCD usually begins with a diagnostic evaluation and administration of normative symptom measures. In clinical practice most therapists use an unstructured clinical interview to determine whether an individual meets diagnostic criteria. However, semistructured diagnostic interviews significantly improve the reliability and validity of diagnostic assessment and so are recommended over unstructured approaches (Miller, 2002; Miller, Dasher, Collins, Griffiths, & Brown, 2001). The following section presents a select number of obsessive–compulsive symptom measures. More thorough reviews are published elsewhere (e.g., Antony, 2001; Feske & Chambless, 2000; Grabill et al., 2008; Taylor, 1995). Although not discussed below, clinicians treating OCD should also administer normative measures of depressive, anxious, and worry symptoms because of their prominence in OCD.

Diagnostic Interviews

The best-known standardized diagnostic interviews for OCD are the Structured Clinical Interview for DSM-IV (SCID-IV; First, Spitzer, Gibbon, & Williams, 1996) and the Anxiety Disorders Interview Schedule for DSM-IV (ADIS-IV; Brown, Di Nardo, & Barlow, 1994; Brown et al., 2001). Both measures have updated versions that correspond to DSM-5 diagnostic criteria (Brown & Barlow, 2014; First, Williams, Karg, & Spitzer, 2016).

Based on earlier versions, the SCID has interrater reliability for OCD that ranges from low (.59) to very high (1.00) kappa values (Steketee, Frost, & Bogart, 1996; Williams et al., 1992). The ADIS, on the other hand, was developed specifically for anxiety disorders and so provides more information on obsessive–compulsive symptom severity, lack of insight, resistance, and avoidance. The ADIS-IV Lifetime version has high interrater agreement for OCD (kappa = .85) as the principal diagnosis (Brown et al., 2001). Although both interview schedules require training and are time-consuming, they provide valuable diagnostic and symptom information. The ADIS-IV might be slightly more reliable than the SCID-IV for diagnosing OCD (Feske & Chambless, 2000; Taylor, 1998). Given the high comorbidity rate in OCD and its influence on treatment response, a structured interview can be indispensable when developing the case formulation and treatment plan. The SCID-5-CV and the ADIS-5 can be purchased from American Psychiatric Association Publishing and Oxford University Press, respectively.

Yale–Brown Obsessive–Compulsive Scale

The original YBOCS is a 10-item clinician-rated scale that assesses the severity of obsessions and compulsions independent of the type (content) or number of symptoms (Goodman, Price, Rasmussen, Mazure, Delgado, et al., 1989; Goodman, Price, Rasmussen, Mazure, Fleischmann, et al., 1989). It is considered the "gold standard" for assessment of obsessive–compulsive symptom severity in treatment outcome studies. The YBOCS consists of three sections. First, the interviewer provides the respondent with a definition and examples of obsessions and compulsions. Second, the client completes a checklist consisting of 64 obsessions and compulsions to provide an overview of past and current obsessive–compulsive symptom content.

The final section consists of 10 core items, a six-item investigational component and 3 global ratings. The 10 core and six investigational items are each rated on a 5-point scale ranging from 0 (none) to 4 (extreme or severe). A descriptive statement is associated with each of the response options. Only the 10 core items are included in the total and subscale scores. Obsessions (items 1–5) and Compulsions (items 6–10) subscales assess five symptom features: (1) duration/frequency, (2) interference in social or work functioning, (3) associated distress, (4) degree of resistance, and (5) perceived uncontrollability of the obsession or compulsion. Two additional items, (1b) and (6b), inquire about the longest time in a typical day that the client is free of the obsessions or compulsions, but these are not included in the total score. The six investigational items assess lack of insight, avoidance, indecisiveness, inflated responsibility, slowness, and pathological doubt.

Interrater agreement on the 10 YBOCS items is excellent, ranging from .76 to .97 across three studies (Goodman, Price, Rasmussen, Mazure, Fleischmann, et al., 1989; Nakagawa, Marks, Takei, De Araujo, & Ito, 1996; Woody, Steketee, & Chambless, 1995). Internal consistency for the two subscales and total score was acceptable in some studies (Amir, Foa, & Coles, 1997; Goodman, Price, Rasmussen, Mazure, Fleischmann, et al., 1989; Richter, Cox, & Direnfeld, 1994), but not in others (Steketee et al., 1996; Woody et al., 1995). Temporal stability is excellent over a 1- or 2-week interval (see Taylor, 1995), although a two-factor obsessions and compulsions solution has not always been found (see Grabill et al., 2008, for review). Convergent validity with other obsessive–compulsive self-report symptom and cognition measures has been inconsistent, and its discriminant validity is weak, given moderate correlations with depression and anxiety measures (e.g., Goodman, Price, Rasmussen, Mazure, Delgado, et al., 1989; OCCWG, 2001, 2003; Woody et al., 1995). The YBOCS is highly sensitive to treatment effects and can distinguish individuals with OCD from other diagnostic and nonclinical groups (Frost, Steketee, Krause, & Trepanier, 1995).

An early attempt to convert the clinician-administered YBOCS into a computer-administered self-report version was reported by Rosenfeld, Dar, Anderson, Kobak, and Greist (1992). Subsequent studies indicate that the self-report YBOCS is highly correlated with the original interview version (Baer, Brown-Beasley, Sorce, & Henriques, 1993; Nakagawa et al., 1996; Steketee et al., 1996). Given their equivalence, most therapists will use the self-report YBOCS (see Antony, 2001, for a copy).

More recently, a second edition of the YBOCS (Y-BOCS-II) was published to address some of the psychometric shortcomings of the original version. Several changes were made that included (1) replacing "resistance to obsession" with an item that refers to "obsession-free interval," (2) increasing item response options to a 0–5 scale, (3) adding probes to elicit "distress if compulsions prevented" and "interference from compulsions" to emphasize active avoidance, and (4) modifying the content and format of the symptom checklist (Storch et al., 2010). The interview version of the Y-BOCS-II demonstrated good reliability, adequate construct validity, and strong correlations with the original YBOCS, although it had weak correlations with the Obsessive–Compulsive Inventory—Revised (OCI-R) and had modest associations with depression and worry measures (Storch et al., 2010). A subsequent OCD study reported high interrater reliability for the Y-BOCS-II total score and subscales and excellent correlations with clinician ratings of OCD severity, although again a modest correlation with self-report depressive symptoms was found (Wu, McGuire, Hong, & Storch, 2016). An Italian translation of the Y-BOCS-II found a different two-factor solution to the original but the measure exhibited significant correlations with obsessive–compulsive self-report measures, although it correlated almost as highly with the Beck Depression Inventory–II (BDI-II; $r = .40$) as with the OCI-R ($r = .45$) (Melli, Avallone, et al., 2015).

The self-report YBOCS is an essential instrument to include in an assessment of OCD because it gives the clinician a measure of symptom severity independent of content, it is sensitive to treatment effects, and it has such widespread use that considerable normative data are now available. Some shortcomings were found that led to the development of the Y-BOCS-II. This second edition holds promise, but its diagnostic specificity is unknown, its treatment sensitivity not yet documented, and its discriminant validity limited in relation to depression.

Obsessive–Compulsive Inventory

The Obsessive–Compulsive Inventory (OCI) is a 42-item self-report questionnaire designed to (1) assess a broad range of obsessive–compulsive symptom content, (2) provide greater symptom severity range, and (3) have widespread applicability to clinical and nonclinical individuals (Foa, Kozak, Salkovskis, Coles, & Amir, 1998). Each item is rated on a 5-point Likert scale for frequency and distress. This yields frequency and distress total scores, as well as separate frequency and distress scores for seven rationally determined subscales: (1) Washing (eight items), (2) Checking (nine items), (3) Doubting (three items), (4) Ordering (five items), (5) Obsessing (eight items), (6) Hoarding (three items), and (7) Mental neutralizing (six items).

In the initial psychometric study (Foa, Kozak, et al., 1998), internal consistency of the frequency and distress total scores and most of the seven subscales (with the exception of mental neutralizing) were within an acceptable range (greater than .70). Two-week test–retest ranged from .68 to .97. Although the OCD group had similar frequency and distress scores, the remaining groups scored significantly higher on the Frequency scale than on the Distress scale. The OCD group scored significantly higher than those with other anxiety disorders and nonclinical controls on all OCI scales except Hoarding, and the scales had strong correlations with the Maudsley Obsessive Compulsive Inventory (MOCI) and Compulsive Activity Checklist (CAC) total scores, but correlations with the interview YBOCS were low.

An 18-item short form of the OCI (OCI-R) was developed that correlated .98 with the 42-item questionnaire (Foa, Huppert, et al., 2002). Analysis revealed six factors (i.e., Washing, Checking, Ordering, Obsessing, Hoarding, and Neutralizing), and subscales based on this factor structure showed acceptable internal consistency and good test–retest reliability. Although the OCI-R correlated moderately with the YBOCS ($r = .53$) and very highly with the MOCI ($r = .85$), it also had substantial correlations with depression measures (BDI, $r = .70$). Individuals with OCD scored significantly higher than those with generalized social phobia and PTSD on all subscales except Hoarding.

Subsequent studies have generally supported the convergent and, to a lesser extent, discriminant validity of the OCI-R (for reviews, see Grabill et al., 2008; Overduin & Furnham, 2012). The OCI-R subscales, excluding Hoarding, are sensitive to the primary obsessive–compulsive symptoms indicated on the YBOCS (Huppert et al., 2007). Findings from receiver operating curve (ROC) analyses indicate that an OCR Total Score cutoff of 12 correctly distinguished 83% of an OCD sample from nonclinical controls (Wootton et al., 2015), whereas ROC analysis by Abramowitz and Deacon (2006) indicated a cut score of 14 best differentiated OCD from other anxiety disorders. ROC analysis on a Spanish translation of the OCI-R suggested that a Total Score of 21 best classified OCD from non-OCD-anxious and nonclinical groups (Belloch et al., 2013), a finding that is consistent with the cut score reported in the original psychometric study (Foa, Huppert, et al., 2002). As well, the OCI-R Obsessions subscale has good diagnostic specificity, with 5 the optimal cut score (Foa, Huppert, et al., 2002; see also Overduin & Furnham, 2012). OCD samples consistently score significantly higher than non-OCD-anxious and nonclinical groups on the Total Score, and the Washing, Checking, Obsessing, and Neutralizing subscales (Abramowitz & Deacon, 2006; Belloch et al., 2013; Foa et al., 2002; Sica et al., 2009). The criterion-related validity for the Ordering and Hoarding subscales has been less consistent but the measure is sensitive to treatment effects (Belloch et al., 2013).

The OCI-R is a psychometrically sound obsessive–compulsive symptom questionnaire with demonstrated reliability and validity for use in screening, diagnosis, and treatment evaluation. It has been validated in many different languages and cultures and has become an established self-report measure in the OCD clinical research literature. CBT clinicians should consider including the OCI-R in their assessment armamentarium for OCD. However, several limitations of the questionnaire must be recognized, including (1) heavy weighting toward compulsions with only three items assessing obsessions, (2) moderate correlations with depression and worry, (3) omission of a separate severity scale, (4) moderate to weak correlations with the YBOCS, and (5) low correlations with obsessive–compulsive cognition measures. The original OCI can be found in Antony (2001), and the OCI-R in Foa, Huppert, and colleagues (2002).

Clark–Beck Obsessive–Compulsive Inventory

The 25-item CBOCI (Clark, Antony, Beck, Swinson, & Steer, 2005; Clark & Beck, 2002) is a self-report measure of obsessive–compulsive symptoms with an item structure and response format identical to the BDI-II (Beck, Steer, & Brown, 1996). Four response option statements are associated with each item and scored on a 0–3 scale. Fourteen items assess core diagnostic, symptom content and cognitive features of obsessions, and 11 items assess similar features relevant to compulsions. CBOCI total score, as well as obsessions and compulsions subscales, are derived by summing across respective items.

The original CBOCI psychometric study reported high internal consistency for the total score and two subscales, and a 3-month temporal reliability measure was adequate (Clark et al., 2005). The OCD sample scored significantly higher on all CBOCI scales than the non-OCD-anxious, depressed, or nonclinical control groups, and the CBOCI total score had a strong association with the self-report YBOCS ($r = .78$) and the Padua Inventory ($r = .77$). However, the questionnaire was also highly correlated with worry, anxiety, and depression symptom measures, although partial correlations revealed that the CBOCI was more closely related to obsessionality than worry. CBOCI obsessions and compulsions have moderate correlations with obsessive–compulsive beliefs and scrupulosity in nonclinical samples (Inozu, Clark, & Karanci, 2012; Inozu, Karanci, & Clark, 2012), and highly religious individuals score significantly higher on the CBOCI subscales than a low religious group (Hale & Clark, 2013).

A Schmid–Leiman analysis revealed a high-order General Distress factor (68% of variance) and two lower-order factors of Obsessions (17%) and Compulsions (15%). This indicates that the CBOCI assesses specific symptom features of OCD (Clark et al., 2005). In an unpublished report, ROC analysis indicated that a CBOCI total cutoff score of 22 yielded high sensitivity (90%) and specificity (78%) for distinguishing individuals with OCD from a student comparison group (Clark, Antony, Beck, Swinson, & Steer, 2003).

The CBOCI provides a fairly even assessment of obsessions and compulsions. It assesses key cognitive features such as responsibility, uncontrollability, mental neutralizing, and perfectionism as part of a brief symptom screener. However, the questionnaire is not often used in the research literature because it is a copyrighted, published instrument. Therefore, it is missing critical psychometric information such as an analysis of its diagnostic specificity and treatment sensitivity. Although highly correlated with depression and worry measures, this might be due to a greater emphasis on obsessions, which respondents can find difficult to distinguish from other types of repetitive negative thought. The CBOCI is available from Pearson Clinical Assessment (*www.pearsonclinical.com/psychology/products/100000201/clark-beck-obsessive-compulsive-inventory-cboci.html*). The instrument has been translated into Spanish and Turkish languages.

Vancouver Obsessional Compulsive Inventory

Development of the Vancouver Obsessional Compulsive Inventory (VOCI) began in 1994 as a radical revision of the MOCI (Hodgson & Rachman,

1977). Initial item construction resulted in a final 55-item questionnaire that assesses six obsessive–compulsive symptom constructs on a 5-point Likert scale (i.e., contamination, checking, obsessions, hoarding, just right, and indecisiveness) (Thordarson et al., 2004). The final validation study indicated that the VOCI had (1) a stable factor structure, (2) good temporal reliability for the OCD sample but not the nonclinical group, (3) high internal consistency for all scales, (4) strong convergent validity with other OCD measures except the YBOCS, and (5) mixed discriminant validity because of a moderate correlation with self-report anxiety, depression, and worry. The OCD sample scored significantly higher than the non-OCD-anxious group on the VOCI total score, and the Contamination, Checking, Just Right and Indecisiveness subscales, but not Obsessions and Hoarding (Thordarson et al., 2004). Similar psychometric properties were reported for a French translation of the VOCI tested on an undergraduate sample (Radomsky, Ouimet, et al., 2006).

Gönner, Ecker, Leonhart, and Limbacher (2010) proposed a 30-item revision to the VOCI that included 24 items from the VOCI and six items from the Symmetry, Ordering and Arranging Questionnaire (SOAQ; Radomsky & Rachman, 2004). Labeled the VOCI-R, the questionnaire consisted of five symptom constructs: contamination/washing, hoarding, checking, harming obsessions, immoral obsessions, and order/symmetry. Gönner and colleagues argued that the VOCI Just Right and Indecisiveness subscales should be removed because they are not core symptom presentations in OCD, and five items from the Obsessions subscale were excluded because they do not refer to harm or immoral content. Confirmatory factor analysis supported the factorial validity of the VOCI-R, and it showed good convergent and discriminant validity. However, the VOCI-R is not ready for clinical use because critical psychometric information is missing, such as its temporal stability, criterion-related validity, ROC characteristics, and treatment sensitivity.

Summary

A clinical assessment of OCD should include (1) a diagnostic interview; (2) brief screening measures of obsessive–compulsive, depressive, anxious, and worry symptoms; and (3) a more detailed self-report measure of OCD, such as the VOCI. The OCI-R, YBOCS self-report, or CBOCI are brief, time-efficient screening questionnaires that provide a snapshot of obsessive–compulsive symptom severity. There are, however, a number of other OCD measures not discussed that clinicians might find helpful: the Dimensional Obsessive–Compulsive Scale (DOCS; Abramowitz et al., 2010), the Padua Inventory—Washington State University Revision (PI-WSUR; Burns, Keortge, Formea, & Sternberger, 1996), Compulsive Activity Checklist (Freund, Steketee & Foa, 1987), and the Florida Obsessive–

Compulsive Inventory (FOCI; Storch et al., 2007). In addition, clinicians may want to include specific symptom measures relevant to certain OCD subtypes. Chapters 10–13 discuss some of these more focused obsessive–compulsive symptom measures.

COGNITIVE ASSESSMENT OF OCD

After completing the diagnostic and symptom assessment, the CBT clinician will want to evaluate obsessive–compulsive-relevant cognitive processes. This information is critical to the cognitive case formulation. Two types of measurement are available for cognitive assessment: normative and idiographic.

Normative Measures of Beliefs and Appraisals

Several self-report measures were developed to assess the appraisal, belief, and neutralizing constructs of the generic CBT model. Although these measures are primarily research tools, they can be utilized in the clinical setting as adjunct measures to help identify key cognitive processes for treatment. The following subsections provide brief descriptions of select cognitive measures.

Obsessive Beliefs Questionnaire

Based on the OCCWG (1997) cognitive conceptualization of OCD, an 87-item questionnaire, the Obsessive Beliefs Questionnaire (OBQ), was developed to assess six belief domains: overestimation of threat, tolerance of uncertainty, importance of thoughts, control of thoughts, responsibility, and perfectionism (Taylor, Kyrios, Thordarson, Steketee, & Frost, 2002). The initial validation study indicated that the OBQ subscales had high internal consistency, moderate test–retest reliability, and convergent validity (OCCWG, 2001, 2003). However, the OBQ subscales correlated as highly with self-reported anxiety, worry, and depression as with obsessive–compulsive symptoms, and the OCD group scored significantly higher than non-OCD-anxious participants only on control of thoughts, importance of thoughts, and responsibility.

A subsequent factor analysis of the OBQ indicated that a 44-item version possessed similar psychometric properties to the original measure (OCCWG, 2005). It consists of three subscales: Responsibility/Threat Estimation, Perfectionism/Certainty, and Importance/Control of Thoughts. Because of its shorter length, the OBQ-44 has been the instrument of choice in subsequent research, although only Importance/Control of Thoughts and, to a lesser extent, Perfectionism/Intolerance of Uncertainty may be specific to OCD (e.g., Fergus & Wu, 2010; Kim et al., 2016; OCCWG, 2005). However, the OBQ-44 subscales significantly correlate with anxiety, depression, and worry measures (e.g., Myers et al., 2008; Tolin et al., 2008) and show sensitivity to treatment effects—which calls into question their trait-like feature and specificity to obsessive–compulsive symptoms (Anholt et al., 2010). Through a series of factorial analyses based on nonclinical samples, Moulding and colleagues (2011) reduced the OBQ-44 to a 20-item questionnaire that assesses overestimation of threat, inflated personal responsibility, perfectionism/intolerance of uncertainty, and importance/need to control thoughts. Fergus and Carmin (2014) found that the OBQ-20 had good psychometric properties, although the Importance/Control of Thoughts subscale did not correlate more strongly with the DOCS total score, and both OBQ-20 Responsibility and Perfectionism had high correlations with self-reported depression and generalized anxiety.

The OBQ-44 is primarily a research instrument and so its clinical utility has not been determined. It could be used in the clinical setting as a preliminary indicator of obsessive–compulsive-relevant beliefs, provided the clinician realizes that these beliefs may not be specific to OCD, and that elevated scores may not be due to the presence of obsessive–compulsive symptoms. As well, the OBQ subscales are highly intercorrelated, so it's questionable whether they measure distinct constructs.

Thought–Action Fusion Scale

The 19-item Thought–Action Fusion (TAF) Scale was developed to assess Rachman's construct of *"psychological fusion,"* which is the tendency to appraise obsessional thoughts as increasing the likelihood of a feared outcome or being morally equivalent to a forbidden action (Rachman & Shafran, 1998). Developed by Shafran and colleagues (1996), the questionnaire assesses three aspects of TAF: moral (12 items), likelihood–others (four items), and likelihood–self (three items). Bifactor confirmatory factor analysis, however, indicates that the TAF items form a TAF–General Factor and a domain-specific TAF–Likelihood factor (Meyer & Brown, 2012).

Individuals with OCD tend to score higher on the TAF—Revised (TAF-R) Scale than do nonclinical groups, and it has good convergent validity with obsessive–compulsive symptom measures, although TAF–Likelihood has a closer relationship with obsessionality than TAF–Moral (Berle & Starcevic, 2005; Shafran & Rachman, 2004; for evidence of TAF–Moral specificity, see Bailey et al., 2014). However, findings are mixed on whether TAF is specific to OCD, and whether the construct fluctuates over time and situations (Amir, Freshman, Ramsey, Neary, & Brigidi, 2001; Coles, Mennin, & Heimberg, 2001; Rassin, Merckelbach, Muris, & Schmidt, 2001; Rassin, Muris, Schmidt, & Merckelbach, 2000; Shafran et al., 1996; Smári & Hólmsteinsson, 2001). If administered during the assessment phase, scores on the TAF-R Scale might indicate whether the TAF bias should be included in the cognitive case formulation (see Chapter 5 for further discussion).

Intolerance of Uncertainty Scale

The 27-item Intolerance of Uncertainty Scale (IUS) assesses emotional, cognitive, and behavioral reactions to ambiguous situations as an indicator of intolerance of uncertainty (Buhr & Dugas, 2002; Freeston, Rhéaume, et al., 1994). Although originally developed for GAD and worry, the IUS shows strong correlations with obsessive–compulsive symptom measures, and individuals with OCD have elevated scores on the IUS or on its shorter form, the IUS-12 (e.g., Fergus & Wu, 2010; Jacoby, Fabricant, Leonard, Riemann, & Abramowitz, 2013; Tolin et al., 2003). As well, the IUS is moderately correlated with obsessive–compulsive beliefs and has a strong correlation with the OBQ-44 Perfectionism/Uncertainty subscale ($r = .66$; Calleo et al., 2010). The IUS demonstrates particular relevance for individuals with pathological doubt and checking rituals (Jacoby et al., 2013; Tolin et al., 2003; see Gillett, Bilek, Hanna, & Fitzgerald, 2018). However, Gentes and Rusico (2011) found that the IUS was more specific to GAD than to OCD, whereas the OBQ-44 Perfectionism/Uncertainty subscale failed to distinguish between OCD and major depression. The shorter 12-item IUS, consisting of two factors labeled *Prospective Anxiety* and *Inhibitory Anxiety,* appears to have similar psychometric properties to the original questionnaire (Carleton, Norton, & Asmundson, 2007). Either the OBQ-44 Perfectionism/Uncertainty or the IUS (short or long form) are useful for determining whether intolerance of uncertainty might be a relevant cognitive process for the cognitive case formulation.

Responsibility Interpretations Questionnaire and Responsibility Attitude Scale

Salkovskis and colleagues (2000) developed two questionnaires to assess appraisals and beliefs of inflated responsibility. The Responsibility Interpretations Questionnaire (RIQ) is a 44-item retrospective self-report measure of the frequency and strength of beliefs associated with statements of interpretations and beliefs about responsibility for harm and the significance and control of unwanted intrusive thoughts. Respondents are instructed to write down "worrying intrusive thoughts which you know are probably senseless or unrealistic" (Salkovskis et al., 2000, p. 353). Individuals rate the RIQ items based on their recall of times when they were bothered by the intrusive thoughts over the last 2 weeks. Four subscale scores are derived: (1) Frequency of High Responsibility, (2) Frequency of Low Responsibility, (3) Percentage of Belief in High Responsibility, and (4) Percentage of Belief in Low Responsibility. The Responsibility Attitude Scale (RAS) consists of 26 statements that assess a general attitude or beliefs about assuming a responsibility toward life.

The original study reported that the RAS total score and the RIQ frequency and belief for high responsibility had acceptable 2-week test–retest reliability, high internal consistency, and a strong association with obsessive–compulsive symptom measures (Salkovskis et al., 2000). As well, individuals with OCD scored significantly higher than non-OCD-anxious and nonclinical controls (see also Cougle, Lee, & Salkovskis, 2007). The RIQ frequency and belief for low responsibility showed less temporal stability, so further analysis was not conducted. Researchers using a Japanese translation of the RAS and RIQ reported similar psychometric properties for clinical and nonclinical samples (Ishikawa, Kobori, Ikota, & Shimizu, 2014). The clinical utility of the measures has not been established, although the RAQ and RIQ could be administered when doubt and checking are present (Cougle et al., 2007; Foa, Sacks, et al., 2002). Moreover, Pozza and Dèttore (2014) concluded from their meta-analysis that responsibility is a transdiagnostic factor, so elevated scores on the measures may not be due to obsessionality.

Thought Control Questionnaire and Metacognitions Questionnaire

The 30-item Thought Control Questionnaire (TCQ) assesses individual differences in use of various thought control strategies when experiencing unwanted, unpleasant, and difficult to control thoughts and images (Wells & Davies, 1994). It consists of four subscales: Distraction, Social Control, Worry, Punishment, and Reappraisal. Correlational analysis indicated that TCQ Worry and Punishment are maladaptive control strategies associated with obsessive–compulsive, anxious, depressive, and/or worry symptoms, whereas distraction and reappraisal are adaptive strategies that show some negative association with symptoms (Ree, 2010; Reynolds & Wells, 1999; Wilson & Hall, 2012). As well, clinical samples score significantly higher on TCQ Punishment than nonclinical controls (e.g., Halvorsen et al., 2015). The TCQ Punishment subscale could be used to determine if excessive self-criticism is present, but the clinical utility of the other TCQ subscales is not known.

The 65-item Metacognitions Questionnaire (MCQ) was developed to assess positive and negative beliefs about worry and intrusive thoughts (Cartwright-Hatton & Wells, 1997). Based on Wells's metacognitive theory of worry, a series of seven studies reported on the development and psychometric properties of the MCQ in clinical and nonclinical samples. Factor analysis revealed five factors: (1) Positive Beliefs about Worry; (2) Negative Beliefs about the Uncontrollability of Thoughts and Corresponding Danger; (3) Lack of Cognitive Confidence; (4) Negative Beliefs about Superstition, Punishment, and Responsibility (SPR); and (5) Cognitive Self-

Consciousness. Except for MCQ Positive Beliefs and Cognitive Consciousness, the other subscales were moderately correlated with trait anxiety and slightly correlated with obsessive–compulsive checking symptoms. Regression analysis found that MCQ Cognitive Confidence made the largest contribution to the Padua Checking score. Discriminant analysis indicated that the MCQ SPR and Cognitive Self-Consciousness subscales may have more specificity for OCD.

In a subsequent study Wells and Cartwright-Hatton (2004) reported that a 30-item short form of the MCQ (MCQ-30) exhibited adequate psychometric properties with a slightly different five-factor structure consisting of (1) Cognitive Confidence, (2) Positive Beliefs about Worry, (3) Cognitive Self-Consciousness, (4) Negative Beliefs about the Uncontrollability of Thoughts and Danger, and (5) Beliefs about the Need to Control Thoughts. Correlational analysis indicated that the MCQ-30 was more closely associated with worry, and to a lesser extent, trait anxiety, than with obsessive–compulsive symptoms, although the MCQ-30 Negative Beliefs about the Uncontrollability of Thoughts, Cognitive Confidence, and Need to Control Thoughts showed some relationship with self-reported obsession symptoms. Consistent findings have been reported by others (e.g., Halvorsen et al., 2015; Wilson & Hall, 2012), and the MCQ-30 has greater relevance for anxiety than for other psychopathological states (Hjemdal, Stiles, & Wells, 2013). More specifically, it will be more useful in the assessment of worry than obsessions.

White Bear Suppression Inventory

The White Bear Suppression Inventory (WBSI), a 15-item self-report questionnaire, was developed by Wegner and Zanakos (1994) to measure individual differences in the use of effortful suppression to control unwanted thoughts. They found a significant correlation between WBSI Total Scores and obsessive–compulsive symptoms, although chronic thought suppression also correlated significantly with other emotional states, such as anxiety, worry, and depression, as well as emotional reactivity (de Bruin, Muris, & Rassin, 2007; Smári & Hólmsteinsson, 2001; Wegner & Zanakos, 1994). However, Rassin, Diepstraten, Merckelbach, and Muris (2001) found that pretreatment WBSI scores did not predict symptom improvement in individuals with OCD who received CBT. Nevertheless, the psychometric properties of the WBSI have been supported in various studies (e.g., Muris, Merckelbach, & Horselenberg, 1996; Wegner & Zanakos, 1994). As expected, higher WBSI scores are related to intrusion frequency and greater effort at controlling unwanted thoughts in thought suppression experiments (Lynch, Schneider, Rosenthal, & Cheavens, 2007; Muris et al., 1996). In addition, Rassin, Merckelbach, Muris, and Stapert (1999) found that students with elevated scores on the WBSI also reported a more intense urge to engage in their rituals, more discomfort from the rituals, and more resistance against their ritualistic urges than low scorers. There were no differences in frequency of actual ritualistic behavior or in success in resisting the urge to ritualize.

Höping and de Jong-Meyer (2003) identified a serious problem with the WBSI. In their factor analysis of the WBSI, two factors emerged: the first was an unwanted intrusive thoughts dimension and the second a thought suppression factor. It was the first factor that accounted for most of the questionnaire's association with negative affect and obsessive–compulsive symptom measures, and not the thought suppression factor. This finding has since been replicated in other studies (e.g., Kennedy, Grossman, & Ehrenreich-May, 2016; Schmidt et al., 2009), indicating that caution should be exercised when using the WBSI as a measure of trait thought suppression.

Intrusion and Appraisal Questionnaires

Research on the cognitive basis of OCD has resulted in the development of numerous self-report measures of unwanted intrusive thoughts and their appraisal and control strategies. Some of the best-known instruments are the Cognitive Intrusions Inventory (CIQ; Freeston et al., 1991), the Revised Obsessional Intrusions Inventory (ROII; Purdon & Clark, 1994b), the Interpretations of Intrusions Inventory (III; OCCWG, 2001, 2003), and the Spanish modification of the ROII (Inventorio de Pensamientos Intrusos Obsesivos [INPOIS]; Garciá-Soriano et al., 2011). Their psychometric properties have been reported in various research articles but differ according to sample characteristics and which appraisal or control variable is under consideration. All of these measures have been used as research tools, so their clinical utility is largely unknown. They should be used only in special cases when the clinician is unable to determine the client's faulty appraisal and control responses through more accurate idiographic methodologies.

Idiographic Assessment of Cognition

Idiographic assessment refers to person-specific methodologies that focus on variability within the individual rather than comparisons across persons. It is concerned with intraindividual change in performance or function across time or situations (Lyon et al., 2017). The clinical utility of idiographic assessment is enhanced because measurement is specifically tailored to capture structures and processes that are uniquely responsible for the persistence of the individual's obsessional state. Thus, the information obtained from idiographic measures make an invaluable contribution to the case formulation, treatment planning, and outcome evaluation. There are two idiographic methods particularly important for cognitive assessment in OCD: self-monitoring and symptom provocation.

Self-Monitoring

Diaries, individualized rating scales, and semistructured logs have been a mainstay of clinical data gathering in cognitive and behavioral therapies for decades. Self-monitoring forms are critical for identifying the client's unique experience of obsessions and compulsions. Forms 7.1–7.4 can be used as baseline measures to provide information crucial to the cognitive case formulation. In addition, Form 3.3 provides important information on the determinants of neutralization.

When completed as pretreatment homework assignments, considerable time is spent in session reviewing the information provided, seeking elaboration and clarification of the data to identify faulty appraisals of significance and neutralization. Self-monitoring is perhaps the most valuable assessment tool for elucidating the cognitive basis of the client's OCD.

Symptom Provocation

Another idiographic approach is behavioral observation of deliberate provocation of obsessive–compulsive symptoms within session. The client is invited to approach a feared object, such as touching the office door handle if physical contamination is present, and ratings of distress and urge to neutralize are obtained. As well, clinicians can question the client in real time about the appraisals, beliefs, and neutralization strategies associated with the obsessive–compulsive symptom provocation exercise.

Using symptom provocation as part of the assessment process raises several issues. First, the provocation exercise needs to be determined collaboratively, with an invitation to participate extended to the client and any concerns discussed fully before attempting the exercise. A symptom provocation that is too intense could cause the client to refuse to continue with the assessment. Second, a solid rationale for the provocation exercise must be present that emphasizes the benefits of behavioral observation for understanding the client's OCD. And third, it's important to debrief clients on their reactions to the exercise. An individual leaving an assessment session still distressed by a provocation may be dissuaded from ever returning. It could also send the wrong message about exposure and turn the individual against the CBT perspective. Thus, caution must be exercised when introducing symptom provocation during the assessment phase. The experience should engender hope and positive expectation for change rather than fear of what might come next.

COGNITIVE CASE CONCEPTUALIZATION OF OCD

Individualized case conceptualization involves the development of a data-driven collaborative hypothesis about the factors responsible for the etiology and persistence of a psychological disturbance, in order to generate treatment goals, identify maladaptive processes for change, and inform the selection of treatment strategies (Beck, Freeman, & Davis, 2015; Key & Bieling, 2015). In one of the most elaborated cognitive-behavioral approaches to case formulation, Persons (2008) noted that it should (1) provide a description of symptoms, disorders, and problems; (2) propose hypotheses about causal mechanisms; (3) identify precipitants or triggers to the disorder; and (4) identify the origins of mechanisms. This latter includes coping mechanisms such as avoidance or compulsive rituals.

Learning how to develop a case formulation is one of the hardest clinical skills to acquire in CBT (Key & Bieling, 2015). There are several aspects to case conceptualization that should be noted:

1. *Tentative.* Developing a case formulation begins with the initial session but continues to evolve and change throughout the therapy process. It is always considered a hypothesis that is subject to change as new information and insights are gleaned from therapy.
2. *Data-driven.* The case formulation is based on the clinical interview, client history, self-report measures, in-session observations, review of homework, and the therapeutic interaction. While guided by the CBT model, the therapist must ensure that the client's experiences provide the primary input into the formulation and its revision.
3. *Individualized.* Although commonalities will be found in the case formulations of individuals with OCD, the conceptualization must be tailored to the unique social and personal characteristics of the client. For OCD, the formulation should capture how faulty appraisals, beliefs, and neutralization efforts are expressed in the client's experience with obsessions and compulsions.
4. *Collaborative.* Development of the case formulation should model the collaborative approach emphasized in CBT. The cognitive-behavioral therapist takes the initiative in proposing the cognitive conceptualization. Individuals are provided with a copy of the formulation, and it is reviewed periodically throughout treatment with client feedback solicited.
5. *Treatment orientation.* The purpose of the cognitive case formulation is to guide treatment. If therapy sessions deviate from the formulation, then either therapy drift must be addressed or the formulation should be revised to align with the current needs and priorities of the client.

Cognitive Formulation

Form 7.5 provides an outline of a cognitive case formulation that can be used to determine treatment goals and guide the therapy process. This outline is based on the generic model presented in Figure 5.1. It begins by listing the client's primary obsessive content. This is readily available from the clinical interview or OCD symptom measures like the YBOCS. Most clients can easily report on their primary obsessions, although individuals with repugnant or embarrassing obsessions may be hesitant to disclose their intrusions. In these cases, it may take several sessions before the therapist can even start on the case formulation. Even then, it may be necessary to write the obsession in an abbreviated and disguised manner to minimize client distress when working on the profile.

Interpretation of Significance

The next step is to delineate the faulty appraisals and beliefs responsible for elevating the emotional significance of the obsession. Clients often struggle to understand this part of the model because their focus is on the emotional quality of the obsession. If the therapist asks, "What makes this obsession so important to you?," they will often respond "Because it makes me feel anxious, guilty, upset." To guide the client toward the faulty interpretations that underlie the emotion, the following questions can be utilized:

- *Overestimated threat.* "What concerns you most about having this unwanted thought pop into your mind? Does the thought represent a threat to you or others? If so, what is this threat?"
- *TAF–Likelihood.* "Are you concerned that the obsession will cause you to do something you'll regret? If so, what is it?"
- *Inflated responsibility.* "Do you feel a greater sense of responsibility or self-blame when you have this thought? If yes, what are you thinking you're responsible for preventing from happening to others or yourself?"
- *Intolerance of uncertainty.* "Does the obsession raise any doubts or uncertainties in your mind? What are you uncertain about? How uncomfortable does this uncertainty make you feel?"
- *Need for control.* "Is it important to stop thinking about the obsession? How much do you try to suppress the obsession or get it out of your mind? Do you try to stop yourself from having the obsession—that is, prevent it from entering your mind in the first place? Are you concerned about losing self-control over the obsession?"
- *Importance of thought.* "Do you think the obsession is personally meaningful? Does it signify something about your personality, your

values, or your morality? Does it cause you to question your integrity or the type of person you are?"
- *Perfectionism.* "Are you disappointed in yourself for having such thoughts? Do you think you shouldn't be thinking this way, that there must be something wrong with you? Does the obsession feel like a violation of your personal standards, of what you expect of yourself?"
- *Ego dystonicity (feared self).* "Does the obsession feel completely opposite to how you see yourself? Does it seem completely unlike you, unlike your personality? Does the obsession involve something you fear about yourself, like your worst nightmare?"

After exploring clients' faulty appraisals and beliefs, it is important to summarize this work in clients' own words. Time is spent exploring the appraisals and emphasizing their relevance to ensure that clients appreciate their relevance to their experience of OCD.

Mental Control Strategies

Compulsive rituals are noted in the mental control strategies step of the profile. Any strategies used to terminate the obsession, reduce associated distress, or prevent a feared consequence should be listed. Avoidance, reassurance seeking, thought stopping, mental ritualizing, rationalization, and the like are a few of the control strategies often evident in OCD. The Checklist of Neutralization Strategies Associated with OCD (Form 3.2) and the Determinants of Neutralization Rating Scale (Form 3.3) are useful resources for highlighting the key control strategies that contribute to the client's obsessional state. In addition, the stop criteria used to signal termination of a compulsion should be noted.

Associated Negative Cognitions

Many individuals with OCD experience other types of negative cognition that contribute to a worsening of their emotional state. These include worry, rumination, and negative self-referential thinking. Often this type of negative thinking is directly related to the individual's OCD. For example, a parent might worry that her children will be negatively affected by her obsessionality, or another person might ruminate over the causes of his OCD. A third person may feel depressed, thinking that she must be stupid or mentally weak to be plagued with such irrational thoughts. Often this negative thinking subsides with remission of obsessive–compulsive symptoms, but in some clients the therapist may need to incorporate this associated thinking into the treatment plan.

CONCLUSION

Effective CBT for obsessions and compulsions begins with a theory-driven, disorder-specific assessment and cognitive case formulation of the client's experience with OCD. The selection of normative and idiographic assessment instruments is guided by the generic CBT model (see Figure 5.1) and the case formulation presented in Form 7.5. The clinician must recognize that various aspects of OCD may present challenges for assessment, such as symptom heterogeneity, concealment, comorbidity, and temporal instability. Individuals with OCD can find the assessment, especially questionnaire completion, threatening because of high anxiety, unrealistic standards of correctness and honesty, pathological doubt, indecision, slowness, and lack of insight. A therapeutic approach that includes validation and encouragement, a clear rationale for the assessment process, and cognitive restructuring of faulty beliefs about the assessment can mitigate its distressing aspects.

A CBT assessment of OCD will include diagnostic and clinical interviews as well as normative self-report questionnaires and/or clinician rating scales that quantify obsessive–compulsive symptom frequency and severity. In addition, various cognitive measures are available that assess faulty appraisals, obsessive–compulsive beliefs, and neutralization efforts, but these may have limited clinical utility because of their research orientation. Ultimately, idiographic tools that allow individuals to evaluate unique aspects of their obsessive–compulsive experience will provide the most valuable data for the cognitive case formulation. Various clinical resource materials were provided that can assist in the idiographic portion of the assessment.

A template of the generic cognitive case formulation is presented in Form 7.5. More tailored templates are presented in the OCD subtype chapters, but each follows the generic format found in this chapter. The individualized case conceptualization must be closely aligned with the CBT model, incorporate features unique to the individual, be developed collaboratively, and be revised periodically. As discussed in the next chapter, the client's cognitive case conceptualization is the basis for goal setting, psychoeducation, and the introduction of cognitive intervention strategies.

FORM 7.1. Obsessions and Compulsions Experience Form

Instructions: Complete this form at the end of each day to summarize your experience of OCD symptoms over the next week.

Day	List Obsessions Experienced	Response to Obsessions (List any compulsions, neutralization efforts, avoidance, or mental control strategies employed.)	Rate Average Distress (From 0 = no distress to 10 = panic-like distress)	Personal Significance (Why did you pay attention to the obsessions? What made them so distressing for you? Note any negative consequences that concerned you about the obsessions.)
Sunday				
Monday				
Tuesday				
Wednesday				
Thursday				
Friday				
Saturday				

From *Cognitive-Behavioral Therapy for OCD and Its Subtypes, Second Edition*, by David A. Clark. Copyright © 2020 The Guilford Press. Permission to photocopy this material is granted to purchasers of this book for personal use or use with individual clients (see copyright page for details). Purchasers can download enlarged versions of this material (see the box at the end of the table of contents).

FORM 7.2. Situation Record and Rating Scales

Instructions: Use the following worksheet to list the situations, objects, or circumstances that most often trigger the primary obsession and then complete the rating scale associated with each situation.

List of Triggering Situations	Distress Rating of Situation (From 0 = none to 100 = extreme, panic-like)	Likelihood of Avoiding Situation (From 0 = never avoid to 100 = always avoid)
1.		
2.		
3.		
4.		
5.		
6.		
7.		
8.		
9.		
10.		

From *Cognitive-Behavioral Therapy for OCD and Its Subtypes, Second Edition*, by David A. Clark. Copyright © 2020 The Guilford Press. Permission to photocopy this material is granted to purchasers of this book for personal use or use with individual clients (see copyright page for details). Purchasers can download enlarged versions of this material (see the box at the end of the table of contents).

FORM 7.3. Record of Anticipated Consequences

Instructions: Use the following worksheet to list and then rate the consequences or outcomes that concern you most if the obsession persisted in your mind.

Negative Consequences/Outcomes Associated with Obsession	Likelihood of Outcome (From 0 = never happen to 100 = certain to happen)	Importance of Preventing Consequence (From 0 = not at all important to 100 = critical to my survival)
1.		
2.		
3.		
4.		
5.		
6.		
7.		
8.		
9.		
10.		

From *Cognitive-Behavioral Therapy for OCD and Its Subtypes, Second Edition,* by David A. Clark. Copyright © 2020 The Guilford Press. Permission to photocopy this material is granted to purchasers of this book for personal use or use with individual clients (see copyright page for details). Purchasers can download enlarged versions of this material (see the box at the end of the table of contents).

FORM 7.4. Control Strategies Worksheet

Instructions: Various strategies that people often use in response to their obsessions are listed in this worksheet. Use the rating scales associated with each strategy to estimate how often you use this strategy and its perceived effectiveness.

Control Strategies	Frequency (0 = never, 1 = occasionally, 2 = often, 3 = frequently, 4 = daily, 5 = several times a day)	Effectiveness (0 = never effective, 1 = occasionally effective, 2 = often effective, 3 = frequently effective, 4 = always effective)
1. Engage in a behavioral compulsion (e.g., wash, check, repeat). [BC]		
2. Engage in a mental compulsion (e.g., say a particular phrase, repeat a prayer, think certain thoughts). [MC]		
3. Think about reasons why the obsession is senseless, unimportant, or irrational. [CR]		
4. Try to reassure myself that everything will be all right. [SR]		
5. Seek reassurance from others that everything will be all right. [OR]		
6. Distract myself by doing something. [BD]		
7. Distract myself by thinking another, possibly pleasant, thought or image. [CD]		
8. Try to relax myself. [R]		
9. Tell myself to stop thinking the obsession. [TS]		
10. Get angry, down on myself for thinking the obsession. [P]		
11. Try to avoid anything that will trigger the obsession. [A]		
12. Do nothing when I get the obsession. [DN]		

Note. Modified from the Structured Interview on Neutralization (see Ladouceur et al., 2000), Thought Control Questionnaire (Wells & Davies, 1994), and Revised Obsessional Intrusions Inventory (Purdon & Clark, 1994b). Coding key: A, avoidance; BC, behavioral compulsion; BD, behavioral distraction; CD, cognitive distraction; CR, cognitive restructuring; DN, do nothing; MC, mental compulsion; OR, other reassurance; P, punishment; R, relaxation; SR, self-reassurance; TS, thought stopping.

From *Cognitive-Behavioral Therapy for OCD and Its Subtypes*, Second Edition, by David A. Clark. Copyright © 2020 The Guilford Press. Permission to photocopy this material is granted to purchasers of this book for personal use or use with individual clients (see copyright page for details). Purchasers can download enlarged versions of this material (see the box at the end of the table of contents).

FORM 7.5. Cognitive Case Formulation Profile

Instructions: This form is completed collaboratively with the client during the case formulation session. Key points of the case conceptualization are noted in the relevant sections of the case formulation profile, and a copy is provided to the client. The profile should be reviewed and reevaluated at various intervals throughout therapy.

Obsessive Thought Content

1. _____
2. _____
3. _____

↓

Interpretation of Significance (faulty appraisals)

_____
_____
_____
_____
_____
_____

↓

Mental Control Strategies (compulsions, etc.)

1. _____ 2. _____
3. _____ 4. _____
5. _____ 6. _____

↓

Associated Negative Cognitions

1. _____
2. _____
3. _____

Note. Adapted from Clark (2018) with permission from New Harbinger Publications.

From *Cognitive-Behavioral Therapy for OCD and Its Subtypes, Second Edition,* by David A. Clark. Copyright © 2020 The Guilford Press. Permission to photocopy this material is granted to purchasers of this book for personal use or use with individual clients (see copyright page for details). Purchasers can download enlarged versions of this material (see the box at the end of the table of contents).

CHAPTER 8

Goals, Education, and Cognitive Interventions

Assuming that the client accepts the cognitive case conceptualization, therapy progresses to goal setting, psychoeducation, and provision of the treatment rationale. The earliest therapy sessions are devoted to cognitive interventions for evaluation and correction of faulty appraisals and beliefs. There is some debate over whether treatment should start with exposure-based interventions or cognitive restructuring. Historically, CBT practitioners preferred to start with ERP and then introduce cognitive interventions in later sessions (e.g., Freeston & Ladouceur, 1999; Steketee, 1999). More recently, it is recommended that clients engage in cognitive work before therapists introduce ERP (i.e., Abramowitz, 2018; Rachman, 2003; Rachman et al., 2015; Salkovskis, 1999). In fact, one prominent CBT researcher argued that cognitive therapy for OCD can be effective without ERP (Radomsky, 2014). In any case, there are several reasons for starting treatment with cognitive interventions:

- Many individuals with OCD find ERP too threatening and overwhelming. Work at the cognitive level provides opportunity for the client to get accustomed to treatment before exposure to more demanding exercises.
- Cognitive interventions reinforce the client's understanding of the CBT perspective.
- They can strengthen a collaborative therapeutic alliance.
- They provide strategies the client can employ during ERP to manage anxiety and thereby encourage persistence with the exercises.

At first glance, cognitive interventions might seem quite ineffective, possibly even counterproductive, in the treatment of obsessional states. Individuals with OCD usually recognize the irrationality of their obsessions and compulsions. As a result, the use of finely tuned arguments about the improbability of an obsessional fear would be futile, because the client already knows the fear has tenuous ties to reality (Salkovskis, 1999; Steketee, Frost, Rhéaume, & Wilhelm, 1998). Even if you could convince a person with OCD that there is, for example, only a one-in-a-billion chance of catching a deadly disease by touching a doorknob, the individual would probably conclude that those slimmest of odds are sufficient reason to continue with compulsive washing and avoidance. Moreover, many individuals with OCD are particularly skilled at using intellectualization and rationalization to support their preoccupation with a primary obsession.

Despite justified skepticism about the utility of verbal therapies for the treatment of OCD, several treatment studies have shown that cognitive interventions can make a significant contribution to symptom improvement (e.g., de Haan et al., 1997; van Oppen, Hoekstra, & Emmelkamp, 1995; Whittal, Woody, McLean, Rachman, & Robichaud, 2010; see meta-analysis by Olatunji et al., 2013). A more recent mediation analysis found that changes in obsessive beliefs during the first 6 weeks of CBT predicted end-of-treatment symptoms (Diedrich et al., 2016). Furthermore, current best-practice guidelines recognize that both cognitive and behavioral interventions should be offered to individuals with OCD (i.e., APA, 2007; National Institute of Health Care and Excellence [NICE], 2005).

This chapter focuses on the first few CBT sessions in which goal setting, psychoeducation, and cognitive restructuring are the primary treatment objectives. It begins by presenting a clinical case composite that illustrates the various therapy ingredients discussed in the chapter. We start with treatment goal setting, which is derived from the cognitive case conceptualization. An individualized, experiential-based psychoeducation protocol is described that is designed to deepen clients' understanding of the cognitive basis of OCD and to foster acceptance of the treatment rationale. Finally, several cognitive intervention strategies are presented that can be used to modify the faulty appraisals and beliefs of significance that are responsible for the persistence of obsessions and compulsions.

CASE ILLUSTRATION

Darren had struggled with OCD since childhood. Initially, his obsessional concerns focused on physical contamination and washing compulsions. Many situations such as bathrooms, school, public places, parks, and the like elicited fears of having touched something dirty, and the belief that he was now contaminated and might spread this to others. As feelings of anxiety and disgust escalated, he would engage in various cleansing rituals such as washing his hands excessively, sprinkling water over "contaminated areas," or spitting. More recently, his obsessive concerns shifted to a focus on bodily secretions, especially semen. He became preoccupied with whether tiny amounts of semen might be on his clothing and transferred to others. He avoided masturbation or any sexual activity because he was afraid of God's disapproval and punishment by eternal damnation. He often felt disgust and a sense of moral filth, thinking that semen and urine may be seeping from his penis. To deal with the thought of unwanted bodily secretions, Darren washed and showered excessively, used an inordinate amount of toilet paper, repeatedly laundered all clothing and bedding, and repeatedly checked where he sat to ensure that he had not left semen or urine stains that would contaminate others.

This case illustrates a mixed-symptom presentation of OCD contamination. There are strong elements of physical contamination that stretch back to his childhood, and more recently aspects of mental contamination and scrupulosity are also present. He primarily relies on washing and cleaning compulsions to neutralize his fear and the probability of contamination, and there are many situations or activities he avoids so as not to elicit his obsessive fears. Figure 8.1 presents Darren's cognitive case conceptualization that is the basis of the clinical discussion in this chapter.

TREATMENT GOAL SETTING

Goal setting has always been an important element of behavioral and cognitive therapies. The therapist can expect to spend an entire session working collaboratively with the client on goals that will guide subsequent therapy sessions. Unless an individual has had previous experience with CBT, it is unlikely that he or she will share the same goals as the therapist. Often, clients enter therapy expecting to learn:

- How to gain effective control over their obsessions and compulsions.
- How to eliminate obsessions and compulsions from their life.
- How to greatly reduce anxiety, guilt, and other negative emotions associated with the obsession.
- How to prevent a return of obsessive–compulsive symptoms.

Clearly, these treatment expectations do not correspond well with the basic CBT perspective. For example, Darren's goal would be the cessation of thoughts about bodily secretion and the associated anxiety, the ability to ignore reddish dirt specks or streaks, and to be convinced that God really didn't care whether he masturbated. Of course, the CBT perspective of Darren's treatment is quite different, emphasizing instead the acceptance of intrusive thoughts about bodily secretions and possible contamination,

---

Obsessive Thought Content

1. Maybe there are traces of semen on my clothing, and they get transferred to a coworker.
2. Maybe that reddish speck on the floor is blood, and if someone steps on it and gets infected, it will be my fault.
3. What if I've been immoral and God punishes me with eternal damnation? here

⬇

Interpretation of Significance (faulty appraisals)

Because I'm so preoccupied with urine and semen, there must be something to it. I'd feel terrible, completely to blame, if someone got sick because they accidentally came in contact with stains that I left behind. It's so gross to think there's even a slight chance someone could come in contact with trace amounts of my semen. I have to make sure I'm clean and have not put others at risk. Any uncertainty about this would be intolerable and cause me to worry that I've inflicted harm on others. Besides, what kind of person is constantly worried about urine and semen? Obviously, I can't be trusted around others.

⬇

Mental Control Strategies (compulsions, etc.)

1. Compulsive washing
2. Repeated checking
3. Self-reassurance
4. Rationalization
5. Thought suppression
6. Cognitive distraction

⬇

Associated Negative Cognitions

1. Rumination focused on postevent processing to convince himself he didn't contaminate others
2. Worry about his future and whether OCD would ruin his life
3. Excessive self-criticalness (thoughts of worthlessness, helplessness, failure)

FIGURE 8.1. Darren's cognitive case formulation.

focused attention to dirt and specks without neutralizing, and embracing the uncertainty and impossibility of knowing the mind of God. It is easy to see how the goals and rationale for CBT could collide with the client's expectations for treatment. When this happens, there is a high probability the client will decide not to continue with CBT.

Figure 8.2 presents a treatment goal-setting scheme based on the cognitive case conceptualization of OCD. It can be reviewed with clients to

Treatment Goal Scheme

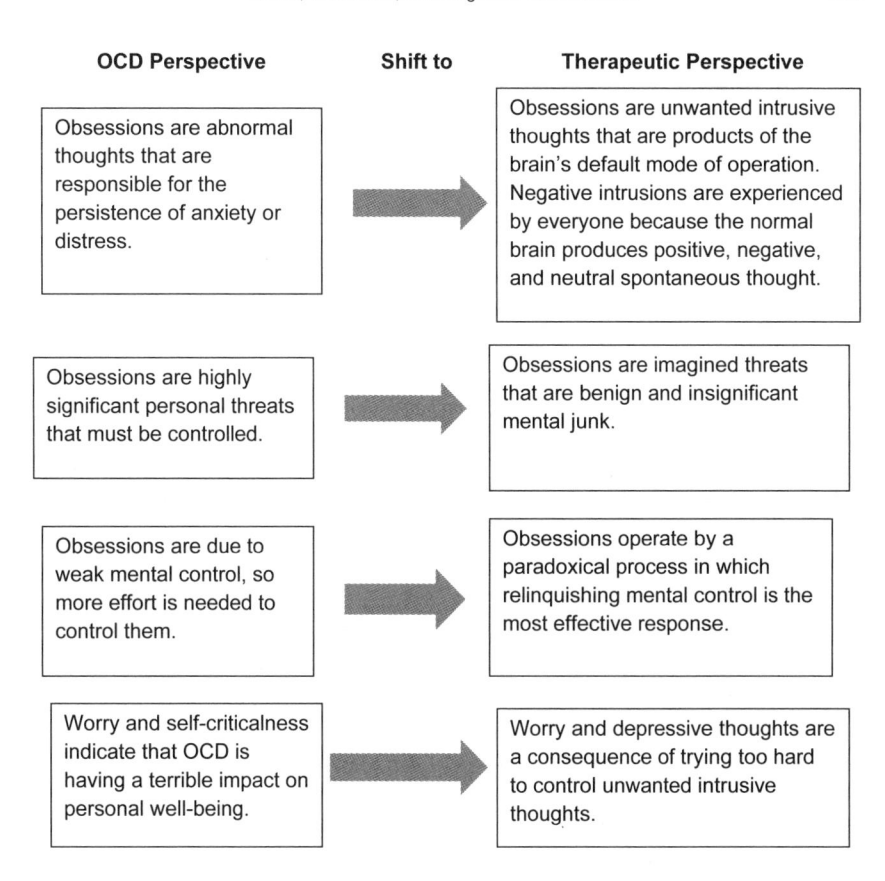

OCD Perspective	Shift to	Therapeutic Perspective
Obsessions are abnormal thoughts that are responsible for the persistence of anxiety or distress.	→	Obsessions are unwanted intrusive thoughts that are products of the brain's default mode of operation. Negative intrusions are experienced by everyone because the normal brain produces positive, negative, and neutral spontaneous thought.
Obsessions are highly significant personal threats that must be controlled.	→	Obsessions are imagined threats that are benign and insignificant mental junk.
Obsessions are due to weak mental control, so more effort is needed to control them.	→	Obsessions operate by a paradoxical process in which relinquishing mental control is the most effective response.
Worry and self-criticalness indicate that OCD is having a terrible impact on personal well-being.	→	Worry and depressive thoughts are a consequence of trying too hard to control unwanted intrusive thoughts.

FIGURE 8.2. Treatment goal scheme.

facilitate their own goal setting and acceptance of the treatment rationale. The left column describes the treatment expectations that many individuals bring to CBT, whereas the right column presents the alternative CBT goals for effective treatment. Clients could be encouraged to write out their own version of Figure 8.2, with particular focus on how they would specify their goals according to the description found in the four right-hand boxes. The therapist could ask, "What do you think is the consequence of thinking in the OCD way?" (left column) and, "What do you think might be the consequence, the outcome, if you truly thought of the OCD in the therapeutic manner?" (right column). This collaborative, Socratic-questioning approach will promote commitment to the treatment and its goals, and provide opportunity to transition into psychoeducation and treatment rationale.

In summary, the focus of CBT can be contrasted with the client's original treatment expectations and stated as follows:

- Learn to relinquish effortful mental control of obsessions and compulsions.
- Learn to tolerate, even embrace, obsessions and response prevent compulsions.
- Strip obsessions of their meaning and significance.
- Learn how to manage a return of obsessive–compulsive symptoms.

PSYCHOEDUCATION

Educating clients about the cognitive model and its treatment is a key therapeutic ingredient that dates to the early days of cognitive therapy. Individuals are introduced to the connection between thought and feeling and provided with a treatment rationale in the first session of cognitive therapy for depression (Beck et al., 1979). Educating the client is again highlighted in cognitive therapy of anxiety disorders (Beck & Emery, 1985), and J. S. Beck (2011) noted the importance of sharing the case conceptualization and collaborating with clients in treatment planning. Several OCD researchers and practitioners also have recognized that education is an important part of treatment (Freeston & Ladouceur, 1999; Rachman, 1998, 2003; Salkovskis, 1996; Steketee, 1999; Whittal & McLean, 1999).

Educating clients about the CBT perspective on OCD is not a distinct phase of therapy but rather an emphasis that begins at assessment and carries through the case conceptualization and goal-setting sessions. In the present context, psychoeducation is defined as *an experiential, individualized learning process that emphasizes the role of faulty appraisals, neutralization, excessive control efforts, and ill-defined stop criteria in the persistence of an individual's obsessive–compulsive symptoms and associated distress*. This definition emphasizes that the learning process in psychoeducation must be tailored to the individual and based on his or her personal experience with OCD. Therapists avoid giving lectures on the model but instead demonstrate to clients how the CBT perspective can explain the onset and persistence of their obsessive–compulsive symptoms, as well as how treatment of underlying cognitive and neutralization processes can lead to symptom remission. Psychoeducation, then, consists of experiential, personalized learning exercises introduced in the collaborative therapeutic style. In the spirit of guided discovery, individuals are invited to test out whether the CBT perspective applies to their daily experience of obsessions and compulsions.

Therapists may find it helpful to work with the generic CBT model (Figure 5.1) or the relevant subtype model found in later chapters, as well as the cognitive case formulation profile (Form 7.5) and the treatment goal-setting scheme of shifting from an OCD to a therapeutic perspective (Figure 8.2). In each of these cases, it is important to make notes on the handouts that describe how these cognitive and behavioral constructs are expressed

Goals, Education, and Cognitive Interventions

in the client's obsessive–compulsive experience. Several aspects of the CBT model are demonstrated when educating the client.

Normalizing Unwanted Intrusions

Educating the client on the normality of intrusive thinking is an important therapeutic element in the treatment. Most clients are not familiar with the term *intrusive thoughts,* so psychoeducation starts with a description of the phenomena. Clients can be asked, "Have you ever had a thought, an image, memory, or impulse suddenly pop into your mind with little or no effort on your part?" If the client answers in the affirmative, ask for an example of a recent spontaneous thought. If the client can't think of an example, sit in silence for 3 minutes and then ask the client to report on his or her stream of thought. Discuss whether all thoughts experienced during the 3-minute interval were effortful and directed, or whether some were spontaneous, distracting thoughts. This exercise should lead into a discussion of four important points:

- Spontaneous thought is a normal feature of human brain functioning and has been called its *default mode* of operation (Killingsworth & Gilbert, 2010).
- Spontaneous or intrusive thinking can be positive, negative, or neutral (i.e., benign, irrelevant, trivial).
- Intrusive thinking is universal, although some people may have more intrusive thoughts or be more aware of them than others.
- Our ability to stop these mental intruders is limited (i.e., we can't stop our brains from generating spontaneous thoughts, even the negative and distressing ones).

Several exercises are provided in *The Anxious Thoughts Workbook* (Clark, 2018) that can increase individuals' sensitivity to and understanding of intrusive thinking. For individuals with OCD, psychoeducation emphasizes the relationship between unwanted intrusive thoughts and obsessions (see also Chapter 2). Individuals can be shown lists of common intrusive thoughts that are relevant for OCD, such as those in Handout 8.1.

Clients are asked to pick an intrusive thought from the list that they have experienced but that didn't bother them, and then an intrusive thought that did bother them. This latter might be their primary obsession. The client can be asked, "Why do you think one thought bothered you but the other didn't?" This question should lead into a discussion of faulty appraisals and the fact that the troubling intrusive thought:

- Was considered highly unacceptable ("I shouldn't be thinking this way").
- Captured attention and disrupted concentration.

- Had an upsetting or distressing quality.
- Was difficult to ignore, suppress or dismiss.

The therapist emphasizes that unwanted intrusions with these qualities can turn into obsessions. Obsessive thinking is like "intrusions on steroids," first beginning as an unwanted, negative involuntary thought, image, or impulse but then developing into a form of mental torment. Most individuals with OCD believe that it is the obsession itself that is the core problem. Hearing that the obsession is rooted in normal thinking is a novel idea to most people. Many clients will then ask, "If my obsessive thinking starts out as a normal way of thinking, why has it become considerably more frequent, distressing, and uncontrollable than other people's intrusive thoughts?" The answer to this question introduces the role of faulty appraisals and neutralization as key cognitive processes responsible for the escalation of unwanted intrusions into clinical obsessions.

Faulty Appraisals

Because individuals with OCD are so focused on the obsessional content and whether it is true and likely to lead to dire consequences, they may have difficulty viewing the obsession from a metacognitive perspective (i.e., recognizing the personal meaning or significance of the obsession). This can be the most challenging part of the psychoeducation process, but cognitive-behavioral therapists have had some success in communicating this distinction by explaining appraisal in terms of the "importance given to the thought" (Freeston & Ladouceur, 1997a), or "what you think about the obsession, its meaning" (Whittal & McLean, 1999). The case formulation section in Chapter 7 provides a list of specific questions that can be used to probe the client's faulty appraisals of significance.

When educating clients about the role of faulty appraisals, it's important to base this material on the client's case formulation (Form 7.5). The following dialogue is a hypothetical exchange between Darren and his therapist that illustrates education about faulty appraisals.

> THERAPIST: Darren, let's take a look at why this intrusive thought about semen on your clothing has become so frequent and distressing. I'd like you to take a look at the second box in your case formulation. Could you read the description out loud so we can both hear it?
>
> DARREN: (*Reads the interpretation of significance description.*)
>
> THERAPIST: Based on what you read, what is it about "thoughts of semen" that draws your attention to them, makes them such a significant and important thought in your mind?
>
> DARREN: Well, I keep thinking how terrible it would be if someone got

sick because of my semen. I don't think I could live with myself. It would be terrible.

THERAPIST: Okay, so you're frightened of the consequence if the thought came true. Anything else?

DARREN: Well, I feel really anxious when I am thinking about semen. I tell myself I'd better stop thinking like this or I'll have to leave work, take a sick day. I just feel so terrible, and I can't concentrate on anything else.

THERAPIST: So another reason why the "semen thought intrusion" is so important is its strong emotional quality and the belief that you have to get it out of your mind. Anything else?

DARREN: Well, if I could be certain that I didn't have semen on my clothing, then I'd stop thinking about it. So I keep thinking I need to do something to deal with the thought.

THERAPIST: Darren, you've identified a few ways in which the "semen thought" has become a significant intrusive thought. You think about it having dire consequences, being emotionally upsetting, creating a terrible state of uncertainty, and needing to be controlled. Can you see from our previous discussion about troubling mental intrusions how the "semen thought" has taken on obsessive qualities. Do you see how the intrusion has been turned into an obsession?

To strengthen the clients' understanding of the role of faulty appraisals, they can be asked to select a negative intrusive thought that they have experienced but that does not bother them, and then their primary obsession. Handout 8.1 or a similar list of intrusions can be used for this purpose. Using Socratic questioning, the therapist can ask, "Why are you not bothered by this negative thought? Why is it not important or significant to you?" Then the client is asked, "How could you turn this into a distressing thought? What would you need to think about in order to become upset by the thought?" Finally, therapists ask clients to consider their primary obsession and ask, "How would you need to think about the obsession in order to turn it into just another unwanted intrusive thought?" More detailed instruction and exercises on this educational approach to faulty appraisals can be found in *The Anxious Thought Workbook* (Clark, 2018), where it is referred to as "toxic" and "nontoxic" interpretations of significance. This rather intensive psychoeducation on faulty appraisals of significance sets the stage for the cognitive intervention strategies discussed later in this chapter.

Neutralization

Psychoeducation into the CBT perspective includes education on the role that compulsions, neutralization, avoidance, and other control strategies play in the pathogenesis of OCD. Once again, the client is asked to review the control strategies listed in his or her case formulation (Form 7.5.) as well as the Control Strategies Worksheet (Form 7.4). Discussion should focus on the perceived short-term and long-term effectiveness of each strategy. Educating Darren about the role of compulsive washing might proceed as follows.

> THERAPIST: Darren, I notice from the case formulation that when you think there might be traces of semen on your clothes, you immediately change clothes, thoroughly wash the "contaminated clothing," and then wash your hands repeatedly to ensure that there is no trace of semen. How effective is all this washing and cleaning?
>
> DARREN: Well, in the short term I feel a lot better knowing that I've gotten rid of any possible semen, although I'm never certain that I'm "semen-free." There's always a little concern that I didn't get it all.
>
> THERAPIST: Have you had days when you seemed to get stuck in compulsive washing? That is, you'd wash and feel a little better, then something else would happen and you'd be right back to washing? Or, have you had times when you still felt anxious even after washing and cleaning?
>
> DARREN: Oh, yes, I've had a few bad days like that.
>
> THERAPIST: On the other hand, have you ever been caught in a situation where you couldn't wash, such as when you were at work or visiting a friend? If so, what happened?
>
> DARREN: Yes, I've had times when I thought I had semen on my clothes, but I couldn't change or spend a long time in the bathroom washing. For a while I was beside myself, but eventually I calmed down and after a couple of hours, I forgot about it.
>
> THERAPIST: If I could summarize, it sounds like most often washing and cleaning bring some relief in the short term, but the relief doesn't last because the "semen obsession" eventually returns. Other times, when you can't wash or clean, it's very stressful in the short term, but in the long term you settle down and the obsession goes away, or at least is tolerable.
>
> DARREN: That describes it quite accurately.
>
> THERAPIST: I'd like to consider whether the washing and cleaning compulsions might be *"feeding your OCD,"* that is, making the semen obsessions worse, and whether preventing yourself from washing and cleaning might *"starve the OCD,"* that is, decrease the frequency and intensity of the semen obsession.

At this point the therapist can introduce ERP, which can be proposed as a series of experiments to observe the effects of delaying the compulsion to determine its effects on the obsession and its associated distress (see Chapter 9 for more details). What clients should be learning is that compulsions, neutralization, avoidance, and other control strategies increase the salience and meaningfulness of the obsession, thereby contributing to its frequency and intensity. Eliminating the compulsion and other neutralization efforts is a tangible way of treating the obsession as a benign, insignificant mental intrusion.

Excessive Mental Control

Educating clients with OCD into the deleterious effects of excessive mental control can be challenging because these individuals often believe that they have weak self-control and so seek treatment to gain better control over the obsession. However, the CBT model asserts that a major problem in OCD is that individuals try *too hard* to exert mental control over their obsessive intrusive thoughts (Clark & Purdon, 1993; Freeston et al., 1996; Rachman, 1998; Salkovskis, 1996). The goal of CBT is to encourage individuals to *give up* their efforts to control the obsession.

Rather than use verbal persuasion or disputation to change the individual's view on control, an experiential exercise, like the white bear thought suppression experiment, is more effective. It is a potent learning exercise for demonstrating the *paradox of mental control*. Derived from experimental research on thought suppression (Wegner, 1994b; Wegner et al., 1987), the white bear thought suppression experiment has become a useful clinical tool in CBT for OCD (Freeston & Ladouceur, 1997b; Clark, 2018). In the first *thought retention* phase of the experiment, individuals are instructed to think about a white bear continuously for 2 minutes with eyes closed to improve concentration on the task. If they get distracted from the white bear thought, they are to signal by raising a finger. The therapist records the number of interruptions in the 2-minute period. This is followed by a brief discussion of the difficulties encountered in holding a specific thought, the limits of mental control, and the brain's natural tendency to generate intrusive, distracting thoughts. In the second phase, *thought dismissal* is introduced, in which individuals are instructed not to think about a white bear for 2 minutes and to signal when the unwanted bear thought intrudes into consciousness. The therapist then uses Socratic questioning to guide the client toward several observations that can be reached about mental control:

- Trying hard to "not think" a specific thought is much harder and less successful than trying hard "to think" about a specific topic or idea.
- Even under the best of circumstances, with a neutral thought, intentional mental control is limited.

- Concentration and attention are constantly shifting from one thought to the next.
- The brain is constantly generating distracting, intrusive thoughts, even though we are trying to concentrate on a single idea.
- Strong mental control effort may be futile at best and counterproductive at worse.

If clients have difficulty accepting this last point, the white bear experiment can be repeated, and the client invited to try really hard to "not think about white bears." Then a comparison is made between the number of "bear intrusions" under normal effort and extra effort conditions. Even if there were fewer intrusions with extra mental effort, the client can be asked whether the difference was worth the effort and whether he or she would be able to sustain this tremendous effort over several hours or days, not just 2 minutes. This aspect of the educational process should conclude with clients' willingness to consider whether excessive mental control effort might be contributing to their OCD.

Stop Criteria

As discussed in Chapter 3, individuals with OCD often use vague, multiple, subjective internal states to determine when a compulsion or neutralization response can be stopped. These criteria should be evident from the assessment and cognitive case formulation. As part of psychoeducation, the therapist needs to discuss the role of stop rules in propagating the obsessive state. For example, Darren used a reduction in anxious feelings and a sense that *"he had done his best"* when cleaning his clothes and washing his hands. Also, if he thought, *"God knows I've done my best,"* then he would feel less guilt and could stop the compulsion. In this case the therapist would explore whether the multiple criteria sometimes conflict with each other, whether the criteria make it more difficult to know when he's done enough, and whether these stop criteria hinder rather than promote a sense of safety and certainty of knowing. Education on stop criteria should conclude when the client is willing to accept that a more specific, sensory-based external criteria might facilitate a reduction in compulsive symptoms.

Treatment Rationale

Psychoeducation should conclude with a discussion of the treatment rationale. Clients are informed that therapy will focus on helping them change their reactions to the obsessions. The following illustrates a possible treatment rationale.

> "As you have seen from the work we've done so far, how individuals react to their unwanted intrusive thoughts and obsessions has a major

impact on their frequency and distress. Treatment will involve a variety of intervention strategies used to explore different ways to interpret or understand the obsession, so you'll learn to assign less importance or personal significance to whether the obsession occurs or not. One goal of therapy is to help you see the obsession as less threatening. A second goal is to develop different ways of responding to the obsession and to reduce the use of compulsive rituals, neutralization, and other mental control strategies. In addition, you'll be learning that it is better to cease trying to control the intrusive obsessions and accept the output of your spontaneous mind. As well, you'll be learning to use different stop criteria so you don't get stuck in compulsive rituals. You can expect to see significant reductions in the frequency of the obsession and in your level of distress, once the thought has become less important to you and you have learned healthier ways to respond. You can expect treatment to take another 15–20 sessions. In addition to the work we will do in the weekly therapy sessions, there will be a variety of self-help tasks you'll need to do between sessions. These are designed to help you develop better responses to the obsession. Do you have any questions about the treatment?"

The treatment rationale for ERP should be provided in later sessions after some of the cognitive work is complete. Chapter 4 presents an extended discussion of how to prepare clients for ERP, address possible compliance issues, and provide a treatment rationale (see also Kozak & Foa, 1997).

COGNITIVE INTERVENTIONS

Appraisal Self-Monitoring

Cognitive treatment begins with an in-depth analysis of a recent obsessional experience. Form 8.1 presents a worksheet that can be used between sessions to self-monitor faulty appraisals and neutralization of the obsession.

The worksheet serves the same function as Thought Records in conventional cognitive therapy for anxiety and depression. It is a clinical resource that is used (1) to increase clients' awareness of their faulty appraisals and neutralization, (2) to strengthen client education on the CBT model, and (3) to provide data for practicing cognitive restructuring interventions. Handouts 8.2 and 8.3 provide further education on faulty appraisals and beliefs. With the aid of these materials, the therapist focuses on the specific faulty appraisals apparent in the client's misinterpretation of significance. With practice, individuals become more adept at identifying the faulty appraisals associated with their obsessive–compulsive experiences. This increased sensitivity to errors of appraisal is a prerequisite to gaining any therapeutic benefit from cognitive restructuring. Breaking down the "appraisals of significance" can be introduced in the following way:

> "Now that you've told me why this unwanted intrusive thought (obsession) is so important to you, I would like to look at this much more closely to see if there are some themes or ways of evaluating the obsession that make it so important. The cognitive-behavioral model assumes that there are certain ways we tend to evaluate our thoughts that can make them more frequent and distressing. I would like to see if these problematic evaluations are evident in your interpretation of the obsession."

Most individuals with OCD have difficulty identifying their faulty appraisals. Self-monitoring homework may need to be assigned repeatedly, and the therapist may need to devote several sessions to working with clients on how to identify the specific appraisals evident in their misinterpretations of the obsession. Eventually, individuals can achieve greater self-awareness of their faulty meta-cognitive processing of their obsessions.

Cognitive Restructuring Strategies

Once clients gain insight into their faulty appraisals, the next step is to provide cognitive skills in challenging their "interpretations of importance." There are three reasons why cognitive interventions are employed to treat OCD:

- To help clients realize that their "automatic" interpretation of an unwanted thought is one of *several possible ways* to react to the thought.
- To demonstrate that appraisals of the importance or significance of the obsession are based on a *possibility inference* (O'Connor & Robillard, 1999). That is, the obsession is considered important not because of "what *will* happen" but "what *could* happen."
- To highlight that an individual's faulty appraisal and overcontrol of the obsession comprise a *highly selective* approach to certain types of unwanted thoughts. Learning that one's reaction to low-frequency, nondistressing intrusive thoughts differs from one's reaction to high-frequency, distressing obsessions introduces the possibility that alternative ways of dealing with the obsession could be beneficial.

The following discussion considers some specific cognitive interventions that can be used with the primary appraisals implicated in the persistence of obsessions. Although cognitive-behavioral therapists may start with these cognitive interventions, they should quickly integrate them with behavioral tasks and experiments. Discussion of specific cognitive interventions for obsession-relevant beliefs and appraisals can be found in various publications (e.g., Clark, 2018; Freeston et al., 1996; O'Connor & Aardema, 2012; Rachman, 2003, 2006; Rachman et al., 2015; Salkovskis, 1999; Salkovskis & Wahl, 2003; van Oppen & Arntz, 1994; Whittal & McLean, 1999, 2002; Wilhelm & Steketee, 2006).

Overestimated Threat

Cognitive work on overestimated threat begins with a clear specification of the client's obsessional fear. For Darren, one of his obsessions was "What if I have traces of semen on my clothing, it spreads to my coworkers, and they get sick?" The therapist asks the client to provide an estimate of the likelihood that the obsessional concern would happen in real life. The estimate should be based on how the client feels rather than a post-hoc rationalization. The following is a possible exchange between Darren and his therapist.

> THERAPIST: Darren, when you are experiencing the "semen obsession" at its peak, how likely is it that your coworker would get sick because of your semen?
>
> DARREN: Well, I know it's extremely unlikely.
>
> THERAPIST: I am sure that it seems highly unlikely as you sit here calmly and talk about the obsession. But in the "heat of the moment," when you are feeling so upset by the obsession, how likely does it feel then?
>
> DARREN: Oh, when the obsession is strong, it feels like 1 in 10 chance that I've infected my coworker.

Once the emotion-based probability has been established, the therapist works with the client to determine the sequence of events or steps that would lead to the dreaded outcome. It is best to document this sequence as a flowchart that ends with the catastrophic outcome. It begins with the therapist explaining the purpose of the exercise: "I would like to understand the sequence of events that would need to happen for the obsessional concern to come true. I'd like to create a flowchart of these various steps with each step leading to the next, so that together they end with the dreaded outcome." Figure 8.3 presents a possible flowchart of Darren's semen obsession.

Often individuals will express embarrassment when seeing the obsessional concern broken down in this manner. However, it is important to continue with the exercise and ask the client to assign a probability estimate that each step could occur. Again, it's important to emphasize that the probability estimate is based on "how it feels" at the time of the

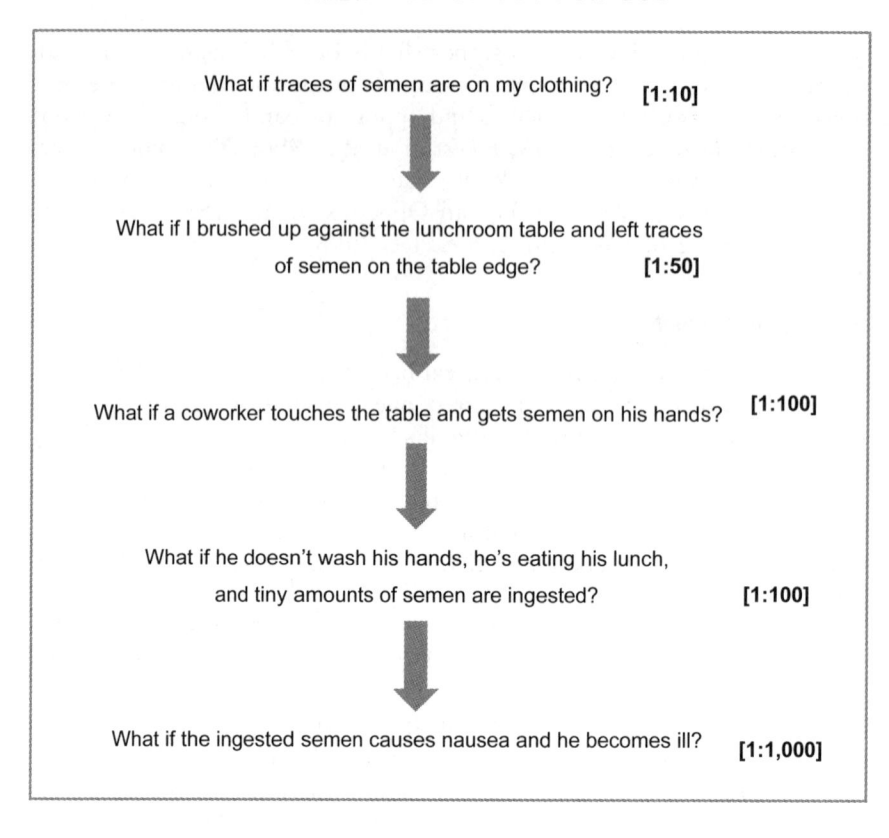

```
What if traces of semen are on my clothing?          [1:10]
                         ↓
What if I brushed up against the lunchroom table and left traces
         of semen on the table edge?                  [1:50]
                         ↓
What if a coworker touches the table and gets semen on his hands?   [1:100]
                         ↓
What if he doesn't wash his hands, he's eating his lunch,
      and tiny amounts of semen are ingested?        [1:100]
                         ↓
What if the ingested semen causes nausea and he becomes ill?   [1:1,000]
```

FIGURE 8.3. Flowchart of Darren's semen obsession.

obsessional episode, rather than basing the estimate on a post-hoc rationalization. This part of the intervention is derived from van Oppen and Arntz's (1994) description of the cumulative probability exercise, in which the client's original estimation is compared with the multiple estimate of each sequence of events leading to the feared outcome (see also Wilhelm & Steketee, 2006). As well, the therapist can compare the cumulative probability for the obsessional concern with the probability associated with a non-OCD daily risk. The point of this intervention is threefold:

- That exaggerating the probability of bad outcomes will increase anxiety and distress.
- That lowering one's estimates of bad outcomes reduces anxiety and distress.
- That therefore, repeatedly correcting one's overestimated threat appraisal will help reduce anxiety and distress associated with the obsessional concern.

To illustrate the application of this cognitive intervention, consider the probability estimates for the sequence of steps involved in Darren's semen obsession (see Figure 8.3). Darren would be asked to "guesstimate" the likelihood that each of these steps could occur in real life. To arrive at a cumulative probability that each of these steps could occur in a sequence that would result in a coworker's becoming sick from contact with Darren's semen, we multiply the probabilities presented in Figure 8.3 ($0.1 \times 0.02 \times 0.01 \times 0.01 \times 0.001$), which comes to 1 in 2 billion. (Of course, all of this is highly imaginative, since it's ludicrous to treat minute traces of semen as if it were anthrax.) The therapist then compares the client's original estimate (1 in 10) with the calculated probability of 1 in 2 billion. In addition, the therapist can compare the client's inflated threat estimate of semen with his deflated threat estimate of having a minor car accident, which is far more likely. The therapist could summarize this intervention as follows.

THERAPIST: As you can see from these calculations, there is a 1 in 2 billion chance that you could infect someone with your microscopic traces of semen, even though you tell yourself it's much more likely, such as 1 in 10. What effect does this information have on you?

DARREN: I know this is all ridiculous, but it seems so real at the time.

THERAPIST: Do you agree that you are exaggerating the probability of causing sickness in a coworker due to accidental contact with your microscopic traces of semen?

DARREN: Yes.

THERAPIST: Do you think that exaggerating the probability makes you more or less anxious about semen?

DARREN: Probably more anxious.

THERAPIST: And when you're driving, you don't think about the chances of having an accident, even though it's somewhat high. Does thinking that the probability of an accident is low make you feel more or less anxious?

DARREN: I feel less anxious.

THERAPIST: So, from this we discover a strategy you can use to reduce your anxiety about semen. When you have the obsession, if you practiced countering the 1 in 10 estimate with the 1 in 2 billion estimate, could this not help reduce the anxiety?

DARREN: Maybe, but I don't see how this will help.

THERAPIST: I agree. At first it may not seem helpful, but it is one of many strategies you can use to deal with the obsession in a healthier manner. With practice and other strategies, like ERP, you can learn to accept the obsessional fear for what it is: a ridiculous, highly imaginative idea.

TAF Bias

Socratic questioning and inductive reasoning are relevant cognitive strategies for addressing the TAF–Likelihood bias because of its basis in threat estimation and a belief in the overimportance of thought. As in the previous discussion, the intervention begins with a clear statement of cause and effect, in which the client expresses a belief that the more often he or she has the obsession, the greater the likelihood of the feared outcome (e.g., "If I think that my boyfriend will have an accident, he is at greater risk of having an accident"). A belief rating is obtained to determine how strongly the person believes that unwanted thoughts can cause unwanted actions with real-life negative consequences. Next, the therapist obtains a specific and detailed account of how the obsession increases the likelihood of the negative event. The following illustrates a sequence of Socratic inquiry employed to challenge TAF–Likelihood bias:

> "In your mind, how does thinking about an accident cause the accident to happen?"
> "Do you think the accident could happen immediately when you think about it, or is there a time delay?"
> "When you think about the accident, does it increase the chances of accidents over a short or long period of time?"
> "Does it increase the likelihood of just a certain type of accident or any accident in general?"
> "Does the length of time you have the accident thought, or the number of accident thoughts, further increase the likelihood of the accident?"
> "Do you think you could be held legally responsible for harm or death to someone because you thought about it?"
> "How many people do you think are killed each year by someone else's thoughts?"

The purpose of this type of Socratic questioning is to guide clients toward realization they are falsely empowering their obsessive thinking with causal effects. If obsessive thoughts can somehow cause bad things to happen, then individuals who believe this will become overly concerned about the thoughts. But if the premise that unwanted thought frequency has real-life consequences is erroneous, then these cognitive intrusions become less meaningful and significant. This intervention is a good way to prepare the client for the empirical hypothesis-testing-prediction experiments discussed in the next chapter.

The TAF–Moral bias is based on the premise that the way we think determines our true moral character; that is, "bad thoughts" are equivalent to "bad deeds." The cognitive interventions for ego dystonicity and TAF–

Moral presented in Chapter 12 are relevant for the present discussion. The following is the type of Socratic questioning useful for helping the client reevaluate the validity of the TAF–Moral premise.

> "Have you ever changed your mind about someone you at first thought was highly moral (a good person) but now you're questioning his or her moral character? What happened that caused you to change your mind? Was it what the person thought or what the person did?" [The therapist could give an example from news reports of a prominent individual accused of a morally reprehensible crime, like murder, rape, violent assault, etc., and ask whether it was the person's thoughts or deeds that were newsworthy.] If morality is mainly determined by what we think, how many bad thoughts must a person have to be deemed immoral? Is one terribly immoral thought equal to 100 slightly immoral thoughts? Is it the number of different types of immoral thoughts or the frequency with which a person thinks a single immoral thought that calls into question the individual's moral character?"

Therapists can use this type of guided inquiry to shift the client's moral reasoning from a rigid, absolutistic system based on mental control of unwanted thoughts to a more adaptive, realistic system based on self-control of behavior.

Another cognitive intervention for the TAF–Moral bias was introduced by Whittal and McLean (2002). Here the client is presented with a continuum, with one end labeled *Best Person Ever* and the other *Worst Person Ever* (see also Steketee, 1999). Next the client is asked to think of someone who would fit either end of the continuum; and then to indicate where that person would place him- or herself on the continuum. The therapist provides examples of people who have either had bad thoughts or have done bad deeds, and they are placed on the continuum (e.g., a person who had an aggressive thought against a friend, versus another person who physically assaulted a friend). Discussion then focuses on why one person is placed closer to the immoral end of the continuum than the other person. Again, this exercise challenges the premise of the TAF–Moral bias by indicating that "bad deeds" are more important criteria of immorality than "bad thoughts."

The therapist can also explore whether a person's will plays any role in moral value. Consider a person who intentionally runs down a pedestrian versus a person who accidentally runs over someone who was jaywalking. Freeston and colleagues (1996) suggest that a mini-survey could be conducted in which close friends or family are asked whether they have ever had "bad thoughts." As well, individuals could be challenged to research whether the most moral person they know has ever had "bad thoughts," and if so, how frequently, and then whether this information calls into question his or her moral character. The opposite could be said of the client's most immoral person: that is, has he or she had "good thoughts," and if so, how often, and do these good thoughts cast the person in a better moral light? Together these cognitive interventions are intended to challenge clients with a TAF–Moral bias to shift their moral self-evaluation from their ability to prevent "bad thoughts" to a morality based on behavioral self-control.

Inflated Responsibility

A cognitive technique often used for inflated responsibility is the pie chart (Abramowitz, 2018; Salkovskis & Wahl, 2003; van Oppen & Arntz, 1994; Whittal & McLean, 2002; Wilhelm & Steketee, 2006). It begins with the therapist asking, "What is the percentage of responsibility you feel for the feared outcome associated with your obsession?" As before, it is emphasized that the initial estimate is based on what it feels like at the peak of the obsessional experience. For Darren and his obsession about contaminating others with bodily secretions, he might state that he felt 85% responsible for not cleaning a reddish speck on the lunchroom counter that could have been blood caused by a scratch on his arm. If coworkers touched this speck, they might get infected and become sick.

Next the client is asked to think about all the possible contributors to the feared outcome. In Darren's case, a coworker might become sick because she (1) caught the flu virus that was going around the office; (2) was caring for a sick child; (3) failed to get a seasonal flu shot; (4) caught it from a friend who had a severe cold; (5) failed to engage in appropriate personal hygiene; (6) had poor physical health related to diet, lack of exercise, or quality sleep; (7) was experiencing heightened stress at work; (8) had a preexisting chronic illness; (9) had a compromised immune system; or (10) was exposed to a reddish speck on the lunchroom counter that Darren failed to clean up.

A circle is drawn (i.e., pie chart), and the client is asked to place all possible contributors in the pie, with an estimate of the percentage of importance or responsibility of each contributor to the obsessional concern. Van Oppen and Arntz (1994) suggest that the client's own contribution should be the last estimate, with all the estimates adding up to 100%. The therapist then compares the client's initial responsibility estimate with the final estimate in the pie chart. Figure 8.4 illustrates a responsibility pie chart for Darren's belief that he is 85% responsible for making his coworkers sick by not cleaning the lunchroom counter after seeing a reddish speck that might be blood.

To obtain the full therapeutic benefit of the responsibility pie, Socratic questioning is employed to highlight what the client has learned from the exercise and how it can be used to counter faulty responsibility appraisals

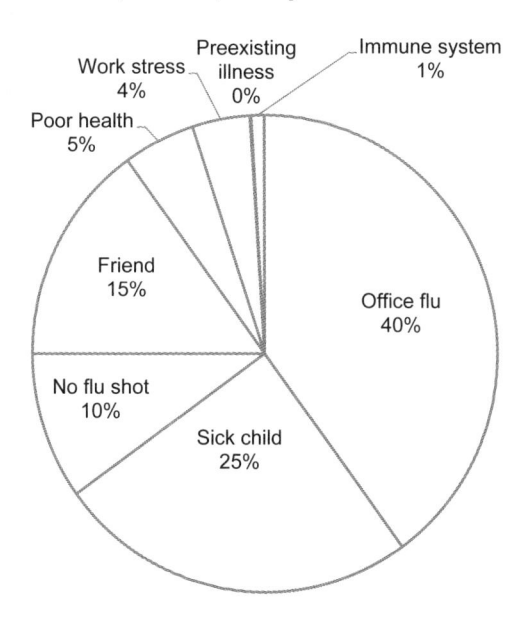

FIGURE 8.4. Darren's responsibility pie chart.

during an obsessional experience. Darren's therapist could pose the following questions:

"What do you make of the enormous difference between your initial responsibility estimate and the responsibility estimate that resulted from the exercise? Which do you think is more accurate, that is, more likely to be realistic?"

"When you think you are 85% responsible for a coworker's illness, how does this make you feel? How does it feed into your obsessive thinking?"

"When you do the responsibility pie exercise and realize your influence on making people sick is miniscule, how does that make you feel? If you reflected on the realistic estimate of your personal responsibility when you're stuck in obsessive thinking, do you think this could be another cognitive tool to lower the intensity of your obsessions and compulsions? Let's consider how you can use the responsibility pie chart effectively to deal with your obsessive–compulsive experiences."

After consolidating the exercise, the therapist could suggest a homework task in which clients record their success or difficulties in using the responsibility pie to correct faulty responsibility appraisals and beliefs.

Another cognitive intervention is the transfer-of-responsibility manipulation in which individuals are asked to temporarily transfer responsibility for their obsessional concern to the therapist for 1 week and then assume full responsibility the following week (Freeston et al., 1996; Rachman, 2003). During each week clients record the frequency, distress level, and their reactions to the obsession on a self-monitoring form. Once again, the therapist uses Socratic questioning to explore the effect of having full versus deferred responsibility on their obsessional experiences.

A third cognitive intervention is the courtroom role play in which clients assume the role of prosecuting attorney, who must use only empirical evidence (i.e., not feelings or speculation) to prove "beyond reasonable doubt" their guilt or responsibility for some negative event (Freeston et al., 1996; Wilhelm & Steketee, 2006). Next, the client (most often with the therapist's help) assumes the role of defense attorney, who argues for the client's "innocence" because the prosecutor failed to prove responsibility beyond reasonable doubt. Then the therapist and client take the perspective of judge or jury and consider the factual evidence presented by the prosecutor and the defense. This should result in an alternative perspective in which guilt or responsibility is assigned based on the factual evidence presented in the role play. This is a good exercise for highlighting the tenuous, even imagined, basis for the client's exaggerated responsibility interpretations. Wilhelm and Steketee (2006) emphasize that the courtroom technique will need to be repeated several times to be beneficial. Also, the role play must be executed in a gentle, empathic manner so there is no hint of a therapist–client debate.

Finally, Wilhelm and Steketee (2006) present two supplementary cognitive interventions for responsibility interpretations. In the double-standard technique, the therapist creates a two-column form on which the client lists all the reasons why he or she is responsible for an obsessional concern in the first column, and then in the second column lists all the reasons why a specific friend or family member would be responsible for the obsessional concern. For example, Darren could list all the reasons why he is responsible for coworkers' sickness, and then list all the reasons why Cynthia, one of his coworkers, is responsible for other people's sickness. The therapist then explores whether the client has one standard for him- or herself and another, more realistic standard for others.

Another intervention, which is a modification of the one described by Wilhelm and Steketee (2006), is the personal responsibility continuum. In this exercise a line is drawn with 0% (no personal responsibility) at the left end, 50% in the middle (moderate, shared responsibility), and 100% (complete personal responsibility) at the right end of the line. Clients are asked to list experiences, especially behaviors or actions, that qualify as 0%, 50%, and 100% personal responsibility. For example, under 0% Darren might list how others drive on his way to work, the mood state of his coworkers, the early morning traffic, etc. For 100% personal responsibility, he could list personal self-care, physical exercise, his diet, etc. Darren would probably discover that most of his experiences revolve around the 50% region of the continuum. Then clients are asked where they should place their obsessional concern on the personal responsibility continuum. This is a good exercise for highlighting the dimensional nature of responsibility, and the dangers inherent in committing the all-or-nothing cognitive error when determining personal responsibility. Therapists can use the exercise to point out the clients' ability to think normally about personal responsibility and assign reasonable responsibility interpretations to most of their daily experience. If clients erroneously place the obsessional concern too high on the responsibility continuum, the therapist can follow this with a cost–benefit analysis of exaggerating personal responsibility or review the responsibility pie chart to determine if clients are being realistic in their responsibility estimate.

Overimportance and Control of Thoughts

The main emphasis in these interventions is that faulty evaluations involve circular reasoning, with the construct being both a *cause* and a *consequence* of thought frequency. When an unwanted intrusive thought is evaluated as personally important, it will become more frequent, but this greater frequency will in turn strengthen the individual's belief that the thought must be important.

An intervention using a comparative list can be used to challenge the belief that "If the thought is frequent, it must be important" (see Whittal & McLean, 2002). The client is asked to generate examples of important nonobsessive thoughts (e.g., thinking about an impending medical test, not having an income tax return completed, the outcome of a job interview), and Socratic questioning is employed to determine how much the person dwells on these thoughts. A second list of unimportant nonobsessive thoughts is generated, and the extent that the individual thinks about these thoughts is noted. A final list of obsessional thoughts is produced, and the client is encouraged to evaluate the importance of these thoughts in comparison to those on the previous lists. The conclusion from this exercise is that the client's own experience indicates that the importance of a thought does not depend solely on its frequency. Because a thought occurs frequently does not mean it's important.

Another cognitive intervention that addresses appraisals of overimportance is based on verbal disputation. Freeston and colleagues (1996) emphasize that overimportance evaluations involve circular thinking based on "distorted Cartesian reasoning." They illustrate this circular thinking with this example: "People buy more of a particular brand of sausage[s] because they are fresh and they are fresh because people buy more" (pp. 437–438).

Using guided discovery, therapists can explore with clients how their experience with obsessions might involve a distorted reasoning process. The therapist asks whether it is more likely that appraisals of importance cause a preoccupation with the obsession, and not the reverse. Note that it is critical that these within-session cognitive exercises be followed by the empirical hypothesis-testing experiments discussed in the next chapter.

Wilhelm and Steketee (2006) discuss several other cognitive interventions that can be used to challenge overimportance appraisals. These include (1) the wise mind technique, in which the therapist helps clients catch their biased thinking and replace it with a more balanced blend of rational and emotional thinking; (2) metaphors illustrating how thinking (i.e., imagine something) can create feeling without being real; (3) the downward arrow technique, in which the therapist explores "what's the worst that can happen" in order to emphasize the irrationality of one's thinking; (4) consultation with an expert on whether the obsessive thought is important; and (5) double-standard, continuum, and cost–benefit exercises. All of these interventions are intended to help clients correct their assumption that the obsession must be significant because it is frequent.

CBT for OCD must include cognitive work on beliefs and appraisals of the need to control obsessions, as well as on the importance and effectiveness of neutralization efforts (Freeston & Ladouceur, 1997a; Salkovskis, 1999; Salkovskis & Wahl, 2003; Whittal & McLean, 2002). Appraisals and beliefs relevant to neutralization were discussed in Chapter 3, along with the role of mental control in OCD. The need to control beliefs and appraisals drives the excessive mental control effort that is a major construct in the generic CBT model (see Figure 5.1). The white bear suppression experiment and its variants, discussed extensively in the next chapter, are the most effective interventions with which to address this need to control thoughts. These interventions can be supplemented with Socratic questioning about the costs and benefits of excessive mental control efforts (Wilhelm & Steketee, 2006).

Another cognitive intervention for overcontrol of thought is to normalize spontaneous intrusive thought (Clark, 2018), as mentioned previously. To reiterate, this begins with a didactic discussion of "how the brain works," emphasizing that over 50% of normal brain function involves spontaneous, stimulus-independent thought (Christoff, 2012). Clients are encouraged to list examples of their positive and negative nonobsessive spontaneous thoughts. The following is an example of how the therapist can apply this cognitive work to an individual's overcontrol of thoughts.

> THERAPIST: I see from your list that you were able to identify a few examples of spontaneous thought. I notice some of these are positive, some are negative, and still others are just random, irrelevant thoughts. Were you aware that your brain generated so much spontaneous thought?

CLIENT: Of course, I've always known that I can be a spontaneous thinker. In fact, I often come up with good ideas that seem to appear out of nowhere.

THERAPIST: Do you think you can stop yourself from having spontaneous thoughts? Do you think it's possible for your brain to think only what you want it to think? In fact, would you even want to lose all your spontaneity?

CLIENT: No, even if it were possible, that might turn me into a type of robot. Maybe spontaneity is what makes us human.

THERAPIST: I agree. But what do you think that tells us about your obsessions and your need to control them? Aren't obsessions a type of very negative, spontaneous thought? Do you think you can stop your brain from generating obsessions? In fact, could you willfully make yourself have only good spontaneous thoughts?

CLIENT: That seems like an impossibility.

THERAPIST: True, but in case you have some doubts, what about doing the following exercise. One of the spontaneous thoughts you listed was "It's such a beautiful day." Over next week, each morning upon waking, remind yourself that you want your brain to spontaneously generate that thought. Now the thought must be spontaneous, so you can't try to think this way. It must pop into your mind automatically, without effort. Let's see what happens.

CLIENT: I already know the outcome. There's no way I can make myself have this spontaneous thought.

THERAPIST: Okay, but I suggest you give it a try. It's a good way to do some work on the limits of mental control.

It is important that work on the "normality of spontaneous thought" is followed by interventions that demonstrate the limits of thought dismissibility (see Chapter 9). Together with the cognitive strategies presented in this section, clients can learn that excessive effort to control their obsessions is counterproductive and only contributes to a persistence of their OCD.

Intolerance of Uncertainty/Perfectionism

Cognitive interventions for intolerance of uncertainty (IU) and perfectionism appraisals and beliefs focus on (1) demonstrating the impossibility of absolute certainty or perfectionism, (2) the negative impact of striving for certainty and perfection, and (3) evidence that individuals actually accept a considerable amount of uncertainty and imperfection in their daily living. Therapists will find treatment manuals on CBT for perfectionism (Egan et al., 2014; Shafran, Egan, & Wade, 2010) and intolerance of uncertainty (Dugas & Robichaud, 2006) helpful for treating these problems in OCD.

Cognitive therapy for IU and perfectionism begins with Socratic questioning to help clients understand both constructs. It is important to encourage individuals to be as specific as possible and to indicate how they know when strict or absolute certainty or perfectionism has been achieved with their obsessional concerns. Often clients have only vague, emotion-based notions of certainty and perfectionism, such as the comment "I just feel like I know it's okay to stop checking" or "It just feels good enough and I send the email" (see Chapter 3 on stop criteria). The therapist can explore whether clients have more lenient certainty and perfectionism criteria that operate in other areas of their life. A comparison of the advantages/disadvantages of strict versus lenient criteria is made, and clients are encouraged to construct more lenient certainty/perfectionism criteria when they experience obsessions and compulsions.

In a second cognitive intervention, clients are asked to recall the most memorable times when they were certain of an action or decision, or when they acted perfectly. Each certain and perfect incident is evaluated in terms of the advantages and disadvantages of such appraisals. In other words:

> "What was the consequence or outcome of that certain or perfect performance?"
> "How much effort was involved to achieve the certainty or perfection you desired?"
> "In retrospect, was it worth the effort?"
> "What advantage or positive outcome was associated with the certainty or perfect state?"
> "Were there any costs or disadvantages associated with striving for certainty or perfection in this specific situation?"

By asking for specific examples of efforts to achieve certainty and/or perfectionism, the therapist is challenging the clients' belief that they can't stand to be uncertain or that it's always better to keep trying until its perfect.

Clients are then asked to recall significant experiences in which certainty or perfection was not achieved and they had to live with doubt. Again, the therapist probes the positive and negative consequences of tolerating uncertainty and imperfection. The therapist should also explore the frequency with which certainty and perfection are achieved, as well as how much effort is involved in striving for these difficult goals. The objective of this intervention is to bring clients to the realization that certainty and perfection are rarely achieved, and so they are tolerating uncertainty and imperfection better than they realized. The cognitive restructuring exercise concludes with a cost–benefit analysis: "Is striving for certainty and perfection really worthwhile?"; "On balance, do the costs far outweigh the benefits?" If clients agree that the appraisals of uncertainty and perfection are not beneficial, their agreement provides additional impetus for constructing a more accepting perspective on uncertainty and imperfection.

Intolerance of Anxiety/Distress

Although the appraisals and beliefs associated with high anxiety or distress sensitivity are transdiagnostic to the anxiety disorders, they do play an important role in the persistence of obsessions and can undermine compliance with ERP (Freeston et al., 1996; Rachman, 1998). Intolerance of anxiety involves beliefs (1) that anxiety will lead to serious or threatening consequences, (2) that one cannot function or perform while anxious, and (3) that anxiety or distress must be kept to an absolute minimum level. Rachman (1998) noted that intolerance of anxiety often involves *ex-consequentia reasoning* (Arntz, Rauner, & van den Hout, 1995), in which a person deduces the presence of threat or danger from the feeling of anxiousness (e.g., "I'm feeling anxious so there must be something threatening about this situation").

The most effective interventions for intolerance of anxiety/distress are exposure-based exercises that generate elevated anxiety levels. Nevertheless, some prior cognitive work is needed to strengthen the client's resolve to tackle his or her intolerance appraisals and beliefs. This work begins with Socratic questioning to discover the client's thoughts and appraisals about experiencing elevated anxiety/distress and its consequences.

> "When you left the house and felt anxious about whether the door was truly locked or not, what were your concerns about being so anxious?"
> "Did the anxiety last as long as you expected?"
> "How did the anxiety affect your ability to function?"
> "Was there any direct consequence for allowing your anxiety to remain elevated longer than normal?"
> "What were you like 2 hours [4 hours, etc.] after leaving the house?"

Individuals can be asked to keep a diary of their obsessive–compulsive-related and non-obsessive–compulsive-related anxiety/distress experiences and how hard they tried to lower or eliminate their negative emotional state versus let the anxiety dissipate on its own. As well, the diary could include a column in which the consequences of the anxiety experience are recorded. The diary becomes the basis for applying the downward arrow technique to determine how close the client came to experiencing his or her catastrophic outcome (Wilhelm & Steketee, 2006). In addition, tolerance of obsessive–compulsive-related and non-obsessive–compulsive-related anxiety can be compared to determine if the client is more resilient to anxiety/distress when it's not related to obsessional concerns. Darren, for example, might feel like the anxiety would "nearly drive him crazy" if he didn't complete his washing compulsion and feel some relief from the distress caused by the "semen obsession." As a homework assignment, Darren could be asked to vary the length of time between the obsession and the washing compulsion to collect data on his ability to tolerate anxiety and its imagined consequences. Socratic questioning is used to explore whether obsessive–compulsive-related anxiety could be tolerated more like non-obsessive–compulsive-related anxiety, knowing that the consequences are not as dire as expected. Discussion could focus on whether the client's strategies for tolerating non-obsessive–compulsive-related anxiety/distress could be transferred to situations involving obsessive–compulsive-related anxiety/distress. At the very least, work on the client's beliefs about anxiety/distress is a useful therapeutic strategy for dealing with heightened anticipatory anxiety and reluctance to engage in ERP homework.

Generating Alternative Interpretations

Cognitive therapy for OCD does not end with cognitive restructuring interventions, followed by exposure-based empirical hypothesis-testing experiments. It is critical that individuals adopt an alternative, more adaptive explanation for their obsessional concerns to obtain maximum benefit from the behavioral interventions. If clients are to accept the idea that their faulty appraisals and beliefs about obsessions are erroneous, then they must adopt a different framework for understanding the persistence of their symptoms.

Cognitive restructuring of faulty obsessive–compulsive beliefs should culminate in a new, less threatening understanding of the obsession, in which it is the *interpretation* of the obsession, rather than its mere occurrence, that is responsible for the persistence of OCD (Salkovskis & Freeston, 2001). In addition, this alternative perspective must be contrary to the faulty interpretation so that accepting one view requires rejection of the other. Handout 8.4 presents alternative explanations that are contrary to the faulty appraisals found in OCD.

The overriding theme of the alternative interpretations is that unwanted intrusive thoughts involving the client's obsessional concerns (e.g., dirt, disease, doubt, unintended harm) are a normal part of brain function that produces spontaneous thought. The unintended and sudden appearance of such thoughts reflects benign, meaningless, and personally insignificant "mental chatter." Its existence can be acknowledged but requires no action. The goal is to accept the mental chatter in the form of unwanted mental intrusion, appraise it as meaningless, and desist from any effort to intentionally control it. The anxiety and distress associated with the intrusion is due to faulty appraisals of significance and neutralization efforts. In this phase of treatment, the therapist works with the client to develop a narrative (or explanation) of the insignificance of the obsession that incorporates unique aspects of the client's experience with OCD (Clark, 2018).

A good alternative explanation will have several characteristics. First, it must be tailored to the idiosyncratic content and meaning of the person's obsession. Standard explanations are less effective in countering the client's faulty appraisals of the obsession. For example, a young woman with harming obsessions believed that her frequent thoughts about whether she could lose control and sexually assault an innocent person were evidence that she might be a "latent rapist" (overimportance of thought appraisal). Her alternative explanation was that she had frequent "rape-related thoughts" because she was an overly sensitive and conscientious person who was especially offended by such thoughts, and so paid more attention to them. Notice that the alternative interpretation fits with the explanation offered in Handout 8.4, but is tailored to the client's obsessional content.

Second, it is important to develop the alternative interpretation/narrative through collaborative guided discovery (see Padesky & Greenberger, 1995). The client is less likely to consider alternative interpretations that are dictated by the therapist. In this regard, it may be useful to do some cognitive and behavioral intervention on the faulty appraisals and beliefs prior to introducing an alternative interpretation. However, at least some of the interventions should involve a test between the adaptive and maladaptive appraisals. In the aforementioned example, a behavioral experiment was set up to gather evidence that the woman had "unconscious motives to rape" versus being "hypersensitive to thoughts of hurting another person." Rachman (2003) provides guidelines on how to collect new information that therapist and client can use to construct alternative interpretations of the significance of obsessions.

Finally, the alternative explanation needs to emphasize that anxiety and distress are caused by misinterpreting the obsessions as a personally significant threat and trying too hard to exert conscious control over them through neutralization and other mental control efforts. If individuals can accept the idea that their unwanted thoughts, images, or impulses are harmless, irrelevant, even silly phenomena that require no response, then a more adaptive perspective is developed that will counter future obsessional tendencies. The following illustrates an alternative explanation for Darren's "semen obsessions":

> "I know that I am a highly creative, imaginative person who has lots of weird, strange thoughts pop into my mind. One of those wild thoughts is that others could become ill because they became exposed to microscopic traces of my bodily secretions, especially semen. If I've had sexual activity, the semen intrusion is rampant in my mind. Of course, what young man hasn't occasionally wondered about semen 'leakage' on his clothing?
>
> "However, I've become totally preoccupied and anxious about this because I completely overthink the dangerousness, importance, and need to control the thought. I've developed cleansing rituals which only make the problem worse because I've convinced myself that I've got to assert control over my mind. In real life, I know it may not even

be possible to get sick from accidental contact with semen molecules. This is just another of my wild imaginative thoughts, like alien abductions, living in an alternate reality, and 'What if I'm a zombie?' Like these other bizarre musings of my mind, I can learn to smile at the 'semen obsession' and say to myself, 'There I go again, that wild imaginative brain.' There is no need to do anything when I have the obsession. In fact, trying to counteract the thought only makes it worse. Better to acknowledge the thought and then get on with living, no matter how anxious I feel."

CONCLUSION

Treatment goal setting, educating the client about the CBT model, and cognitive restructuring interventions are critical treatment components that are implemented before introducing exposure-based behavioral interventions. Each is a key element of standard cognitive therapy for the emotional disorders but modified and refined to address unique features of OCD. Treatment goal setting may be more challenging in OCD because individuals often enter therapy with expectations that are contrary to the goals and objectives of the CBT perspective. It is important that therapists address these conflicting expectations to minimize client resistance, homework noncompliance, and risk of premature treatment termination.

Educating clients about the CBT perspective involves Socratic questioning, didactic illustrations, and experiential exercises that highlight key elements of the CBT model: the normalization of unwanted intrusive thoughts or obsessions, the role of faulty appraisals and beliefs, the deleterious effects of neutralization, and the futility of excessive mental control. Psychoeducation dominates the early therapy sessions but is less emphasized as treatment progresses. The educational phase of therapy seeks to provide clients with a solid treatment rationale that will promote greater engagement in the therapy process.

Once the CBT model and treatment rationale are understood, clients are introduced to appraisal self-monitoring to increase their sensitivity to and awareness of faulty appraisals and beliefs in the pathogenesis of obsessions. This new awareness sets the stage for cognitive restructuring interventions that focus on modification of obsessive–compulsive appraisals and beliefs. Several sessions of cognitive restructuring culminate in the adoption of a healthier, acceptance-based perspective on obsessions and cessation of the compulsion. By weakening the faulty obsessive–compulsive appraisals and beliefs through cognitive interventions, a therapeutic context is created that boosts the effectiveness of exposure-based empirical hypothesis-testing experiments, which is the topic of the next chapter.

FORM 8.1. Cognitive Appraisal Worksheet

Instructions: Use this worksheet to record actual experiences of the obsession in your daily life. Consult your case formulation and the questions your therapist asked to determine what made the obsession an important, highly personal threat in each instance. You can also refer to the Obsessions and Compulsions Experience Form to review your OCD experiences (Form 7.1).

Date	Trigger (situation)	Unwanted Intrusion (i.e., obsession)	Importance, Personal Significance of the Intrusion	Control Response (e.g., compulsion, neutralization)

From *Cognitive-Behavioral Therapy for OCD and Its Subtypes, Second Edition*, by David A. Clark. Copyright © 2020 The Guilford Press. Permission to photocopy this material is granted to purchasers of this book for personal use or use with individual clients (see copyright page for details). Purchasers can download enlarged versions of this material (see the box at the end of the table of contents).

HANDOUT 8.1. Selected List of Unwanted Intrusive Thoughts

- When leaving the house/apartment, thoughts of not turning off the stove, leaving lights on, not locking the door, etc.
- While driving, a sudden impulse to veer into oncoming traffic.
- The thought that I could get or give someone a sexually transmitted disease from something I touched (e.g., toilet seat, door handle).
- The thought of blurting out a rude or insulting comment to someone I'm talking to (i.e., tell the person what I really think).
- The thought or image of having sex in a public place.
- While driving, the thought "Did I accidentally hit another car, pedestrian, or cyclist?"
- When seeing a sharp knife, the thought of stabbing the person next to me.
- When in a public place, the thought that I'm becoming dirty or contaminated from touching things other people touched, like door handles, chairs, tables, benches, etc.
- The thought of losing control and doing something embarrassing, like exposing myself or yelling profanities.
- An unwanted thought or image of having unwanted sex with an authority figure (e.g., teacher, manager) or someone disgusting.
- The impulse to jump in front of a car or train even though I'm not suicidal.
- While holding a baby, the thought of accidentally dropping him or her.
- The thought that something terrible is going to happen because of a mistake or omission on my part.
- The thought that I could make a friend or family member sick because of a careless act.
- The thought that I've forgotten something important.
- A repulsive, disgusting, or immoral thought or image of sex or violence that pops into my mind.
- A blasphemous or profane thought against God, the Bible, or other sacred texts.
- A sudden thought or impulse to violently attack or even kill someone.
- A sudden thought of being in danger even though I'm in a safe place.

Note. Based on Clark (2004) and Steketee and Barlow (2002).

From *Cognitive-Behavioral Therapy for OCD and Its Subtypes, Second Edition,* by David A. Clark. Copyright © 2020 The Guilford Press. Permission to photocopy this material is granted to purchasers of this book for personal use or use with individual clients (see copyright page for details). Purchasers can download enlarged versions of this material (see the box at the end of the table of contents).

HANDOUT 8.2. Examples of Faulty Appraisals Involved in the Persistence of Obsessions

Obsession	Interpretation of Obsession	Specific Appraisals
I have a strict routine and sequence of activities that must be followed before going to bed. If this routine is not followed, I will redo until correct.	"The thought of following a strict bedtime routine is important because if I don't, I become quite anxious and can't fall asleep. If I don't get my sleep, then I am more likely to get sick and vomit. If I'm sick, then I'll miss a lot of school and be a burden on others."	1. *Overestimation of threat.* "If I lose sleep, I'll get sick." 2. *Perfection.* "Specific bedtime routine must be followed." 3. *Responsibility.* "I need to avoid getting sick so as not to burden others." 4. *Intolerance of anxiety.* "I can't let myself get anxious."
The thought that my boyfriend could be harmed and so I engage in repeating rituals.	"If something were to happen to him, it would be my fault for thinking that he would be harmed. Also, these thoughts make me feel so anxious. In the past I worried a lot about people getting hurt, so it's important I don't let my thoughts get that bad again."	1. *Thought–action fusion.* "Thinking about harm seems to make it more likely to happen." 2. *Responsibility.* "I need to do something to ensure that harm does not come to my boyfriend." 3. *Need for control.* "I need to control these thoughts so they don't get worse."
The thought of whether I had been sexually touched by a teenage babysitter when I was a preschooler. In response, I would repeat verbal phrases over and over or redo activities again and again (e.g., retrace my steps).	"The thought makes me suffer great anxiety, and so I need to repeat whatever I am doing at the time I have the thought. If I can repeat the action over and over until I don't have the obsession, then the connection between the thought and my action is broken. If I don't do this, more and more things will trigger the thought, causing me to have more obsessions. Eventually, I'll become so absorbed in the obsession and overwhelmed with anxiety that I'll have a nervous breakdown."	1. *Overimportance.* "A thought of the possibility that I was touched sexually as a child becomes my most important thought." 2. *Need for control.* "I need to ensure that the thought does not become more frequent." 3. *Neutralization.* "I need to cancel out the effects of the thought by repeating the action associated with it." 4. *Overestimated threat.* "The thought will escalate until I have a nervous breakdown." 5. *Intolerance of uncertainty.* "I have to repeat a phrase or action over and over until I'm certain that I've done it perfectly without having the obsession."

From *Cognitive-Behavioral Therapy for OCD and Its Subtypes, Second Edition*, by David A. Clark. Copyright © 2020 The Guilford Press. Permission to photocopy this material is granted to purchasers of this book for personal use or use with individual clients (see copyright page for details). Purchasers can download enlarged versions of this material (see the box at the end of the table of contents).

HANDOUT 8.3. Definitions of Faulty Appraisals

Type of Appraisal	Explanation	Examples
Overestimated threat	To overestimate the severity and/or likelihood that a highly negative, even catastrophic, consequence of the obsession could occur. As a result, the obsession represents a serious threat to personal well-being.	1. "If I shake a stranger's hand, then I will contract a fatal disease." 2. "If I leave the car unlocked, then someone will steal it." 3. "If I feel even a little physical discomfort, this means I must be getting seriously sick."
Thought–action fusion	To assume that thinking about a negative event increases the likelihood that the negative event will happen, or that "bad" thoughts are morally equal to "bad" deeds.	1. "If I think something evil, it is more likely to happen." 2. "If I think (or imagine) that a person is having an accident, he or she is more likely to have one." 3. "Thinking that I might have sexually touched a child is almost as bad as doing it." 4. "If I think I've made a mistake, it is more likely that I really have made a mistake."
Inflated responsibility	To hold oneself responsible to prevent a perceived negative outcome that could have a real or imagined consequence for the self or for others. The person believes that he or she has influence over the negative outcome and therefore is responsible for that outcome.	1. "If I see a piece of broken glass on the road, I must pick it up. If I don't, it would be my fault if a car ran over the glass and had an accident." 2. "If I do something wrong, God will punish me by making other people sick." 3. "I must make sure that I don't contaminate other people."
Overimportance of thought	To assume that a highly persistent unwanted thought must have some significance for the self because it occurs so frequently against one's will.	1. "I must be very susceptible to disease and illness because I am preoccupied with avoiding contamination." 2. "If I have violent and aggressive thoughts against people, maybe deep down I want to harm them." 3. "Because I so frequently have blasphemous thoughts against God, I must be an evil person or demon possessed." 4. "If I continually wonder if I've done things in the right and correct way, maybe it is because I have to be extra concerned about carelessness."

(continued)

From *Cognitive-Behavioral Therapy for OCD and Its Subtypes, Second Edition*, by David A. Clark. Copyright © 2020 The Guilford Press. Permission to photocopy this material is granted to purchasers of this book for personal use or use with individual clients (see copyright page for details). Purchasers can download enlarged versions of this material (see the box at the end of the table of contents).

Definitions of Faulty Appraisals *(page 2 of 2)*

Type of Appraisal	Explanation	Examples
Control of thoughts	To assume that it is possible and highly desirable to have near-perfect control over unwanted thoughts in order to avoid negative consequences.	1. "If I don't get better control over these obsessions, I will become overwhelmed with anxiety." 2. "If I do a better job of controlling my obsessions, this means I am less likely to act on them." 3. "If I don't control these thoughts, they will eventually drive me 'crazy.'"
Intolerance of uncertainty	To assume that it is critical to achieve almost absolute or perfect certainty in thought or action in order to maximize predictability and control. Ambiguity, newness, change, or not knowing should be avoided because they can increase anxiety and stress.	1. "If I feel any doubt about a decision, I must keep going over and over it until I am convinced beyond doubt that the decision was the right one." 2. "I must have proof, a guarantee that I am a peaceful person and not capable of rape." 3. "I need to be certain that I did not make a mistake on that form." 4. "It is critical that there is no possibility of contamination in my house (or apartment)."
Perfectionism	To assume that it is possible and highly desirable to strive for the one best response to each problem or situation. Even minor mistakes and inaccuracies must be avoided because they can lead to serious consequences.	1. "It is important that I find the 'perfect' gift for every special occasion." 2. "I can answer 'yes' to a questionnaire item only if it describes me perfectly in every situation." 3. "I should never have a bad or sinful thought against God or other people." 4. "I must ensure that there is not even a speck of dirt in my room that could contaminate me."
Intolerance of anxiety or distress	To assume that anxiety or distress is bad because it may have harmful consequences. Therefore, every effort should be made to avoid feeling anxious or to reduce anxiety as soon as it occurs.	1. "I can't stand this anxiety much longer." 2. "If I am bothered or upset by an unwanted intrusive thought, then I have to do something to relieve the anxiety." 3. "I'm afraid the anxiety and distress will get worse if I don't deal with these reactions when I first feel them."

HANDOUT 8.4. The Alternative Perspective

Type of Appraisal	Faulty Interpretation	Adaptive Alternative Interpretation
Overestimated threat	Anything that elicits the obsession will increase the possibility of highly undesirable consequences.	Situations are safe unless there is external, real-life evidence of actual threat or danger. Having thoughts and feelings about the possibility of imagined negative consequences does not mean that real-life negative outcomes are more certain.
Thought–action fusion (TAF)	*Likelihood TAF.* The occurrence of the obsession increases the probability that a negative event will happen. *Moral TAF.* Having "bad" thoughts is as immoral as acting on these thoughts.	*Likelihood TAF.* Thoughts cannot have a direct causal influence on events in the real world. *Moral TAF.* Moral character is based on what we do and not on what we think.
Inflated responsibility	Because a person thinks about the possibility of the occurrence of harm, that person is primarily responsible for preventing the possible harm occurring to self or others.	All real-life negative events involve multiple factors that cause them to happen. As a result, responsibility is distributed across many contributing factors, with one person's contribution to the event often playing a very minor, practically insignificant role. Because an individual's influence over a possible negative event is so limited, his or her responsibility to prevent that event is minimal, if not practically nonexistent.
Overimportance of thought	Persistent obsessions must be very important because they signify some undesirable inner motive or potential.	Because obsessions involve themes that are completely contrary or alien to a person's cherished values and inclinations, a person tends to give them undue attention. Just dwelling on a thought can raise its perceived importance.

(continued)

From *Cognitive-Behavioral Therapy for OCD and Its Subtypes, Second Edition*, by David A. Clark. Copyright © 2020 The Guilford Press. Permission to photocopy this material is granted to purchasers of this book for personal use or use with individual clients (see copyright page for details). Purchasers can download enlarged versions of this material (see the box at the end of the table of contents).

The Alternative Perspective *(page 2 of 2)*

Type of Appraisal	Faulty Interpretation	Adaptive Alternative Interpretation
Control of thoughts	Failing to exert strong and effective control over the obsession will lead to highly undesirable negative consequences.	Great effort at controlling an unwanted thought will cause an increase in its frequency, salience, and associated distress. By relinquishing effort to exert mental control over the obsession, ultimately less attention is devoted to the thought and the personal importance of the thought is downgraded.
Intolerance of uncertainty	One must strive to achieve absolute certainty in thought and/or action to reduce doubt, ambiguity, and the possibility of negative outcomes, which, in turn, elicits anxiety or distress.	Uncertainty is inevitable and cannot be completely eliminated. It is the striving for certainty (or the complete eradication of doubt) that elevates anxiety and perceived dangerousness rather than the presence of some degree of uncertainty.
Perfectionism	One must strive to achieve a perfect response or solution to every problem or situation to avoid the serious consequences that occur because of minor mistakes and inaccuracies.	Minor mistakes, inaccuracies, or flaws are an inevitable aspect of all human endeavors and do not result in serious negative consequences. Anxiousness and distress are products of striving for that which cannot be attained—absolute perfection. The alternative is a person's best performance that meets the requirements of a situation.
Intolerance of anxiety/distress	If anxiety or distress is not reduced or eliminated, it will lead to harmful consequences.	Anxiety and fear are natural human emotions that are integral to being alive. A person can adapt to varying levels of short-term anxiety without harmful long-term consequences.

CHAPTER 9

Empirical Hypothesis-Testing Experiments

CBT therapists recognize that experientially based interventions must be included in the treatment protocol for effective treatment of OCD. Most of these interventions involve varying elements of ERP, which was discussed extensively in Chapter 4. This chapter presents specific behavioral exercises designed as hypothesis-testing experiments to evaluate dysfunctional obsessive–compulsive appraisals and beliefs, as well as their healthier alternatives. When integrated with cognitive interventions, empirical hypothesis testing is often the most potent ingredient in creating significant therapeutic change. CBT therapists often use cognitive restructuring to prepare clients for the crucial exposure-based hypothesis-testing experiments described in this chapter.

BEHAVIORAL EXPERIMENTATION

Empirical hypothesis testing is the backbone of CBT for OCD. Beck and colleagues (1979) noted that behavioral interventions are introduced to the client as mini-experiments that test the validity of dysfunctional thoughts and beliefs to bring about cognitive change. In CBT for obsessions and compulsions, behavioral experiments are introduced along with cognitive restructuring, once clients learn how to identify their faulty appraisals and beliefs. Table 9.1 summarizes 25 experiential experiments often utilized in CBT for OCD.

Behavioral interventions are always introduced in a collaborative manner (see Chapter 6) and tailored to the client's idiosyncratic obsessional concerns. Experientially based experiments that provide disconfirming

TABLE 9.1. Select Empirical Hypothesis-Testing Experiments for Obsessive–Compulsive Appraisals

Type of appraisal	Hypothesis-testing experiment
Overestimated threat	*Risk assessment.* Record real-life evidence of increased risk after threat exposure.
	Threat prediction. Write down the anticipated (expected, predicted) adverse consequence associated with exposure to an obsessional concern, engage in exposure, and then record the real-life consequence of the exposure.
	Threat survey. Interview acquaintances and/or do an online search of information concerning actual harm or danger related to the primary obsession.
	Atypical exposure. Engage in exposure that involves some unusual behavior outside normal activity to test a specific belief about negative consequences (see also Chapter 4 on inhibitory learning).
TAF	*Premonitions experiment.* At the beginning of the day, imagine that a specific person will contact you during the day and then record whether there is an increase in contacts from this person throughout the day.
	Intrusions survey. Conduct a survey of trusted friends and family on the types of unwanted intrusive thoughts they experience.
	Power of thoughts. Begin the day by forming a specific thought about a positive or neutral event and record whether the event occurs. This is followed by thinking about bad things happening to therapist, friends, or self and recording the outcome.
	Cognitive risk. Increase the frequency and duration of ruminating on unwanted thoughts and record any evidence of increased tendency for negative outcomes.
Inflated responsibility	*Responsibility manipulation.* Record frequency of obsession and associated distress during a high- versus low-personal-responsibility week.
	Responsibility gradient. Exposure to a hierarchy of successively greater responsibility for tasks involving the primary obsessional concern.
Overimportance of thoughts	*Artificial importance.* For 1 week attend closely to some innocuous external stimulus (e.g., HOUSE FOR SALE signs) and then refrain from attending to the target stimulus the following week.
	Importance manipulation. Select a nonobsessional intrusive thought, give it full concentration for 30 seconds, and then rate its perceived importance and distress. Repeat the exercise, but this time embellish its significance, and again rate its importance and distress.

(continued)

TABLE 9.1. *(continued)*

Type of appraisal	Hypothesis-testing experiment
Overimportance of thoughts *(continued)*	*Inflated significance.* Deliberately think about the obsession for a short interval (10 seconds) and rate its perceived importance and distress. Then think about the obsession a second time for a longer interval (60 seconds) and again rate its perceived importance and distress.
	Attentive days task. On alternate days attend closely to the obsession, recording its frequency, associated anxiety, and any other outcomes. On the remaining days let the obsession go, as if it were an unimportant intrusive thought.
Control of thoughts	*White bear experiment.* This begins by suppressing a neutral thought for 2 minutes and recording the number of thought occurrences. Next, a non-obsessive–compulsive but important thought (e.g., current worry) is suppressed for 2 minutes, and thought recurrences are recorded. Finally, suppression is attempted on the primary obsession for the same time interval, and thought recurrences are recorded.
	Alternate control days. On alternate days intentional mental control of an obsession is suspended and compared to remaining days when engaged in usual obsessive–compulsive controlled responses.
	Mental control holiday. Take a 1-day break from vigilance and control of the obsession in order to focus on more productive activities (Rachman, 2003).
Intolerance of uncertainty	*Certainty survey.* Conduct a survey of friends, family, and work colleagues on their certainty about remembering whether routine actions were performed (e.g., stove turned off, door locked).
	Certainty manipulation. Record level of certainty and remembering for routine non-obsessive–compulsive activities (e.g., brushed teeth, vacuumed house completely). Then select one of these tasks and increase the effort to be certain, recording success of certainty and associated distress throughout the exercise.
	Uncertainty exposure. Obsessive–compulsive-related tasks are performed, or decisions made, in a manner that results in low, moderate, or high levels of uncertainty. The costs and benefits associated with exposure to varying levels of uncertainty are noted, as well as one's ability to tolerate uncertainty.
Perfectionism	*Cost–benefit analysis.* Several key tasks at work or at home are selected that elicit perfectionism. Task completion is assigned, and ratings are obtained on levels of perfectionism, effort, and distress associated with each occurrence. A "calculation" is made of the extra time and effort needed to obtain a specified increment in perfection.

(continued)

TABLE 9.1. *(continued)*

Type of appraisal	Hypothesis-testing experiment
Perfectionism *(continued)*	*Perfectionism observation.* A friend or work colleague admired for their productivity and success is selected and his or her level of perfection in key tasks is observed and rated. The therapist explores whether the gold standard of "absolute perfection" was achieved and how often. Were flaws or shortcomings evident? If so, what effect did these flaws or shortcomings have on the final outcome? Did the person focus on absolute perfection or settle for a lower standard, such as meeting the requirements of the situation?
	Intentional errors. Obsessive–compulsive-related tasks are performed with the intentional inclusion of some minor flaw or inaccuracy. The consequences of the flawed performances are recorded.
	Instructed checking. Perform tasks associated with obsessional concerns with varying levels of repeating and redoing, and rate the accuracy of the task performance and the certainty of achieving a flawless outcome.
Intolerance of anxiety or distress	*Anxiety survey.* Friends or family members are interviewed about their experiences with feeling anxious, nervous, or fearful. How common was anxiety in this survey? What was it like for your interviewees? How did they cope with it and what were the outcomes?
	Anxiety monitoring. People are observed in a variety of situations and a judgment is made about their anxiety level. What was observed that suggested a person was anxious? What was the intensity level of the anxiety? What effect did it have on the person's performance or the outcome of the task?
	Anxiety comparison. A comparison is made between the anxiety experienced while performing a nonobsessional but anxious task (e.g., giving a work presentation) and the obsessional task.
	Anxiety prediction. Prior to exposure, a prediction is made about anticipated anxiety and its effects. Next, the exposure exercise is implemented and the actual anxiety and its effects are recorded. Comparisons are made between predicted and actual levels of anxiety.

Note. Material based on Freeston and Ladouceur (1997a), Freeston et al. (1996), Rachman (1998), Salkovskis (1999), and Whittal and McLean (2002).

evidence for the faulty appraisal and support for the alternative explanation will be the most effective interventions. It is important that therapists spend time in the follow-up session exploring the client's experience with a behavioral assignment to maximize its therapeutic benefit. In fact, therapists often return to the client's experience with an assignment in subsequent sessions so that significant insights gained through behavioral experimentation can be reinforced (e.g., "Recall the experiment you did a few weeks ago, in which you tried to suppress the obsession on some days and not on other days. Do you remember the outcome of that experiment?"). The behavioral exercises summarized in Table 9.1 are briefly described in the following sections (see also Abramowitz, 2018; Clark, 2018; Rachman, 2003; Wilhelm & Steketee, 2006).

Overestimated Threat

Exposure-based interventions are well suited to evaluate the exaggerated probability and severity of negative consequences associated with obsessional concerns and to determine whether obsessive–compulsive situations are safer than assumed. Table 9.1 includes four types of hypothesis-testing experiments that may be particularly effective with this type of faulty appraisal. The *risk assessment exercise* involves gathering real-life evidence of increased risk or danger after completing an exposure task. For example, those with physical contamination obsessions could be asked to push elevator buttons or hold a stairwell rail with their bare hands and then abstain from any handwashing behavior afterward. Clients are asked to record any signs of feeling sick or unwell that might suggest contamination (e.g., sore throat, coughing, aches, or pains). The therapist emphasizes that the absence of empirical evidence of danger indicates that the client is using "emotion-based criteria" for determining risk, which leads to the exaggerated threat appraisals that contribute to obsessive–compulsive symptom escalation. By shifting to empirically based evidence, the client can downgrade the threat and arrive at a more balanced interpretation that recognizes safety as the more likely outcome in otherwise obsessive–compulsive situations.

Threat prediction interventions are often used in CBT for anxiety disorders (Clark & Beck, 2010). In this intervention clients are asked to make a prediction of what they think will happen if they engage in an exposure task. (This is similar to the modifications to ERP discussed in Chapter 4 under inhibitory learning.) In the case of physical contamination, clients could be asked to describe what they think will happen if they hold onto public staircase railings with their bare hands. For maximum effectiveness, it is better that the anticipated narrative is generated in a prior therapy session. The therapist keeps this record, asks clients to engage in the exposure, and then has them write down their actual experience (Forms 4.5 and 4.6 can be used for this purpose). In the subsequent therapy session, the anticipated and actual records can be compared. When the anticipated or predicted outcome is much worse than the actual experience, this becomes evidence that the client is exaggerating the threat or danger associated with the obsessive–compulsive concern. The following is a hypothetical dialogue illustrating how the threat prediction experiment can be interpreted in a therapeutic manner.

> THERAPIST: I see from the two records that you expected a much worse outcome from holding the handrail with your bare hands than you experienced. What do you make of the fact that your anxiety and urge to wash your hands were much less than you expected?
>
> CLIENT: Yeah, I surprised myself. I did a lot better than I expected.
>
> THERAPIST: Absolutely. I congratulate you on doing so well with this assignment. Clearly, you're really determined to break the cycle of OCD. Given how you responded in this experiment, do you think it's possible that you're anticipating more problems than you'll experience in real life? If so, what effect do you think this negative anticipation is having on your OCD?
>
> CLIENT: Sure, I get it. I probably anticipate the worst all the time and then I really feel anxious.
>
> THERAPIST: I agree. This is a good example of exaggerating the danger, and when we exaggerate danger, it drives up our anxiety. In OCD it also makes the urge to wash stronger and harder to resist. So one of the skills you'll want to learn is to catch yourself when you're exaggerating some upcoming danger and replace it with more realistic expectations so you'll feel less anxious and more likely to do exposure experiences. Is this an important lesson to take away from this exercise?
>
> CLIENT: I agree that my negative expectations are a problem, but I think this will be a hard habit to break. I seem to do this all the time and not just with my OCD.
>
> THERAPIST: Breaking the habit of exaggerated threat predictions *is* difficult, but I've helped others with this problem. It takes awareness of the problem and lots of willingness and practice. Do you want to get started?
>
> CLIENT: Sure.

Forms 9.1A and 9.1B are worksheets specifically designed for the threat prediction experiment. They contain detailed instructions and questions that clients can use to generate their predicted experience and then record their actual experiences with an exposure assignment.

A third experiment, the *threat survey,* is useful for individuals with harm and injury obsessions and checking compulsions (see Rachman, 2003; Steketee, 1999). In this intervention clients are asked to interview acquaintances and/or do web-based searches for statistics or other recorded information on, for example, the number of houses burglarized because of unlocked doors, houses that catch fire because of leaving lights on, cancer that is contracted by using public toilets, children who are stabbed by their mothers using a kitchen knife, children or strangers sexually assaulted by persons who suddenly lose control of themselves, and the like. Even if the client finds evidence that on very rare occasions an obsessional concern led to the feared outcome, data can be collected on the most likely route to the negative event (e.g., most frequent cause of house fires, etiology of cancer, characteristics of sexual predators). Evidence can also be gathered on the frequency with which the obsessional concern does not lead to the negative outcome (e.g., number of times people shake hands without getting a disease, how many times lights are left on and houses don't catch fire, how often drivers back out of driveways and don't run over a pedestrian). The therapist uses threat survey data to highlight the client's exaggerated threat appraisals of the obsessional fear and its consequences. If the client starts to debate about whether the survey results indicate that the obsessional concern could happen, the therapist returns to the main purpose of the experiment: "Would you agree that the survey indicates that you are overestimating the probability and severity of the obsessional fear, and when this happens, you end up feeling more anxious and your OCD gets worse?"

A final threat-based experiment is an *atypical exposure,* in which the client performs an exposure task to test a specific obsessional belief. For example, a person with harming obsessions had a highly disturbing violent obsessive thought of attacking his wife with a hammer. He sincerely loved her, and there was absolutely no hint of domestic violence or abuse of any kind (a necessary assessment before assigning this exercise). In this case, the therapist suggested that an ordinary carpenter's hammer, which was normally kept in the basement, be moved to different locations in the house. The client was asked to rate "urge to engage in violent behavior" associated with varying levels of accessibility to the hammer (e.g., when the hammer is moved to the kitchen, living room, bedroom). By increasing exposure to the hammer, the person was testing the exaggerated threat belief "I have to avoid hammers because I might snap, lose control, and become violent." Specific exposure tasks can be designed to test whether negative outcomes are as likely as the client assumes, even when going slightly beyond the usual bounds of normal behavior (e.g., leave the house unlocked for an hour, rub a speck of dog feces on your pant leg, leave the trunk of the car open and then shut it without looking inside).

TAF Bias

Whittal and McLean (2002) describe a *premonitions experiment* in which clients are asked to think repeatedly about a specific person or situation and then record the number of times they hear from that friend or the number of times the situation occurs in the following week (see also Rachman, 2003). The point of this exercise is to test TAF–Likelihood that merely thinking about things can influence whether they happen. A variation on this exercise is to test whether the more one thinks about an event, the more likely it is to happen. For example, a client could be asked to occasionally think about his mother phoning for 1 week, and the next week to think a great deal about her phoning. Predictions can be made about the number of times she will phone each week, and then a record kept on the actual number of phone calls. This experiment tests another aspect of TAF–Likelihood, which posits a direct link between number of thought occurrences and increased frequency of behavioral or event occurrences.

To test TAF–Moral, an *intrusions survey* can be conducted in which trusted people are interviewed on the types of "strange thoughts" they experience (Freeston et al., 1996; Rachman, 2003). The client may use a list of typical unwanted ego-dystonic intrusive thoughts, such as those in Handout 8.1, to prime individuals' recollection of their own mental intrusions. Freeston and colleagues (1996) note that this can be a useful exercise for normalizing obsessions and challenging the basis of the TAF–Moral bias.

Form 9.2 is a Moral Values Survey that can be used to gather more specific information on the role of thoughts and behavior in defining individuals' moral code. The therapist begins by asking the client to complete the survey within the session, which is then kept in the client's file. Next, several copies of the survey are given to the client to distribute to close friends and family. At the following session, the surveys are collected, and the therapist tallies up the scores for the cognitive (a) versus behavioral (b) stems of each item. The results are compared with the client's completed survey. Several points can be highlighted:

- Which contributed most to individuals' evaluations of moral character: thoughts or behavior?
- Did the client put more weight on thoughts as a determinant of moral character than the others who took the survey?
- Do people believe that moral people can have immoral thoughts? Can an immoral person have moral thoughts?
- If thoughts are a poor indicator of morality, isn't it erroneous to assume that how people think determines their moral character? Isn't this exactly what is happening in OCD and the TAF–Moral bias?

- Could individuals become less moral if their main concern is how they think? That is, could they be so concerned about having "bad thoughts" that they ignore the importance of "good *behavior*," which is the basis of people's moral code?
- Finally, is the client's moral code or values based on the assumption that behavior is more important than thoughts? If so, then why not realign the OCD concern so that it is consistent with the client's moral code (i.e., that bad thoughts are not equivalent to bad deeds)?

A third experiment, labeled the *power of thoughts exercise,* is useful for challenging the TAF–Likelihood belief that thinking about an outcome can influence the probability of its occurrence (Rachman, 1998, 2003; Whittal & McLean, 2002). The therapist begins with a positive event, such as winning the lottery, or even something more mundane, such as the number of compliments about one's physical appearance one might receive at work in a week. The client is asked to record a baseline occurrence of these events (winning the lottery would probably have a baseline of near zero; receiving a compliment might have a baseline of, let's say, 3). Over the subsequent week the client is asked to begin each day by imagining the positive event of receiving compliments and then to frequently think about the outcome during the day. Predictions are made on whether there will be an increase in the occurrence of compliments during the "mentation week." All occurrences of receiving compliments are recorded during the baseline and mentation weeks. The therapist then discusses the outcome and whether there is any evidence that thinking about receiving compliments caused an increase in compliments. Often, obsessional clients hold an asymmetrical "theory of mind," in which they believe that positive thinking cannot influence positive events, but negative thoughts can influence negative outcomes. When this belief is expressed, the following hypothesis-testing experiment is needed.

Rachman (1998) first described what could be labeled the *cognitive risk exercise,* in which clients intentionally think about adverse or fearful outcomes and note whether there is an increased occurrence of the negative outcome. The therapist can start with a nonobsessional negative thought and record whether increased mentation results in greater likelihood of the event (e.g., thinking about being criticized at work results in more criticism). If this exercise goes well, then the therapist can progress to mild, and then moderate, obsessional concerns (e.g., thinking more about feeling sick and noting whether the person actually gets sick, thinking more about friends in minor mishaps and noting whether they have such mishaps). Not only can these exercises be used to challenge TAF–Likelihood, but they can also reinforce the alternative explanation that thoughts do not have direct causal effects on real-life events. Completing these exercises may also improve the client's acceptance of more threatening ERP exercises.

Inflated Responsibility

In Chapter 8, the transfer of responsibility and the responsibility pie chart were the main cognitive interventions used to modify inflated responsibility beliefs and appraisals. In addition to these interventions, the *responsibility gradient* is another useful behavioral exercise. Here individuals are exposed to a hierarchy of obsessional situations that involve assuming successively higher levels of responsibility for previously avoided or anxiety-provoking tasks. For example, a person with a checking compulsion can be asked to leave the house, lock the door, and check the doorknob once for no more than 3 seconds. Initially, the client's spouse might stand beside him or her as he or she locks the door, observing that the door is locked but not reassuring the client that the door is secure. Next, the spouse could stand at the bottom of the steps as the door is locked. Then the spouse can sit in the car and watch the client lock the door. Finally, the client locks the door but the spouse purposely looks away so as not to attend to the task. Notice that, as the assignment progresses, more responsibility for the locked door is shifted from the spouse to the client. Not only is this a good exercise for directly modifying faulty beliefs about responsibility, but it is also a useful modification of ERP that may improve client compliance.

Overimportance of Thought

Empirical hypothesis testing for an overimportance of thought is intended to challenge the belief that the obsession must be significant because of its high frequency. The alternative belief supported by these exercises is that it's the increased attention to an unwanted thought that contributes to its perceived importance and significance. Together with the cognitive interventions described previously, these exercises reinforce the idea that there is no inherent significance to the obsession, but rather the problem is one of misplaced attention.

The first behavioral exercise, initially proposed by Whittal and McLean (2002), can be called the *artificial importance task*. In this exercise, clients first estimate the number of times in a week they see an innocuous target stimulus, such as a sign advertising "HOUSE FOR SALE." Then, for a 1-week period, they are to attend closely to the target stimulus and record the number of sightings. In the following week clients no longer seek out the stimulus but simply record the number of times the target is sighted. The usual finding with this exercise is that merely attending to a neutral stimulus increases its perceived frequency, even in the week when attention to the target stimulus is discontinued. (A similar experience is that of buying a certain type of car and then experiencing an increased sighting of similar models on the road.) This task highlights the circularity of overimportance and attention by showing that the more we attend to or think about an unwanted topic, the greater are its perceived frequency and importance.

Rachman (1998) proposed an *importance manipulation* that again demonstrates a link between the individual's response to the obsession and its perceived importance. Clients select a statement from a list of unwanted intrusive thoughts that is not their current obsessional concern. They focus on this negative intrusive thought for 2 minutes and then rate its subjective importance and associated distress. Both should be rated quite low at this point. Next, Socratic questioning is used to discover how a person might think about the intrusive thought to increase its importance. The following example illustrates the exercise:

> "I can tell from your ratings that you are not particularly bothered by the thought 'Maybe I'll be contaminated from using a public toilet.' Obviously, this is not an important thought to you, but some people become very upset by thoughts like this. What do you imagine they think that makes this an upsetting thought? Let's write down some ideas of how a person might inflate the importance attached to this thought."

Once an "inflated importance scenario" is developed, the client is again asked to think about the intrusive thought for 2 minutes and to use the "importance scenario" in order to think as deeply and vividly as possible the intrusive thought content. Importance and distress ratings are again completed after the 2-minute interval. Ratings from the first and second thought intervals are then compared to determine the effects of artificially inflating the perceived importance of the thought. This exercise not only highlights the negative effects of overimportance appraisals, but also demonstrates how perceived negative implications for the self are central to this faulty appraisal.

Rachman (1998) suggests that if manipulation of the significance of a nonobsessional thought goes well, then the therapist can progress to deliberate formation of the obsessive thought. The *inflated significance task* listed in Table 9.1 is a variation on Rachman's protocol. Clients are asked to form the obsession for a short interval (i.e., 10 seconds) and then again for a much longer interval (i.e., 60 seconds). Ratings of the perceived importance and distress of the obsession are completed after each interval and compared. The aim of this exercise is to test whether more sustained attention to the obsession increased its perceived importance.

A final empirical hypothesis-testing experiment for overimportance appraisals is the *attentive days task* (Rachman, 1998, 2003; Salkovskis, 1999; Whittal & McLean, 2002). Form 9.3 is a worksheet that can be used with this exercise. For 3 alternating days individuals are asked to attend closely to their obsession, recording its frequency, associated distress, and "felt importance" for that day. *Felt importance* refers to the client's emotion-based evaluation of the obsession, rather than a post hoc rationalization of its actual significance. These "high-attention" days mirror clients' usual obsessive approach. On the other 3 days, clients are instructed to "let the thoughts come and go as if they were unimportant" (Whittal & McLean, 2002, p. 424). Prior to the exercise clients are asked to predict which days would have the most frequent and distressing obsessions. Finding that the unwanted thoughts are less problematic on the "low-attention" days is strong evidence of the negative effects of overimportance appraisals and the positive therapeutic benefits of paying less attention to the obsessions.

The Need to Control Thoughts

Two behavioral exercises are presented in Table 9.1 that challenge appraisals and beliefs about the need to exert greater mental control. Most individuals with OCD think they have poor mental control and so believe that they need to try harder to control their unwanted intrusive thoughts. The purpose of these exercises is to (1) demonstrate the futility of heightened efforts to control intrusive thoughts, (2) challenge beliefs about the need for greater control, and (3) highlight the benefits of letting go of effortful mental attempts to control the obsession.

One of the most effective experiential exercises is the *white bear experiment*. This is based on Wegner and colleagues' (1987) classic thought suppression experiment, which is modified to demonstrate the deleterious effects of intentional mental control (see also Rachman, 2003). The white bear suppression test is first conducted as a within-session experiment but subsequently assigned as homework. Clients are asked to think about a neutral thought (i.e., a white bear) for 2 minutes and to signal with a raised finger each time their concentration is interrupted by a thought intrusion. After this thought formation period, the therapist spends a few minutes in Socratic questioning on the difficulty of holding one's attention on a single thought. Next, the client is asked to suppress the same neutral thought (i.e., not think of a white bear) for 2 minutes and to signal each occurrence of the unwanted thought. The therapist records the number of white bear intrusions and explores with clients their perceived self-efficacy and outcome of the mental control efforts. It is important to emphasize the greater difficulty associated with preventing a thought versus maintaining a single thought in conscious awareness.

The experiment can be repeated with a nonobsessional worry (e.g., failing an exam) as the to-be-suppressed thought. Again, discussion centers on perceived success and efficiency of control. A third trial of thought suppression is attempted with the primary obsession. It is expected that the client will have greater difficulty suppressing the primary obsession than the nonobsessional thoughts. This last iteration of the experiment can be assigned as homework. The white bear experiment and its variants are simple but effective exercises for demonstrating the futility of heightened mental control effort. It forces the client to consider whether "letting go of control" is the best response to obsessive thinking.

A second behavioral experiment, *alternative control days,* is a variation of the attentive days task discussed previously. Instead of instructions to attend closely to the obsession, clients are asked to exert strong intentional mental control of the obsession on 3 days, and then low mental control on alternate days (Clark, 2018). They are encouraged to make note at day's end of the frequency, intensity, and distress associated with the obsession on the high- versus low-control days, as well as any other costs–benefits in terms of their daily mood and level of functioning. For high-control days, clients are invited to use their normal response to the obsession, including any compulsive rituals. On low-control days, individuals are asked to "let the obsession come and go on its own" without any intentional effort to prevent, suppress, or dismiss the thought. The following is a hypothetical example of how findings from the alternative control days experiment can be utilized in the therapy session.

> THERAPIST: Kayla, I notice from your diary that there wasn't much difference in the frequency and intensity of the obsession on high- and low-control days. Were there any other differences between the two types of days that are not as obvious from your diary?
>
> KAYLA: Well, I did find it really hard to simply ignore the obsession on low-control days. I was afraid that it might not go away and that I'd feel anxious all day.
>
> THERAPIST: But what actually happened to the obsession and the anxiety on the low-control days?
>
> KAYLA: Eventually, other things distracted me, and the anxiety decreased. So, I guess my worst fear didn't materialize.
>
> THERAPIST: Overall, what do you think? Were you better off with low control or high control? What were the costs–benefits of each? Taking everything into consideration, was the extra effort put into trying to control the obsession worth it? Could there be some long-term personal benefits if you relinquished mental control every day?
>
> KAYLA: [After completing a cost–benefit analysis of high vs. low control] I can see from this exercise that any short-term benefits of my control efforts are outweighed by the long-term negative effects. I think I'll feel better if I do something to deal with the obsession right now, but I also feel frustrated that so much of my time is spent in obsessive thinking. I think you're right: All this effort at

controlling my obsessions is exhausting. It's just not worth the effort.

THERAPIST: Sounds like you've learned a lot from this exercise. Let's work on a low-control strategy that might be more beneficial and less tiring for you—something like acceptance, focused distraction, or mindfulness.

KAYLA: Sounds good. I realize I need a new approach to my obsessive thinking.

Clients who are reluctant to engage in the alternative control day exercise could be encouraged to take a holiday from their obsessive thinking (Rachman, 2003). A special day, like the weekend or a national holiday, could be designated a "no-control day." An individual could be encouraged to do some low-level exposure to obsessive triggers, refrain from consciously searching for the obsession, simply acknowledge its presence when it intrudes into conscious awareness, but then refrain from effortfully preventing, suppressing, or dismissing the obsession. Instead the person could focus on planned, deliberate, and productive daily activities. Individuals should be encouraged to keep a diary of their "holiday experiences," with the therapist reviewing the diary at the next session to highlight obstacles and benefits to relinquishing control of the obsession. Naturally, the objective is to encourage the client to take a "holiday approach" to the obsession every day.

Intolerance of Uncertainty

Empirical hypothesis testing for the construct *intolerance of uncertainty* (IU) challenges the belief that one can and must eradicate all doubt and uncertainty about the accuracy and correctness of one's actions and decisions to avoid an imagined negative outcome. Like other faulty interpretations, survey methods can be used to provide important information on the impossibility of certainty. A *certainty survey* of trusted friends and family is conducted to determine how well they actually remember instances of doing certain routine tasks like locking the car or house door, washing their hands, turning off the stove burners, and the like (Whittal & McLean, 2002). Before doing the interviews, clients make predictions about how much confidence people have in their memories. As Whittal and McLean (2002) note, clients are often surprised that most people do not remember doing these routine tasks and that even though uncertainty is common, it rarely leads to a negative outcome. In fact, the survey indicates that people live their daily lives with a considerable degree of uncertainty about their routine experiences. Tolerance of uncertainty is the norm, not striving for absolute certainty in all actions and decisions.

The *certainty manipulation* is a possible follow-up exercise to the survey. Clients select a number of daily activities that are not the focus of obsessional concerns (e.g., brushing teeth, vacuuming the house, coming to a full stop at stop signs, putting stamps on envelopes, returning email, texts, or voice messages). Estimated ratings are made of the certainty that these activities are performed correctly and completely on a daily basis. One of these activities is selected, and clients are asked to keep detailed records on level of certainty that the activity was performed completely over the coming week. Again, clients rate their levels of confidence and distress while performing the task, as well as 1–2 hours after completing the behavior.

There are a number of findings that can be drawn from this exercise. Individuals with OCD learn that they perform many "nonobsessional" tasks on a daily basis with some level of uncertainty that does not lead to negative consequences. In addition, the exercise highlights the near impossibility of maintaining a level of absolute certainty over an extended period of time. The task also demonstrates that striving for certainty increases distress even for nonobsessional activities. In addition, the therapist can discuss whether there was any benefit or reduced risk associated with being more certain about performing the nonobsessional task.

A more direct therapeutic intervention involves exposing clients to varying levels of uncertainty for obsessional concerns. *Uncertainty exposure* involves completing various obsessive–compulsive-related activities in a manner that generates moderate levels of doubt and uncertainty. The client is instructed to wait a few hours or even days, and then check to determine whether there were any negative consequences associated with the behavior. For example, a person with checking compulsions may be instructed to quickly (impulsively) buy a friend's birthday card. The client then writes a couple of lines of greetings in the card without rereading what is written. The card is placed in the envelope, sealed, stamped, and mailed without checking. A few days later the client is to call the friend and ask to see the card to determine the outcome. This is a useful intervention for providing evidence that tolerance of uncertainty, even with obsessional tasks, does not necessarily increase the risk of negative consequences, threat, or danger. However, it is also important for the therapist to ensure that "delayed checking" does not become entrenched as reassurance-seeking behavior.

Perfectionism

Because appraisals of perfectionism and IU overlap, behavioral exercises listed under each appraisal are mutually applicable. The *cost–benefit analysis* that Whittal and McLean (1999) used to challenge the "need-for-certainty" appraisals can be modified to deal with perfectionism. Various obsession-related tasks at work or home are selected, and the client rates levels of (1) perfection achieved in performing these tasks, (2) effort to perform perfectly, and (3) associated distress. In the following week clients are asked to attempt to improve their performance of the task, thereby increasing the perfectionism rating. The therapist then discusses the costs and benefits associated with putting extra effort into doing the task even better.

For example, a person with compulsive checking indicates that he achieves 85 out of a 100 on a perfectionism scale when he writes letters because he rereads and rewrites them over and over. In the following week, the client is asked to try to boost his letter-writing perfectionism rating to 95. Effort and distress are noted, as well as time taken to write letters and the outcome. The therapist can use data collected from this exercise to determine whether striving for perfection is associated with significant increased cost (i.e., delayed task completion, more distress) and only slight, if negligible, benefits.

Often, individuals with perfectionistic tendencies assume that their perfectionism is admirable or an adaptive characteristic that will lead to greater success in life. They may erroneously focus on the perceived benefits of perfectionism and overlook its negative consequences. To address this issue, the therapist can suggest that the client engage in a systematic *perfectionism observation exercise,* in which a friend or work colleague is selected who is admired for his or her high productivity level. In the following week the client can be asked to record various tasks completed by this person and the outcome of the tasks, and to give the performances a perfection rating. Strengths and weaknesses of the performances should be noted. For example, a client may indicate that he or she is particularly impressed with how well the director in the office leads departmental meetings. The client could be asked to observe the director's performance at the next meeting and rate the level of perfection. The aim of this exercise is to demonstrate that even people we admire can perform imperfectly and yet achieve very positive outcomes. Thus, perfectionism is not necessary to ensure good performance or a desired outcome.

Once less threatening perfectionism exercises are completed, the therapist can progress to a more direct challenge to perfectionism, using a modification of the uncertainty exposure task. Certain obsession-related tasks are selected, and the client is instructed to perform the tasks in a way that includes a minor flaw or inaccuracy. The consequences of these *intentional errors* are recorded for discussion at the following session. Clients with obsessional doubts about whether they said something embarrassing while conversing with a friend could be encouraged to say something that has potential for slight embarrassment. For example, the client could say to the friend, "I'm sorry, my mind wandered, and I wasn't paying attention. Would you please repeat what you just said to me?" The client would later record the outcome of this "flawed conversation," including the friend's reaction to the request and any perceived long-term or actual consequences.

The aim of this exercise is to test the belief that minor mistakes must be avoided because they will lead to serious negative consequences.

A final behavioral exercise is *instructed checking,* which is based on the cognitive theory of compulsive checking (Rachman, 2002; see also Chapter 12). In this exercise a preplanned number of checks, redoing, rereading, etc., is conducted with a primary obsessional concern. For example, a client believes her email correspondence must be written perfectly to convey a full understanding of the recipient's issue and to communicate her opinion with perfect clarity and insight. The client is asked to check her emails (1) just once or twice, (2) a moderate number of checks (three to five times), and (3) a high rate of checking (10–20 times). After completing each check routine, the client rates her level of confidence that the task was completed perfectly (see Egan et al., 2014). At the subsequent session, the therapist uses Socratic questioning to highlight the negative impact of repeated checking on confidence that a task was performed perfectly.

INTOLERANCE OF ANXIETY OR DISTRESS

The behavioral exercises listed under intolerance of anxiety or distress focus on providing evidence that anxiety is common and that individuals can tolerate and function quite well under anxious conditions. Once again, a *survey method* can be used in which clients interview trusted friends about their experiences with feeling anxious, nervous, or fearful. Most individuals will report anxious symptoms at varying levels of intensity in situations such as giving a speech, going for a job interview, taking an exam, going to the dentist, and the like. This information should help clients realize that feelings of anxiety are common even among nonanxious individuals and that these individuals experience some of the same anxious symptoms that the client feels in obsessive–compulsive-related situations.

A complementary *anxiety monitoring exercise* can be used, in which clients are asked to observe people at work or in public settings for signs of anxiety. Notes are taken on the situation and the specific behaviors that indicated a person was anxious. In addition, an anxiety rating is made and the outcome of the person's anxious performance noted. These exercises are intended to show that anxiety is common, that people function even when they are anxious, and that negative consequences resulting from anxious performances are rarely significant.

The final two behavioral exercises focus on the client's own experience of anxiety. An *anxiety comparison task* provides evidence that the client can tolerate anxiety in nonobsessional situations. Data are collected on the experience of anxiety in a non-obsessive–compulsive-anxious situation (e.g., preparing for an exam, taking a trip to a new city, making a speech, going to the dentist) and in an obsessive–compulsive-relevant context. Socratic questioning is used to explore the similarities and differences in the anxiety in both contexts. As discussed previously, ERP exercises can be modified to directly challenge the belief that one cannot tolerate being anxious. When an *anxiety prediction* feature is added to ERP, individuals can compare their predicted level of anxiety before exposure and the actual anxiety level after exposure (Rachman, 2003). Often individuals with OCD anticipate higher anxiety or distress than is actually experienced in the fear situation.

CONCLUSION

This chapter presented a series of behavioral interventions used in CBT for obsessions and compulsions. Many of these exercises are exposure-based and so require some familiarity with ERP (see Chapter 4). They are specifically designed to directly challenge the faulty appraisals and beliefs proposed in the generic CBT model (see Chapter 5). And yet, for treatment to be effective, individuals with OCD must have repeated opportunities to face their obsessional fears without engaging in compulsions or other neutralizing responses. Symptomatic improvement is possible only through cognitive change: that is, when individuals learn that the dreaded consequence associated with the obsession will not occur and that their efforts to control their obsessional thinking are futile. The most effective way to achieve this cognitive change is through empirical hypothesis-testing experiments.

FORM 9.1A. Threat Prediction Form

Instructions: This exercise has two parts. Part A involves collaborating with your therapist on developing an exposure exercise you would be willing to do to test the threatening aspects of your OCD. With your therapist's help, write in the space provided what you expect would happen if you engaged in the exposure task. Several questions are provided that you can answer when creating your description of what you think will happen to you, and others, if you did the exposure exercise.

1. Description of exposure task: _____
   _____
   _____
   _____
   _____
   _____

2. Questions to guide your expectation/prediction narrative:
   a. How anxious, guilty, distressed, or upset do you expect to feel? How long will the distress last before it begins to fade?
   b. Will the obsessive thoughts get worse? Will you be able to ignore them, or will they completely occupy your mind? Will you be able to think about other things?
   c. Will you be able to resist doing a compulsion or other neutralization behavior? Will the urge be too strong to resist? How long before you give in to the urge? Will you get stuck in the compulsion or be able to stop yourself?
   d. What negative effects will the exposure have on you or other people? Will you be able to function in your daily activities?
   e. How likely is the worst outcome or catastrophe? For example, do you expect any harm, injury, or other adverse consequence to happen to you or to others around you?

3. Expected/predicted consequence of the exposure task: _____
   _____
   _____
   _____
   _____
   _____
   _____
   _____
   _____

From *Cognitive-Behavioral Therapy for OCD and Its Subtypes, Second Edition,* by David A. Clark. Copyright © 2020 The Guilford Press. Permission to photocopy this material is granted to purchasers of this book for personal use or use with individual clients (see copyright page for details). Purchasers can download enlarged versions of this material (see the box at the end of the table of contents).

FORM 9.1B. Threat Prediction Form (Continued)

Instructions: Below is Part B of this exercise. It begins by recording the exposure you actually completed. Where did you do the exposure? What did you do? How long did the exposure last and how often did you do it? What obsessive thoughts and compulsive actions did it trigger?

1. Description of exposure completed: _____

   _____
   _____
   _____
   _____
   _____

2. Questions to guide your description of the actual outcome:
   a. How anxious, guilty, distressed, or upset did you feel? How long did the distress last before it began to fade?
   b. Did the obsessive thoughts get worse? Were you able to ignore them, or did they completely occupy your mind? Could you think about other things?
   c. Could you resist doing a compulsion or other neutralization response? Was the urge too strong to resist? How long before you gave in to the urge? Did you get stuck in the compulsion? Were you able to stop the compulsion?
   d. What negative effects did the exposure have on you or other people? Were you able to function in your daily activities?
   e. What was the worst thing that happened because you did the exposure? For example, did any harm, injury, or other adverse consequence happen to you or others around you?

3. Actual consequence of the exposure task: _____

   _____
   _____
   _____
   _____
   _____
   _____
   _____
   _____
   _____
   _____
   _____

From *Cognitive-Behavioral Therapy for OCD and Its Subtypes, Second Edition*, by David A. Clark. Copyright © 2020 The Guilford Press. Permission to photocopy this material is granted to purchasers of this book for personal use or use with individual clients (see copyright page for details). Purchasers can download enlarged versions of this material (see the box at the end of the table of contents).

FORM 9.2. Moral Values Survey

Instructions: Below is a series of hypothetical scenarios involving thoughts and actions. Read each statement and circle the immoral/moral rating you would give to each situation.

Note. Rating key: –3 = highly immoral, –2 = moderately immoral, –1 = slightly immoral, 0 = neither moral nor immoral, +1 = slightly moral, +2 = moderately moral, +3 = highly moral.

1. (a) Person thinks about being generous but isn't generous toward others.	–3 –2 –1 0 +1 +2 +3
(b) Person acts generously toward others.	–3 –2 –1 0 +1 +2 +3
2. (a) Person wonders if s/he has been dishonest toward others.	–3 –2 –1 0 +1 +2 +3
(b) Person acts dishonestly toward others.	–3 –2 –1 0 +1 +2 +3
3. (a) Person wonders if s/he has accidentally caused harm or injury to others.	–3 –2 –1 0 +1 +2 +3
(b) Person causes harm or injury to others and doesn't care.	–3 –2 –1 0 +1 +2 +3
4. (a) A very clean and hygienic person has intrusive thoughts that s/he might have an offensive odor or contaminated others in some way.	–3 –2 –1 0 +1 +2 +3
(b) Person gives no care to personal hygiene and so is frequently offensive to other people.	–3 –2 –1 0 +1 +2 +3
5. (a) A careful and meticulous person frequently doubts whether s/he has made a mistake that would negatively affect others.	–3 –2 –1 0 +1 +2 +3
(b) Person is careless and often makes mistakes that negatively affects others.	–3 –2 –1 0 +1 +2 +3
6. (a) A conscientious person who has concerns that s/he may have been rude or offensive to others.	–3 –2 –1 0 +1 +2 +3
(b) Person who is often rude and offensive to others.	–3 –2 –1 0 +1 +2 +3
7. (a) Person has unwanted, disturbing thoughts/images of deviant sexual contact with children.	–3 –2 –1 0 +1 +2 +3
(b) Person is a known child molester.	–3 –2 –1 0 +1 +2 +3
8. (a) Person wonders if he or she accidentally stole something.	–3 –2 –1 0 +1 +2 +3
(b) Person often steals things.	–3 –2 –1 0 +1 +2 +3
9. (a) Person thinks about being positive and complimentary toward others.	–3 –2 –1 0 +1 +2 +3
(b) Person often is complimentary toward others.	–3 –2 –1 0 +1 +2 +3
10. (a) Person thinks s/he should be polite and respectful toward others.	–3 –2 –1 0 +1 +2 +3
(b) Person is polite and respectful toward others.	–3 –2 –1 0 +1 +2 +3

From *Cognitive-Behavioral Therapy for OCD and Its Subtypes, Second Edition*, by David A. Clark. Copyright © 2020 The Guilford Press. Permission to photocopy this material is granted to purchasers of this book for personal use or use with individual clients (see copyright page for details). Purchasers can download enlarged versions of this material (see the box at the end of the table of contents).

FORM 9.3. Alternate Days Worksheet

Instructions: This exercise examines the effects of attention on frequency, distress, and perceived importance or significance of unwanted intrusive thinking. There are two parts to this exercise. First, select a nonobsessional but potentially anxious thought, such as failing an exam, getting a poor work evaluation, being publicly embarrassed by a friend, getting bad news about your health, being alone, losing your job, etc. On alternate days, pay close attention to the thought, and on the remaining days just let the thought go—don't pay attention to it. Record the effects of "high attention" versus "low attention" on the frequency, distress, and perceived importance/significance of the thought in the respective columns. Repeat the exercise over 6 days using your primary obsession as the target thought.

High-Attention Days: When the anxious intrusive thought pops into your mind, think deeply about it. Spend a few minutes dwelling on the thought, thinking about its effects on your life, how much the thought upsets you, and all the possible reasons why the thought popped into your mind.

Low-Attention Day: When the anxious intrusive thought pops into your mind, acknowledge that it is there but then proceed with your work or other daily activities. Let yourself be naturally distracted by other thoughts. The goal during low-attention days is to "let go of the thought" or "let it sit in your mind" without intention or effort.

Days	Estimated Obsession Frequency/Day	Level of Distress (0–10 scale, with 0 = no distress and 10 = most) distress)	Felt Importance/Significance of Intrusive Thought
Monday (high attention)			
Tuesday (low attention)			
Wednesday (high attention)			
Thursday (low attention)			
Friday (high attention)			
Saturday (low attention)			

From *Cognitive-Behavioral Therapy for OCD and Its Subtypes, Second Edition*, by David A. Clark. Copyright © 2020 The Guilford Press. Permission to photocopy this material is granted to purchasers of this book for personal use or use with individual clients (see copyright page for details). Purchasers can download enlarged versions of this material (see the box at the end of the table of contents).

PART IV
Subtype Treatment Protocols

CHAPTER 10

Contamination OCD

CASE ILLUSTRATION

Cynthia, a law student, had been concerned about dirt and cleanliness since childhood, making sure her clothes, room, and belongings were kept neat and tidy. She considered anything handled by other people to be dirty and disgusting, and so would avoid touching public items as much as possible. She'd had this heightened concern about cleanliness for as long as she could remember and cringed whenever she came into close proximity to others. Cynthia coped reasonably well with these concerns and minimized their impact on daily living until she experienced a troubling incident while on vacation.

It was during a midterm break with a couple of university friends that Cynthia's life dramatically changed. They had driven late into the night and when they finally stopped, the only hotel available was seedy. Cynthia was horrified at the condition of the room, but she felt too embarrassed to say anything. She slipped into the bed and fell asleep due to sheer exhaustion. However, when she awoke in the morning, she was instantly alarmed. The bed sheets were stained and yellow, and the pillowcase was a grimy gray color. Cynthia panicked. Never before had she slept in such filth. Some of the spots on the bed looked like dried semen, and there were other specks that Cynthia thought might be blood stains. Her mind was filled with images of dirty, sick, older men sleeping in this same bed, leaving behind their bodily fluids. She imagined them drooling on the pillowcase and then her face lying in the same spot. She felt panic-stricken and rushed to the bathroom to shower. She recalls spending over an hour, scrubbing herself over and over in an attempt to cleanse herself of the contamination.

After that incident, Cynthia's fear of dirt and contamination intensified. Her core fear is contracting a sexually transmitted disease

(STD) through contact with human blood, urine, semen, or even saliva by touching things other people have touched. She now worries frequently throughout the day about becoming contaminated, and the fear has now generalized to a concern that she'll infect others. She avoids many public places, and she closely inspects seats, tables, doorknobs, and the like for any unrecognizable specks that could be the remnants of bodily fluids. She feels intense anxiety around others for fear of exposure to minute traces of bodily secretions. If she feels contaminated, Cynthia will engage in excessive handwashing and showering, use large quantities of disinfectant in her apartment, and repeatedly wash her clothes even after a single wear. She firmly believes that handwashing can prevent STDs, and at times of intense anxiety she is convinced she is HIV+. Although she regularly looks up symptoms of STDs on the Internet and has had several blood tests indicating that she is symptom-free, any relief is short-lived. Over the last several months Cynthia has become so preoccupied with contamination, that it is causing significant interference in her life. She is finding it difficult to attend classes, she can't concentrate on her studies, her friends are not calling anymore because of her "unusual behavior," and her long-term romantic relationship came to an end because of her fear of intimacy. Alone and abandoned by others because of her self-imposed quarantine, Cynthia has become increasingly depressed as the prospect of dropping out of law school becomes more likely.

This chapter focuses on the nature and treatment of contamination OCD. It begins with a discussion of clinical features and the role of disgust, as well as an exploration of *mental contamination,* an entirely new perspective on contamination fear. A modified CBT model is presented that emphasizes the role of inflated responsibility in the pathogenesis of contamination OCD. The remainder of the chapter offers specialized CBT strategies, homework assignments, and other resource tools for this OCD symptom subtype as well as a brief overview of the treatment outcome literature.

CLINICAL FEATURES OF CONTAMINATION FEAR

Approximately 50% of individuals with clinical OCD have a fear of dirt or contamination and associated washing and/or cleaning compulsions (Rasmussen & Eisen, 1992, 1998). This finding has been replicated globally, with dirt/contamination fears and cleaning/washing compulsions especially prevalent in OCD samples drawn from religious countries that emphasize cleanliness (e.g., Akhtar, Varma, Pershad, & Verma, 1978; Karadağ, Oguzhanoglu, Özdel, Ateşci, & Amuk, 2006). Contamination and cleaning/washing compulsions may be more prevalent in women, although the proportion of cases with this subtype of OCD may be overrepresented in clinical samples (Fullana et al., 2010).

There is evidence that the contamination/cleaning subtype has higher comorbidity with eating disorders than other obsessive–compulsive symptom dimensions (Hasler et al., 2005), and several reviewers concluded that ERP is more effective for contamination/cleaning (Mataix-Cols, Marks, Greist, Kobak, & Baer, 2002; Starcevic & Brakoulias, 2008). No doubt this conclusion is due to an overrepresentation of physical contamination fear in the treatment groups, in which perceived threat arises from physical contact with a tangible object, organism, or substance. The most common physical or contact contamination fears concern (1) bodily secretions such as urine, feces, saliva, or blood; (2) dirt; (3) germs, viruses, or bacteria; (4) sticky substances or residue; (5) household cleaning agents, chemicals, or detergents; (6) environmental or industrial chemicals or materials such as asbestos, radiation, pesticides, or toxic waste; and (7) animals or insects. Contact contamination fear can be subdivided into concerns that focus on feeling dirty or disgusted by contaminants (disgust-based) and those that fear the contamination could cause harm (harm-based; Williams, Mugano, Franklin, & Faber, 2013). In her review, M. T. Williams and colleagues (2013) noted that disgust-based contamination may be more difficult to treat than harm-based contamination fears.

Given the creativity of the human mind, practically anything can become a contaminant by proxy. Cynthia, for example, became frightened of contamination if she touched a set of car keys that her brother had taken with him into a public toilet. It is not uncommon for the list of contaminants to either expand or switch from one object to another because of this "association by proxy." Often this occurs when a previously neutral object comes into close proximity to a contaminant, but other times the association may be entirely imagined. Whatever the case, it can be challenging for the therapist, who seems to be chasing one new perceived contaminant after another. As the fear over one contaminant fades with treatment, the client may report several new perceived contaminants because of some experience over the past week. In Cynthia's case, ERP effectively reduced her fear and avoidance of public toilets, but she remained fearful of touching the car keys.

A normal fear of excessively dirty, disease-ridden, or decay-infested objects is highly adaptive, preventing us from exposure to contaminants that could cause deadly disease or sickness. Even the fear of contaminating others is an adaptive response that contributes to the safety and survival of the larger community. Thus, contamination fear is a dimensional construct, with irrational and excessive OCD contamination fear on the extreme end of a continuum with milder, circumscribed fears found in the general population at the other end.

Research on unwanted intrusive thoughts supports this dimensional perspective. Purdon and Clark (1993) found that one-third or more of their student sample reported an irrational thought or image of doors or telephones being contaminated, or of contracting a fatal disease from a stranger. These findings have been replicated in other studies, such as the prominence of contamination intrusions in Lee and Kwon's (2003) reactive obsessions subtype (see also Moulding, Kyrios, Doron, & Nedeljkovic, 2007; Radomsky, Alcolado, et al., 2014). Although Rachman and colleagues' (2015) differentiation of clinical contamination fears as "unyielding, expansive, persistent, commanding, contagious and resistant to ordinary cleaning" (p. 8) is helpful, the continuity between normal and abnormal contamination fear presents two major challenges for the therapist:

1. How to accurately distinguish clinically significant contamination fears from a heightened preoccupation with disease and cleanliness that might fall in the high-normal range.
2. What standards of normal attitudes and practices toward hygiene should be set as treatment goals for individuals who have spent years washing and cleaning excessively.

Rachman and colleagues (2015) discuss four features that are helpful in distinguishing clinical contamination fear from its normal, nonclinical variant. Table 10.1 presents these key characteristics, along with an explanation and clinical illustration. Rachman (2006) offers other features of clinical contamination fear that can be helpful in their identification, such as (1) a primary focus on the skin, especially the hands; (2) concern about transmission to others; (3) a fear that other people are vulnerable to the contaminant; (4) anxiety activated by a memory of the contaminant; (5) absence of a moral element; and (6) compulsive checking in the presence of an inflated sense of personal responsibility.

Treatment Considerations

During assessment, the therapist can determine whether a concern about dirt or contamination is clinically significant by its rapid acquisition, persistence beyond fear exposure, ease of generalizability, and resistance to safety information. Given the strong phobic orientation toward contamination fear, exposure will play a central role in its treatment. The contagious feature of these fears means that often therapists are faced with treating a succession of new contaminants that become proxies by their real or imagined association with the original fear stimulus. The provision of health and safety information about disease and contamination will have minimal impact in alleviating a clinically significant contamination fear.

WASHING AND CLEANING COMPULSIONS

As one would expect, washing and cleaning are the most obvious forms of neutralization associated with contamination fears. Excessive handwashing is the most common ritual, but neutralization efforts can also include

TABLE 10.1. **Primary Features of Clinical Contamination Fear**

Feature	Explanation	Clinical illustration
Rapid acquisition	Immediate rise in anxiety after touching or coming in close proximity to a perceived contaminant	Cynthia notices a used syringe next to the sidewalk and instantly feels a surge of intense anxiety.
Nondegradability	Once activated, the contamination fear remains elevated, despite escape from the contaminant or attempts to neutralize with a reasonable level of washing or cleansing.	Despite inspecting her shoes carefully to ensure there is no evidence of puncture by the syringe, Cynthia's anxiety remains elevated for days over the incident.
Contagious	Once activated, the contamination fear spreads to other objects, situations, or people through proximity or some imagined association.	Cynthia became fearful of contamination whenever she passed the street where she had seen the syringe. She also stopped running on the park trails for fear of finding another syringe.
Asymmetry	Contamination fear can expand and spread exponentially, whereas a sense of safety has little benefit beyond a specific situation.	Cynthia soon became fearful of most outdoor public places for fear of finding a used syringe, whereas the many times she failed to encounter syringes and the nonoccurrence of skin poking by a syringe made no difference in reducing her anxiety.

Note. Based on Rachman, Coughtrey, Shafran, and Radomsky (2015, p. 5).

long showers or baths, repeated laundering of clothes, excessive cleaning of bathrooms or bedrooms, heavy use of antiseptics and detergents, and so on. Avoidance can be extensive, and individuals with contamination fear often engage in excessive reassurance seeking. Sometimes the person can neutralize the fear by imagining a clean or contamination-free environment, but usually the neutralization is behavioral because the contaminant is thought to reside in the external world.

For years, cognitive-behavioral researchers focused on identifying the determinants of excessive washing and cleaning. The early behavioral research of Rachman and colleagues established that cleaning and washing compulsions are associated with a reduction in subjective anxiety or discomfort, or, less often, are believed to prevent the occurrence of some undesirable outcome (Rachman & Hodgson, 1980). More recently Rachman and colleagues (2015) recognized that dysfunctional beliefs, such as the following, contribute to compulsive washing and cleaning:

"To feel safe, I must keep everything perfectly clean."
"It's possible to remove all contamination by washing and cleaning."
"If I wash enough, I can keep myself from getting sick."
"The more you wash, the less likely you'll get sick or spread contamination."
"Contagious diseases can be prevented by practicing the highest standards of hygiene."
"People who are hygienic have less illness and probably live longer, healthier lives."

As discussed in Chapter 3, research on stop rules has discovered several criteria that individuals use to terminate compulsive washing/cleaning. Bucarelli and Purdon (2015) found that compulsive experiences classified as "uncertain episodes," of which 25% involved washing/cleaning, were associated with a greater number of repetitions, more doubt, and longer compulsive duration. An analogue study by Taylor and Purdon (2016) found that high-trait inflated responsibility predicted longer handwashing after a contamination induction and individuals in the high contamination fear/high responsibility group exhibited an ironic decrease in sensory but not memory confidence with longer handwashing duration. In another study intensity and total number of "not just right" experiences predicted longer handwashing in students who previously immersed their hands in a disgusting dirt mixture (Cougle, Goetz, Fitch, & Hawkins, 2011). An earlier study found that individuals with compulsive washing relied more on an internal criteria such as the attainment of a "feeling of rightness" to terminate washing, compared to nonwashing obsessional and nonclinical controls (Wahl et al., 2008). In addition, those with washing compulsions reported that the decision to stop the ritual was more deliberate and took more mental effort than the two control groups. Together, these studies indicate that the decision to stop a compulsive washing episode is more than a function of anxiety reduction. It may also involve active efforts to attain a perceived sense of certainty that a rather nebulous internal state of "feeling right" has been reached. At the same time other factors like decreased confidence in one's sensory experience might contribute to prolonged compulsive washing, although momentary states of perceived responsibility may have less effect on length of handwashing than previously thought (Taylor & Purdon, 2016).

Szechtman and Woody (2004) argue that OCD represents a dysfunction of a biologically based security motivation system that functions to acquire information that signifies the possibility of potential danger. The performance of preventive behaviors, such as washing or cleaning, that normally provide negative feedback that terminates the security motivation fails in the person with contamination OCD. For these individuals washing does not provide a satiety-like experience that signals task completion, so the security motivation system remains activated. In other words, there is a failure to attain a "feeling of knowing" (i.e., the satiety-like experience) that the potential danger (i.e., of contamination) has passed because the security motivation system is open-ended and disconnected from immediate environmental control. Washing compulsions, then, persist longer and are repeated because of individuals' difficulty in achieving a "feeling of knowing" that the threat has been removed and they have achieved safety, a state that Szechtman and Woody (2004) call "yedasentience."

In three experiments based on nonclinical samples, Hinds and colleagues showed that a mild harm stimulus (e.g., placing your hands in a pail of supposed dirty diapers) could activate the security motivation system and that the activation persisted until individuals washed their hands, that is, engaged in corrective behavior (Hinds et al., 2010). In a similar induction experiment conducted with OCD samples, individuals with contamination OCD were significantly less able to use a fixed handwashing interval to reduce their initial contamination fear caused by the "dirty diaper" task than individuals with checking OCD (Hinds, Woody, Van Ameringen, Schmidt, & Szechtman, 2012). Together these studies provide support for the security motivation model of OCD, suggesting that the persistence of compulsive washing and cleaning may be due to failure to attain the feeling state that signals that preventive behavior has been completed.

Treatment Considerations

Although washing/cleaning compulsions are strengthened by success in reducing anxiety, they are also generated and maintained by faulty appraisals and beliefs. Thus, effective CBT for contamination fear needs to incorporate cognitive restructuring of dysfunctional neutralization beliefs along with ERP. As well, individuals with contamination OCD falsely rely on internal states to determine when to stop the compulsion. Treatment should focus on developing a more external standard for preventive behaviors. For example, therapists could collaborate with clients on an acceptable handwashing procedure that would be used only at select times, such as after using the toilet or before meals. Thus, rather than wash until a certain sense of safety or "feeling right" is attained, the client is taught to rely on purely external criteria of task completion. Of course, individuals with contamination fears will need strategies to cope with the prolonged distress associated with not having attained the desired internal state.

DISGUST AND CONTAMINATION SENSITIVITY

Since Darwin (1872/1965), emotion researchers (e.g., Ekman & Friesen, 1975; Izard, 1971) have considered disgust to be a basic emotion that has evolutionary significance by promoting cleanliness and transmitting cultural values that admonish avoidance of ingesting dangerous substances that threaten disease and infection (Rozin & Fallon, 1987; Rozin, Haidt, & McCauley, 2008). Concern about contamination is a core feature of disgust, and so the emotion has considerable relevance to contamination OCD. Rozin and colleagues (2008, p. 759) noted that "core disgust" involves (1) a sense of potential oral incorporation (e.g., tasting soiled food), (2) offensiveness, and (3) contamination potency. A broad range of disgust-eliciting stimuli include (1) spoiled food; (2) animals that are slimy or dirty; (3) body products like feces, mucous, etc.; (4) body mutilation; (5) dead bodies; (6) deviant sex; (7) violations of hygiene; and (8) sympathetic magic or stimuli that resemble contaminants like feces-shaped fudge (Rozin et al., 2008; Woody & Tolin, 2002). It was proposed that disgust contributes to the onset and persistence of contamination-related obsessions and compulsions (Power & Dalgleish, 1997). Several studies found a relationship between disgust and OCD contamination fears and washing compulsions (i.e., Mancini, Gragnani, & D'Olimpio, 2001; Olatunji, Williams, et al., 2007; Woody & Tolin, 2002).

The possibility that disgust is a vulnerability factor for OCD contamination requires a distinction between disgust sensitivity and disgust propensity. *Disgust sensitivity (DS)* refers to "the degree to which a person feels disgusted in response to a variety of stimuli" (Woody & Tolin, 2002, p. 544), or the extent of negative evaluation and affectivity elicited when experiencing disgust (Goetz, Lee, Cougle, & Turkel, 2013; Ludvik, Boschen, & Neumann, 2015). On the other hand, *disgust propensity* (DP) refers to individual differences in proneness or the ease with which one has an experience of disgust (Ludvik et al., 2015). Olatunji (2010, p. 314) further clarified the distinction between these two constructs by noting that DP concerns "elevations in the perceived frequency/intensity of experiencing disgust," whereas DS refers to "elevations in the perceived negative impact of experiencing disgust." In sum, DS is to DP as anxiety sensitivity is to trait anxiety (Goetz et al., 2013). Goetz and colleagues (2013) suggested that DP may be more relevant for contamination OCD than DS, because the former reflects an avoidance of repulsive materials.

Early studies suggested that DS may play an important role in the maintenance and persistence of contamination fear and washing compulsions in clinical and nonclinical samples (e.g., David et al., 2009; Deacon & Olatunji, 2007; Moretz & McKay, 2008; Woody & Tolin, 2002). However, more recent studies have concluded that DP has a more specific relationship with contamination OCD than DS (e.g., Inozu, Clark, & Eremsoy, 2015; Melli, Bulli, Carraresi, & Stopani, 2014; Melli, Gremigni, et al., 2015). Likewise, Olatunji, Tart, Ciesielski, McGrath, and Smits (2011) found that DP but not DS was specifically elevated in OCD compared to a GAD sample.

One reason for the differences between the early and more recent research on disgust stems from a methodological problem. The Disgust Scale and its revisions are the most widely used measures of disgust. The developers of the original 32-item Disgust Scale (Haidt, McCauley, & Rozin, 1994) as well as the more recent 25-item revision (Olatunji, Cisler, Deacon, Connolly, & Lohr, 2007) considered the instrument a measure of DS. Others, however, concluded that the Disgust Scale and Disgust Scale—Revised assess DP rather than DS (van Overveld, de Jong, Peters, & Schouten, 2011). Although most researchers now agree that the Disgust Scale—Revised is a measure of DP, confusion can still be found because high scores on the Disgust Scale or Disgust Scale—Revised have been interpreted as DP in one study but DS in another.

Greater clarity occurred with the publication of a new self-report questionnaire, the Disgust Propensity and Sensitivity Scale (DPSS; van Overveld, de Jong, Peters, Cavanagh, & Davey, 2006), which measures disgust propensity (DPSS-P) and sensitivity (DPSS-S) as distinct constructs. The two subscales of the DPSS are moderately correlated ($r = .59$; van Overveld et al., 2006) and the DPSS-P ($r = .49$) and DPSS-S ($r = .40$) are both moderately associated with the Disgust Sensitivity–Revised (DS-R) Total Score (van Overveld et al., 2011). In an initial study based on a student sample, regression analyses revealed that a revised DPSS-S had a more specific association with contamination-related safety seeking as indicated by the Padua Inventory Contamination subscale (Olatunji, Cisler, et al., 2007). However, a more recent nonclinical study found that a revised DPSS-P but not DPSS-S was significantly associated with self-reported washing symptoms, and that only DP predicted avoidance and subjective disgust on a contamination-based Behavioral Avoidance Test (BAT; Goetz et al., 2013). In another study, only the revised DPSS-P subscale was uniquely elevated in OCD, with revised DSPP-S equally high in both OCD and GAD samples (Olatunji et al., 2011). Olatunji and colleagues (2011) used multilevel mediational analysis to show that reduction in DP was associated with changes in OCD symptoms with exposure-based treatment.

Finally, an experimental study based on a small student sample found that an implicit measure of DS was associated with avoidance on a contamination-based BAT (Nicholson & Barnes-Holmes, 2012). Although these results suggest that DS, not DP, may be more specific to contamination symptoms, the study did utilize a novel measure of implicit cognitions for disgust and a small nonclinical sample. Another novel study found that high DP was not associated with greater difficulty controlling disgust-related thoughts in a thought suppression experiment (Ólafsson et al., 2013). In sum, DP might be the better candidate for vulnerability to contamination OCD, although it is clear that the mechanisms of disgust vulnerability are not well known, and that reactions to specific disgust stimuli (i.e., disgust sensitivity) should be considered.

Rachman (2006) proposed a vulnerability construct closely related to DS that he called *contamination sensitivity* and that he defined as a "general sensitivity to feelings of contamination/pollution" (p. 83). Rachman proposed that contamination sensitivity is an enduring personality trait in which a generalized heightened sensitivity to acquire feelings of contamination would be a vulnerability factor for acquiring contamination fears. Individuals with high contamination sensitivity would be more prone to overestimate the probability and seriousness of perceived contaminants. Rachman could only speculate on the origins of elevated contamination sensitivity, but its core feature was endorsement of exaggerated, unrealistic beliefs and appraisals about contamination, its source, consequences, and prevention. (See Rachman, 2006, pp. 90–94, for a list of contamination sensitivity beliefs.)

Rachman developed the 24-item Contamination Sensitivity Scale (CSS; see Rachman et al., 2015, for a copy of the measure) to assess individual differences in contamination proneness. The initial psychometric study based on an OCD sample indicated that the CCS had strong correlations with the VOCI Mental Contamination and Contamination subscales, and correlated .45 and .57 with the Disgust Scale and Anxiety Sensitivity Scale, respectively, (Radomsky, Rachman, Shafran, Coughtrey, & Barber, 2014). Moreover, individuals with OCD contamination scored significantly higher than the noncontamination OCD sample. In a nonclinical experiment heightened contamination sensitivity predicted greater increases in subjective ratings of disgust in response to a negative mood induction (Armstrong, Tomarken, & Olatunji, 2012). The authors concluded that individuals with high contamination sensitivity may have a lower threshold for feeling disgust when experiencing a negative mood. This finding is consistent with Rachman's (2006) contention that high-contamination-sensitive individuals might be at elevated risk of developing a contamination fear during periods of low mood or depression. Clearly, there is a close interplay between contamination sensitivity and disgust sensitivity that may confer vulnerability to contamination OCD.

Treatment Considerations

The numerous studies on disgust indicate that this emotion has considerable relevance for contamination OCD. Clinicians would be well advised to include measures of disgust when assessing treatment change in contamination OCD. As well, it would be expedient to build in exposure to disgust stimuli as part of the exposure hierarchy. Therapists might consider developing two exposure hierarchies: one based on fear avoidance and the other based on disgust avoidance. The two hierarchies could then be integrated, so that the contamination-fearful client learns to tolerate both fear and disgust elicitors. From a cognitive perspective, modifying dysfunctional beliefs about disgust and its tolerance would be an important element of the treatment plan.

As noted earlier, M. T. Williams and colleagues (2013) concluded that disgust-based contamination may be less frequent but harder to treat than harm-based contamination. Several studies found that fear declines more quickly than disgust with repeated exposure in a controlled setting (McKay, 2006; Olatunji, Wolitzky-Taylor, Willems, Lohr, & Armstrong, 2009; Smits, Telch, & Randall, 2002). Ludvik and colleagues (2015) concluded there was strong evidence that exposure alone is ineffective or less effective in reducing disgust reactions. They suggest that counterconditioning may be more effective than exposure. On the other hand, there is evidence that exposure-based treatment of OCD can produce significant reductions in DP (Olatunji et al., 2011). In a one-session treatment of spider phobia, de Jong, Vorage, and van den Hout (2000) found that exposure alone was equally effective to exposure plus counterconditioning in reducing the disgust feelings associated with spider stimuli. At the very least, clinicians should determine whether cases of contamination OCD are primarily disgust- or harm-based. If the former, then a longer course of treatment tailored to disgust stimuli may be needed.

An assessment of contamination sensitivity should be done prior to treatment. Rachman (2006) lists various core beliefs about contamination, based on heightened contamination sensitivity, which could be included in the treatment plan. As well, the exposure hierarchy could be tailored to the individual's level of contamination sensitivity, with highly sensitive individuals needing a more finely graduated hierarchy with extended exposure periods. Whatever the case, clinicians treating contamination OCD should be cognizant of clients' heightened propensity for disgust and greater contamination sensitivity when planning treatment for contamination-based obsessions and washing/cleaning compulsions.

MENTAL CONTAMINATION

Rachman (2006) proposed a novel form of contamination, *mental contamination*, which he defined as "a feeling of dirtiness/pollution/danger provoked by direct or indirect contact with an impure, soiled, harmful, contagious, immoral human source" (p. 19). It is a state of internal uncleanness associated with a range of negative emotions such as disgust, fear, anger, shame, guilt, and revulsion. Mental contamination is typically an obscure, generalized feeling that is difficult to comprehend or control, and is often triggered in the absence of physical contact with a contaminant. Frequently, it involves a moral element, such as violation of one's integrity, dignity, or virtue. When heightened moral violation is present, the term *mental pollution* more aptly describes the person's contamination experience.

Rachman and colleagues (2015) noted that a variety of experiences can give rise to mental contamination, such as physical or sexual assault, as well as experiences that involve degradation, humiliation, or betrayal. The distinct features of mental contamination include the following:

1. Physical contact is unnecessary.
2. The contamination feeling can be generated internally.
3. Usually a perceived violation has occurred.
4. The contaminant is usually a person.
5. There is less generalization.
6. There is a focus on one's unique vulnerability to the contaminant rather than to other people.

In mental contamination, the feeling of inner dirtiness or pollution activates core selfhood beliefs of being a bad, dangerous, dirty, or defiled person (Rachman et al., 2015).

Similar to contact contamination, individuals with mental contamination attempt to rid themselves of this internal dirtiness by compulsive washing and cleaning. Even though there is a powerful urge to wash, cleaning rituals are quite ineffective because the contaminant is inherently internal, abstract in nature (Rachman et al., 2015). The individual who compulsively washes to rid herself of the sense of guilt and disgust from the sexual betrayal of her spouse, for example, has little chance of feeling even transient relief from her inner state of filth by engaging in an external ritual. Despite this functional disconnection between the obsessional fear and neutralizing ritual, the urge to wash or avoid can be as intense as in contact contamination.

Rachman's (2006) proposed four types of mental contamination that are presented in Table 10.2. The first type of mental contamination, labeled *moral violation*, occurs after physical or psychological violation of the person, like a physical or sexual assault, or experiences of degradation, humiliation, or betrayal. A feeling of *mental pollution* is often common in which the individual reports an inner sense of dirtiness (Rachman, 2006). Morally violated individuals personalize the contamination, believing that only they, and not others, can be contaminated by the perpetrator of the violation. Rachman noted that the contamination feelings can decline or even disappear if reconciliation is achieved with the perpetrator, but will flare up again if a breach occurs. Furthermore, the intensity of moral violation will vary with the individual's feelings and attitudes toward the perpetrator. Prominent beliefs are "If an immoral person touched me, I need to wash thoroughly" and "Contact with immoral people causes me to feel unclean" (Rachman et al., 2015).

Self-contamination is a sense of inner dirtiness or impurity caused by having unwanted, repugnant intrusive thoughts, images, or urges that

TABLE 10.2. **Forms of Mental Contamination**

Type	Explanation	Clinical illustration
Moral violation	A feeling of inner dirtiness or pollution caused by a perceived experience of physical, psychological, or emotional violation of moral or personal integrity.	An individual who is the victim of a sexual assault develops extensive bathing and washing rituals in response to feeling profoundly dirty and violated.
Self-contamination	Feeling of contamination caused by contact with one's own bodily products or repugnant intrusive thoughts or repulsive actions.	An individual who is fearful of his or her urine splashing on his or her clothes or body and then contaminating others.
Visual contamination	Feeling of contamination caused by the mere sight of individual(s) perceived as disreputable. Normally reserved for people perceived as despicable, bizarre, possibly threatening, or disgusting.	The person feels contaminated just seeing a homeless individual who is acting in a bizarre or unconventional manner on the street.
Morphing	The fear that one will be transformed or could even absorb undesirable characteristics by close proximity to a perceived human contaminant.	A young man with OCD became anxious in the presence of an older individual he intuitively felt was different and might transfer her declining cognitive ability to him, thereby stifling his youthful creativity.

Note. Based on Rachman (2006) and Rachman, Coughtrey, Shafran, and Radomsky (2015).

are a violation of personal moral values (Rachman, 2006). Often self-contamination is associated with repugnant sexual, blasphemous, violent, or racist mental intrusions. Rachman (2006) noted that self-contamination can be associated with a feeling of mental pollution, and it can occur after engaging in what is perceived as an immoral act, like masturbation or viewing pornography. Guilt and self-disgust are prominent negative feelings, with individuals engaging in compulsive washing to deal with their violated state. Representative beliefs are "I must be an immoral, filthy person to have such nasty, repugnant thoughts" and "I need to cleanse and purify myself for such wicked thinking."

Visual contamination is not as well articulated by Rachman and colleagues (2015). In this case the mere sight of a person perceived as immoral, strange, or somehow unacceptable to the person evokes an inner sense of dirtiness. Rachman and associates noted that visual contamination is closely linked to "morphing," with beliefs such as "Even the sight of a disgusting person makes me feel dirty" and "If I see someone who appears strange or unusual, I will feel so violated and disgusted that I must avoid that person at all cost."

Morphing is the most unusual of the various types of mental contamination. Rachman (2006) defined *morphing* as "a fear that one might be tainted or changed by proximity to particular 'undesirable' people or classes of people" (p. 45). Individuals believe that close proximity to the undesirable person will cause them to be transformed (i.e., morphed) into a person like the undesirable individual. There is a belief that the undesired characteristic, such as mental illness, low intelligence, poverty, sexual orientation, race or ethnicity, etc., is contagious, although it is often personalized in such a way that individuals believe only they are susceptible to acquiring the undesired characteristic. In addition, individuals with "morphing" contamination OCD often hold bizarre ideas about how undesired characteristics might get transferred from one person to another, such as believing that everyone has a personal energy field so that close proximity to the undesired person will cause a transfer of "negative energy" from the undesired person that could transform the "victim's" energy field so that they become more like the undesired person. Rachman noted that people tend to be ashamed of their fear of morphing and so attempt to conceal it from others. Prominent beliefs might be "Mental instability is contagious" and "I must be cautious and avoid weird or distasteful strangers" (Rachman et al., 2015).

Mental contamination may be more common than first assumed. In a study of 177 individuals with high obsessive–compulsive symptoms, 10.2% reported mental contamination alone, 36.1% reported both mental and contact contamination, and 15.3% reported contact contamination alone (Coughtrey, Shafran, Knibbs, & Rachman, 2012). The authors conducted a second study on a subset of the sample that received a formal diagnosis of OCD ($N = 54$). Over half of the sample had contamination fear ($n = 32$), and of this group, 56.5% reported both mental and contact contamination, 18.75% had only mental contamination, and 25% had only contact contamination (Coughtrey et al., 2012). Moreover, significant correlations have been found between self-reported mental contamination and obsessive–compulsive symptoms and beliefs, TAF, and contamination sensitivity in both clinical and nonclinical samples (Coughtrey et al., 2012; Cougle, Lee, Horowitz, Wolitzky-Taylor, & Telch, 2008; Radomsky, Rachman, et al., 2014). In a study of 50 women who had experienced a sexual assault (Fairbrother & Rachman, 2004), 60% reported some feelings of mental contamination after the assault, and 70% had an urge to wash. Feelings of mental contamination were related to the severity of PTSD symptoms and post-assault washing. In addition, deliberate recall of the assault memory was associated with stronger feelings of dirtiness and urges to wash than recall of a pleasant memory. These findings indicate that mental contamination is fairly common in OCD samples and among individuals who have experienced a traumatic physical violation. As well, mental contamination is a prominent feature of obsessive–compulsive symptomatology that can be overlooked if not deliberately assessed.

Mental contamination is thought to occur on a continuum, with normal variants of the phenomena evident in the general population and its more extreme form evident in OCD. The pathological form of mental contamination causes more distress, interference in daily living, misinterpretation of perceived violation, and dysfunctional compulsive behavior than its milder, tolerable, and intermittent nonclinical form (Radomsky, Coughtrey, Shafran, & Rachman, 2018). Radomsky and colleagues (2018) state that clinical mental contamination is distinguishable by several characteristics: (1) uncontrollability, (2) internal distress triggered by violation reminders, (3) recurrent mental intrusions of violation, (4) presence of a strong moral element or guilt, (5) high frequency, (6) powerful compulsive urges, and (7) significant interference in daily living.

Based on the continuity assumption, experimental research indicates that nonclinical individuals can experience feelings of inner dirtiness and urge to cleanse after imagining a personal violation. Zhong and Lijenquist (2006) found that participants who recalled a past unethical deed generated more words related to cleansing in a word fragment test than individuals who recalled ethical deeds. In Study 2 an implicit threat to moral purity resulted in higher desirability ratings of cleansing products, whereas participants in a third study who recalled a past unethical deed were more likely to take an antiseptic wipe than participants recalling an ethical deed. These findings suggest a causal relationship between threats to personal morality and urge to engage in physical cleansing.

The ability of unwanted mentation and moral violation to induce inner feelings of contamination and urge to wash is evident in studies using the "dirty kiss paradigm." In the original study, 121 female undergraduates imagined an audiotaped vignette that described experiencing a consensual kiss at a party and then one of three versions of a nonconsensual kiss incident (Fairbrother, Newth, & Rachman, 2005). Participants in the nonconsensual condition reported feeling more internally unclean, heightened moral violation, and a greater urge to wash compared to imagining the consensual kiss. Many of the participants in the nonconsensual condition reported using several neutralization strategies to reduce discomfort caused by the nonconsensual kiss. Other experiments have replicated this basic finding, with appraisals of perceived personal responsibility for the kiss and ratings of personal violation by the kiss associated with significantly greater feelings of mental contamination and urge to wash (Elliott & Radomsky, 2009; Radomsky & Elliott, 2009). In addition, individuals who imagined themselves as the perpetrator of a nonconsensual kiss also experienced an increase in mental contamination feelings and, to a lesser extent, an urge to wash (Rachman, Radomsky, Elliott, & Zysk, 2012; Waller & Boschen, 2015).

However, most of these studies do not find an increase in physical cleansing behavior after imagining a nonconsensual kiss. Waller and Boschen (2015) found that physical washing, mental washing, and atonement were not effective in reducing mental contamination, and the Zhong and Lijenquist (2006) findings of increased preference for, or use of, cleansing in response to recalling an unethical deed were not replicated in a larger sample (Fayard, Bassi, Bernstein, & Roberts, 2009). In sum, the "dirty kiss" studies indicate that thinking about moral violation can induce a sense of inner dirtiness or mental contamination, with a probable increase in a subjective urge to neutralize (i.e., clean). However, the evidence is weak, at best, that induced mental contamination in nonclinical samples will elicit actual cleaning behavior.

Treatment Considerations

Rachman and colleagues (2015) published a treatment manual, the *Oxford Guide to the Treatment of Mental Contamination,* which provides new insights into its treatment based on the cognitive theory of mental contamination. In a pilot single-case study, Warnock-Parkes, Salkovskis, and Rachman (2012) showed that cognitive therapy, adapted for mental contamination, had a stronger therapeutic effect on a case of treatment-resistant OCD that developed after a betrayal experience than did ERP and high-quality CBT.

Rachman and colleagues (2015) describe eight elements to the cognitive-behavioral treatment of mental contamination.

1. *Psychoeducation.* The client is provided with information on mental contamination, based on the cognitive-behavioral formulation, with a particular emphasis on the difference between contact and mental contamination. Individuals are taught that their fears emanate from an exaggerated misinterpretation of the personal significance of unwanted thoughts or images related to psychological or physical violation (Radomsky et al., 2018). The goal of CBT is to help individuals accept more benign alternative interpretations of these unwanted violation thoughts.

2. *Monitoring.* On a daily basis, clients self-monitor their inner feelings of dirtiness and violation, along with associated unwanted intrusive

thoughts and images, in order to gain insight into their mental contamination.

3. *Surveys.* Family and friends are surveyed on matters related to morally based standards, beliefs, and behavior that may be pertinent to the client's mental contamination. For example, self-contamination clients who feel dirty because they have an unwanted sexual thought could ask close friends for their response to such thoughts, or they could consult an authority figure whom they hold in high regard, like a priest, minister, rabbi, or imam, about the morality of these intrusions.

4. *Utilizing survey information.* The therapist carefully reviews the survey responses with the client, draws out conclusions from the responses, determines whether the results support or refute the client's maladaptive beliefs, and then collaboratively constructs an alternative interpretation that fits with the survey data.

5. *Cognitive restructuring.* The therapist focuses on correcting the faulty appraisals and beliefs responsible for the persistence of intrusive thoughts or images causing the sense of mental contamination. Rachman and colleagues (2015) present a "contrasting explanations" method in which two possible explanations for a problem are contrasted. For example, a person suffering from mental contamination based on moral violation might believe that "I need to wash thoroughly whenever I am reminded of my husband's affair with my best friend because it brings me comfort" (Explanation A). A competing explanation could be posed, such as "Washing may feel nice at the moment, but it does nothing to weaken the hurt and humiliation I feel when reminded of the affair" (Explanation B). The therapist then works with the client in collecting information and evidence for and against the two explanations, with the goal being the client's acceptance of the healthier explanation. The authors note that inflated responsibility, TAF bias, and *ex-consequentia* bias are particularly important to correct in mental contamination. Compared to contact contamination, individuals with mental contamination may need more cognitive work on core beliefs, such as being bad, sinful, defiled, or dangerous.

6. *Behavioral experiments.* These are exercises the client carries out to collect specific information on the veracity of a maladaptive contamination belief and its more adaptive alternative. Normally these experiments are conducted only once in order to gather the necessary information. For example, a person with a morphing contamination could be asked to maintain close proximity to a highly desirable person and then determine if there has been a noticeable transfer that resulted in a boost in some positive attribute. (Note that this type of experiment cannot be done when psychosis is present.) This would test out the belief that a transfer or transformation can occur when we experience close proximity to an individual.

7. *Imagery rescripting.* This involves changing the content and outcome of an unwanted distressing intrusive image associated with the mental contamination. The therapist can use *test probes* in which clients are asked to imagine various types of images relevant to their mental contamination and to rate their degree of contamination. An image that evokes at least 50/100 points of contamination is selected for rescripting. Once the rescripted image is constructed, clients are encouraged to use it daily, whenever they begin to feel a sense of dirtiness or contamination. For example, a person with mental contamination involving violation might use a rescripted image of personal strength and victory over an individual who humiliated him or her in a profound manner.

8. *Relapse prevention.* Like all CBT protocols, treatment ends by specifying the maintenance factors of mental contamination, the intervention strategies that were helpful, triggers for potential setbacks, and ways to deal with future difficulties.

A COGNITIVE-BEHAVIORAL MODEL OF CONTAMINATION

Figure 10.1 presents a cognitive-behavioral model of contamination OCD based on the generic model presented in Figure 5.1 (p. 118). Several psychological processes particularly important in the pathogenesis of contamination OCD are discussed in this section.

Rachman (2006) proposed that heightened sensitivity to disgust and contamination is a vulnerability factor for OCD contamination, with elevated anxiety sensitivity a generalized vulnerability for anxiety disorders. Disgust or fear elicitors are situations, objects, substances, and experiences associated with dirt, disease transmission, poison, contamination, and violation that trigger contamination-related mental intrusions. In contact contamination the elicitors are external to the person, whereas in mental contamination the elicitors are unwanted intrusive thoughts or images of past physical or psychological violation.

Rachman (2006) proposed that five faulty appraisals were especially important in the maintenance of contamination OCD. With contact contamination, threat overestimation is clearly evident. Cynthia, for example, might sit at a table in the cafeteria and notice a reddish-brown speck on the corner of the table. Instantly she would think "Could that be dried blood?!" Anxiety would begin to build as she thought about the possibility of contracting HIV by sitting so close to the unidentified speck. Such thinking involves an exaggerated appraisal of the probability and severity of danger associated with a reddish-brown speck.

TAF biases are also prominent, especially in self-contamination (Rachman, 2006). Here the intrusion is interpreted as increasing the likelihood of

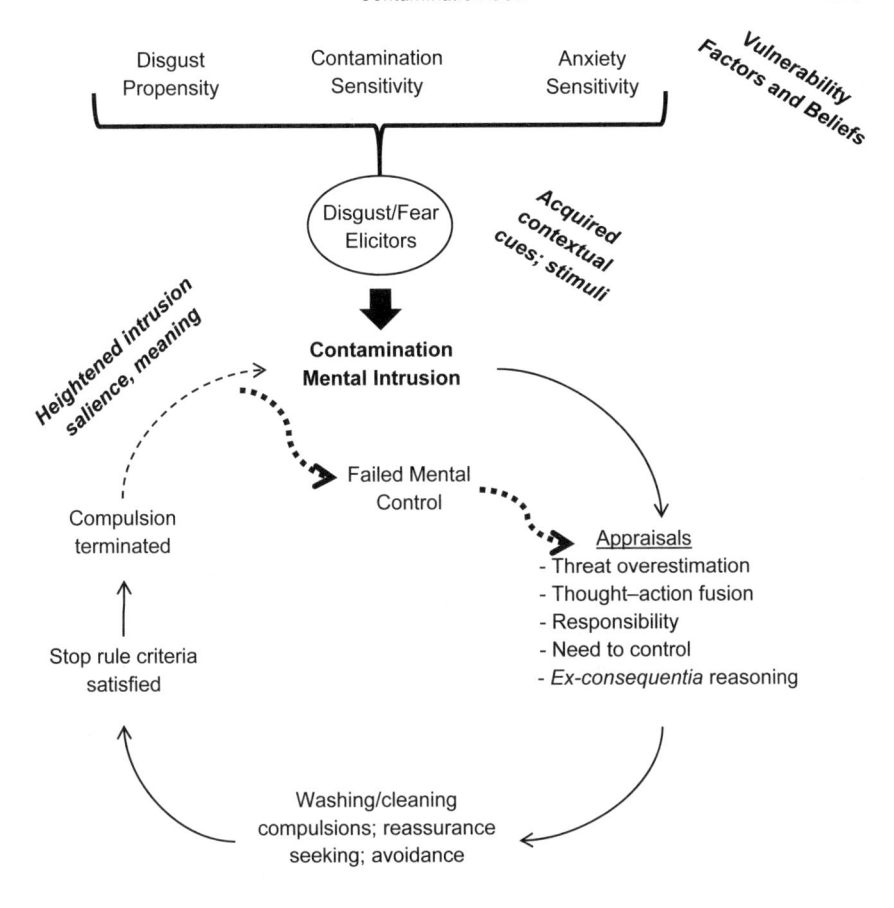

FIGURE 10.1. Cognitive-behavioral model of contamination OCD.

contamination or causing a moral violation. For Cynthia, the mere fact that she was thinking about HIV contamination increased the probability that she could be infected. She got tested for STDs several times simply because she kept thinking about it. With self-contamination, a TAF–Moral bias is present in which having sexually repulsive thoughts, for example, are morally as bad as acting on the thoughts.

Responsibility bias will vary in emphasis depending on the nature of the contamination fear. In some cases, in which the core fear concerns the spread of disease and contamination to others, inflated responsibility bias is paramount in the maintenance of obsessive–compulsive symptoms. Martin, for example, struggled with contact contamination, but his fear focused on whether he might pass his contaminated state on to others, especially his pregnant wife, and therefore be responsible for people getting sick. In self-contamination, in which the person is repulsed by "dirty thoughts," responsibility appraisals are less evident, unless one defines responsibility so broadly that it becomes synonymous with the concept of agency (Clark & Purdon, 2016). Rachman (2006) noted that the central element to the responsibility bias is the assumption that the possibility of preventing misfortune increases the likelihood that it will occur. So if Martin fails to wash thoroughly to prevent the spread of contamination, then his wife is more likely to get sick because of his negligence.

Rachman (2006) noted that need to control unwanted intrusions is present in most cases of OCD contamination. Individuals attempt to block, suppress, or dismiss the unwanted cognitions. The need for mental control becomes an imperative in OCD contamination because individuals are convinced that their thinking means the danger of deadly contamination is imminent. If they can stop the thoughts or images, the danger subsides. As well, calm and safety are strongly desired but impossible to achieve as long as one is thinking about contamination.

A final cognitive bias is *ex-consequentia* reasoning. Although this form of reasoning is common in all emotional disorders, Rachman (2006) offered the following summary in stating its relevance to OCD contamination: "When the patient encounters a perceived contaminant, it evokes fear and this is interpreted as a signal of present danger" (p. 121). Any clinician with experience treating OCD has encountered *ex-consequentia* bias. Cynthia, for example, occasionally went to parties, got intoxicated, and engaged in some reckless sexual behavior that involved an exchange of bodily fluids—which most would consider a moderately risky contamination situation. And yet, Cynthia processed these situations more normally as long as she didn't feel anxious. However, noticing a reddish-brown spot on a chair would cause her to consider this situation dangerous if she felt fearful or anxious. In both cases evaluations of danger or safety are driven by the whether she felt anxious or calm.

In contamination OCD, washing and cleaning rituals are the primary responses for reducing fear and disgust. However, avoidance and reassurance seeking will also be prevalent control strategies. Given their heightened contamination and disgust sensitivity, individuals with OCD contamination will avoid a host of situations, objects, and substances that evoke their OCD fears. Seeking reassurance from others will be a secondary control strategy, in which individuals may ask for help in determining whether they are contaminated or sufficiently clean to eliminate the risk of contamination. However, research on reassurance seeking in the maintenance of OCD is relatively recent (see Chapter 3). Thus, its prevalence and functional significance in OCD contamination are largely unknown.

Figure 10.1 includes stop rules that determine when a washing compulsion is terminated. As discussed previously, a reliance on internal or inferred states such as anxiety reduction, or the attainment of a desired state like safety, calm, and/or certainty, are critical factors in perpetuating the vicious cycle of OCD contamination. The faulty appraisals and beliefs, the excessive use of neutralization, and the erroneous stop rules conspire to ensure an increase in the frequency, salience, and meaningfulness of contamination-related thoughts, images, and memories. Like the generic model in Chapter 5, a perceived failure in mental control provides a secondary pathway that reinforces faulty appraisals of significance. The challenge for the cognitive-behavioral therapist is to bring about change at these critical junctures of the vicious cycle, in order to reduce the emotional intensity of the contamination thoughts and their associated urge to clean.

SPECIAL TREATMENT CONSIDERATIONS

Rachman and colleagues (2015) noted that standard ERP will be more appropriate for contact contamination but that cognitive therapy will be needed for mental contamination because of the frequent absence of external contaminants. Since many cases of contamination OCD have elements of both contact and mental contamination, some combination of ERP and cognitive therapy will be necessary. This relationship is depicted in Figure 10.2. If the primary emphasis is contact contamination, therapists will devote most of their time to ERP, whereas a much greater emphasis will be placed on the cognitive treatment of faulty appraisals and beliefs if the obsessive–compulsive symptomatology is dominated by concerns about mental contamination.

Rachman's (2006) observation of the importance of *ex-consequentia* bias in contamination OCD suggests that therapists should spend extra

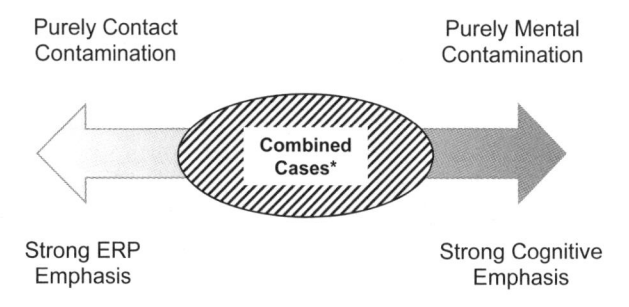

FIGURE 10.2. OCD contamination continuum. *Coughtrey et al. (2012) found that 56% of individuals with contamination fear had both contact and mental contamination concerns.

time on this bias. Drawing the client's attention to *ex-consequentia* reasoning through psychoeducational exercises can be effective. Having individuals self-monitor variability in their fear intensity will help illustrate the close relationship between fear and perceptions of danger. Many clients are prescribed tranquilizers on an as-needed basis. The therapist could ask clients to compare their danger ratings at times when the tranquilizer is taken versus at times when it is not taken. A discussion on how medication can reduce a perceived external threat or danger can then ensue. Clients can also be asked to conduct a survey to determine whether people's judgments of threat or danger vary with their level of subjective anxiety. The goal of these interventions is to encourage clients to evaluate and then correct their automatic threat estimations even when feeling highly fearful or disgusted.

CBT protocols for contamination OCD should emphasize the modification of stop or termination rules. Washing and cleaning compulsions play a major role in most contamination fears. Faulty stop rules mean that individuals with OCD wash and clean much longer when feeling dirty or contaminated compared to non-OCD individuals. One important consideration is to help the client shift from an internal to an external stop criterion. For example, Cynthia would wash her hands until she felt safe; that is, she washed until she felt that the possibility of contracting an STD was reduced to an acceptable level. Of course, this vague criterion shifted considerably depending on her appraisals of the situation and how she felt. As a result, she would occasional get stuck in washing and cleaning. After providing psychoeducation on the importance of stop rules, the therapist and client could collaborate on a more reasonable set of external criteria (e.g., "After using the toilet, I will spend no more than 30 seconds, using hand soap, to wash my hands"). Exposure exercises are developed that incorporate the new external stop criterion.

Finally Rachman and associates (2015) developed a special interview, rating scales, and questionnaires that assess various aspects of contamination OCD. The clinician will find the Contamination subscale of the VOCI helpful in determining elevations in contamination fear (Thordarson et al., 2004). In addition, Rachman (2006) provides a standardized 44-item interview for assessing various aspects of contamination. Several contamination-specific self-report measures also are available, including the specially developed Mental Contamination subscale of the VOCI, Contamination Thought–Action Fusion Scale, and Contamination Sensitivity Scale (see Rachman et al., 2015). The Morphing Fear Questionnaire (MFQ) was developed to assess thoughts and behaviors that suggest that the personal self will be tainted by close proximity to an undesirable person (Zysk, Shafran, Williams, & Melli, 2015). The initial psychometric study found that the MFQ is a single-factor measure with adequate convergent and divergent validity, as well as satisfactory temporal reliability. The clinician will find these measures helpful when assessing contamination OCD.

TREATMENT EFFICACY

Only a few treatment outcome studies have investigated the effectiveness of ERP or CBT for contamination fears. In their multicenter randomized controlled trial of computer-assisted versus clinician-guided ERP, Mataix-Cols and colleagues (2002) concluded that ERP was especially effective for contamination OCD, a conclusion echoed by Starcevic and Brakoulias (2008) and M. T. Williams and colleagues (2013). In their ERP outcome study, Abramowitz, Franklin, and colleagues (2003) found that ERP was significantly effective in all OCD subtypes, although a much higher percentage of individuals in the contamination (70%) and symmetry (76%) subtypes reached clinically significant improvement than participants in the other subtypes.

Jones and Menzies (1997) introduced a type of cognitive therapy for contamination OCD called *danger ideation reduction therapy (DIRT)*. It focuses on decreasing exaggerated likelihood estimates of danger associated with contaminants. No other faulty appraisals, such as inflated responsibility or control of intrusions, are addressed by DIRT. The treatment protocol utilizes the provision of corrective information, cognitive restructuring, "microbiological experiments," attentional focusing, and a probability de-catastrophizing task to modify the client's exaggerated expectancies of contamination danger. Jones and Menzies (1998) provide a more extensive description of the microbiological experiments, which involve actual measurement of the presence of potentially pathogenic organisms on a hand that touched a perceived contaminant (e.g., shaking hands with people, touching the lining of a garbage bin) versus the "control" hand that did not touch the contaminant. The tests, of course, show that none of the contamination tasks resulted in actual exposure to pathogens. Jones and Menzies (1997, 1998) state that direct or indirect exposure, response prevention, or behavioral experiments are not components of the treatment package. Thus, DIRT can be viewed as a more purely cognitive treatment for contamination OCD.

A small outcome study of 11 individuals with contamination OCD treated with eight sessions of DIRT showed significant symptom reduction compared to a wait-list control, although there was no further improvement at 3-month follow-up (Jones & Menzies, 1998). A second outcome study in which individuals with contamination OCD received 12 sessions of DIRT did significantly better on some posttreatment outcome measures than a group treated with ERP, and both conditions showed that symptom change was correlated with change in threat expectancy (Krochmalik, Jones, Menzies, & Kirkby, 2004). A subsequent study of five individuals with treatment-resistant contamination OCD found that 14 weekly individual sessions of DIRT achieved clinically significant improvement in four cases (Krochmalik, Jones, & Menzies, 2001). This is particularly encouraging since all of these individuals had at least 10 years of excessive washing/cleaning, had failed to respond to serotonergic medication and ERP, and had poor insight into their contamination fear. Although there are some unique features to DIRT, its distinction from more conventional CBT for OCD may be overstated (O'Connor, 2009). However, the clinician will find the innovative experimental demonstrations and corrective information useful in modifying the overestimated threat that is so central to contamination OCD. A detailed clinician treatment manual for DIRT has been published by the originators of the therapy (St. Clare, Menzies, & Jones, 2008). Finally, there is some indication from case studies that mindfulness and ACT may have some promise for contamination OCD (e.g., Singh, Wahler, Winton, & Adkins, 2004; Twohig, Hayes, & Masuda, 2006; Wilkinson-Tough, Bocci, Thorne, & Herlihy, 2010).

CONCLUSION

Fear of contamination and cleaning/washing compulsions are the most common OCD symptom subtype, affecting approximately 50% of individuals with OCD. Further distinctions have been proposed for this subtype, such as contact versus mental (Rachman, 2006) and disgust-based versus fear-based (M. T. Williams et al., 2013) contamination. Three cognitive vulnerability factors may be central to the etiology of contamination OCD: DP, contamination sensitivity, and anxiety sensitivity. A cognitive-behavioral model of contamination OCD was presented (see Figure 10.1) in which disgust or fear elicitors, faulty appraisals, and internalized stop rules play a critical role in the pathogenesis of the disorder. Moreover, the various types of mental contamination, which may be evident in most people with contamination OCD, require a greater emphasis on the cognitive substrates of contamination OCD. Violations of morality and a sense of "vicarious contamination" characterize mental contamination.

Conventional ERP is the recommended treatment for individuals with prominent contact contamination symptoms. However, as the symptom presentation moves closer toward mental contamination, cognitively based interventions will take precedence. Although there is considerable empirical evidence that ERP is effective in reducing washing/cleaning compulsions, systematic research is lacking on the effectiveness of cognitive interventions for treating mental contamination. As well, there is some indication that mindfulness and ACT may be helpful, but the necessary empirical evidence is lacking at this time. Finally, treatment process research is needed to determine if change in faulty appraisals, beliefs and stop criteria is needed to bring about significant and lasting relief to those struggling with contamination OCD.

CHAPTER 11

Doubt, Checking, and Repeating

CASE ILLUSTRATION

Mateo doubted just about everything in his life, from the most mundane action like switching off a light to major life decisions. He was in the midst of planning his wedding and a honeymoon when, once again, he was seized with doubt over the relationship. Should he marry Valerie? Did he really love her? Was she the right one for him? Was he really committed to her? At the same time, after agonizing months of indecision he had finally purchased his first home and had secured permanent employment at a promising engineering firm. The future couldn't look brighter, and yet Mateo's incessant doubt was threatening to derail his life. For years he had struggled with obsessive doubt that varied in severity depending on the demands and stresses of life; now was a highly stressful period, with many new beginnings.

Mateo experienced a daily struggle with doubt, questioning even the most rudimentary, mundane of actions or decisions. For example, walking upstairs, leaving a room, getting ready in the morning, shutting the door, turning off taps, leaving the house, answering email, shutting down his computer, and so on, all had to be done correctly. If a doubt intruded into his mind—"Did I do that correctly or completely?"—he immediately felt uncomfortable. This discomfort arose because Mateo wondered if he could be the cause of "bad luck" in the form of some tragedy happening to himself, his fiancée, or his parents due to performing an action incorrectly or making a wrong decision. Often he wasn't even sure how bad luck would manifest itself; it could be physical injury or death, but it could also be a significant financial loss or some ill-defined misfortune. Whatever it was, Mateo was convinced he had to repeat his actions or check something several times to ensure it was done correctly. If not, he experienced intense discomfort and a strong urge to check or repeat.

Mateo spent hours each day checking and redoing his actions and decisions. Although at first praised for his conscientiousness and perfectionism, he was missing deadlines at work. He would sometimes get caught in a check that would cause him embarrassment. His fiancée was becoming increasingly frustrated with his excessive reassurance seeking over daily actions and decisions. Lately the doubt had become so bad that Mateo called in sick because he could not finish his morning routines. He started to doubt what he said to people, worried that he might have offended them in some way. He had even worried that he had run over a pedestrian, and circled the neighborhood repeatedly checking for an injured bystander. It was after one of these extreme doubting incidents that Mateo's family insisted he seek mental health treatment.

This chapter discusses the CBT approach to pathological doubt and compulsive checking, repeating, and redoing rituals. Distinct clinical features of compulsive checking and doubt are considered that include an extensive contrast between normal and pathological doubt. This is followed by a discussion of Rachman's (2002) cognitive self-perpetuating theory of compulsive checking and the inference-based approach to doubt (O'Connor, Aardema, & Pélissier, 2005). An elaborated CBT model of compulsive checking is presented that recognizes the unique features of pathological doubt and associated neutralization efforts. The chapter concludes with a consideration of several treatment issues pertinent to CBT for doubt and compulsive checking.

CLINICAL FEATURES

Compulsive Checking

Compulsive checking is the second most common OCD symptom, ranging in prevalence from 28 to 81% in OCD samples (Antony et al., 1998; Foa et al., 1995; Rasmussen & Eisen, 1992, 1998). Checking, redoing, and repeating compulsions can be found in all OCD subtypes, such as checking to ensure that objects are clean, that one has counted correctly, or that objects are properly placed (Radomsky, Asbaugh, Gelfand, & Dugas, 2008). The same pervasiveness can be seen in the cognitive component of compulsive checking: that is, pathological doubt. In fact, O'Connor, Aardema, and colleagues (2005) contend that doubt is evident in all forms of OCD. Thus, the clinician would be well advised to assess for doubt and checking rituals in all clients with OCD, even if compulsive checking is not the primary compulsive symptom.

Compulsive checking is future-oriented, most often performed to prevent some perceived possible harm from occurring to self and/or significant others (Rachman & Shafran, 1998). Rachman and Hodgson (1980) concluded that checking rituals also occur as an attempt to ensure safety or well-being of self, others, or animals, and to avoid criticism or guilt. They differ from cleaning rituals in focus, with obsessional checking aimed at *prevention* and cleaning at *restoring* a former state. In their experimental research, Rachman and Hodgson found that provocation resulted in less anxiety/discomfort in compulsive checking than in cleaning, and that performance of the ritual produced more variable reductions in anxiety/discomfort. They concluded that checking rituals are associated with more doubt and indecision, take longer to complete, have a slower onset, are less effective in reducing anxiety/discomfort, and tend to be accompanied by anger or tension (see also Rachman & Shafran, 1998). Clearly, checking is a less satisfactory form of neutralization for doubt than washing is for contamination.

In this chapter repeating and redoing rituals are included under compulsive checking because of their substantial phenomenological overlap. Repeating and redoing rituals involve actions such as retracing one's steps until a correct state of mind is achieved, entering a room several times in order to prevent harm from occurring to a family member, rereading a passage until certain it is completely understood, or repeating an expression over and over to make sure a person understands completely. In each of these instances the repeating and redoing ritual is triggered by doubt and is motivated by a desire to prevent a negative consequence or to achieve a feeling of safety. However, repeating and redoing rituals are also highly relevant to order, symmetry, and rearranging OCD (see Chapter 13). Various factor analyses of the YBOCS Symptom Checklist (Goodman et al., 1989a, 1989b) have found that repeating rituals load with symmetry obsessions and with ordering and counting compulsions, rather than with checking compulsions (Bloch et al., 2008).

Treatment Implications

The cognitive-behavioral research on compulsive checking has implications for its conceptualization and treatment. A wider range of negative emotional states must be assessed and treated, including frustration, anger, guilt, and tension. Checking appears to provide a less satisfactory solution to obsessional concerns, as noted, than washing or other compulsive rituals. Thus, the emotional state achieved by repeated checking may not be much better than the emotions evoked during provocation. More cognitive intervention may be needed because of the influence of doubt, indecision, fear of criticism, future perspective taking, and focus on prevention. And finally, the paradoxical nature of checking must be considered; that is, that repeated checking does not reduce the urge to check. As well, it may be difficult to operationalize "normative checking" for individuals with chronic forms of excessive checking.

Pathological Doubt

Doubt is the central cognitive feature in compulsive checking (Rachman & Hodgson, 1980), but it also has strong links with normal human cognitive functioning. Who can credibly claim they have never experienced a sense of doubt or uncertainty about some act of omission or commission (Ciarrocchi, 1995)? For example, one could doubt whether one came across as genuinely friendly to an acquaintance (act of omission) or whether one may have offended this person by a curt remark (act of commission). We all can experience doubt over the most mundane activities (e.g., "Did I lock the door?") to major life decisions (e.g., "Am I really in love and able to make a lifelong commitment to this relationship?").

O'Connor and Aardema (2012) consider doubt to be "an inference about a possible state of affairs in reality" (p. 29). Any thought that contains *maybe, what if, perhaps, the possibility that,* or *could be* is a doubtful statement. So, when Mateo thinks, "Maybe I didn't turn the faucet completely off," this is a doubt because he is inferring a possible state of affairs (i.e., the water faucet is dripping badly, the sink could fill with water, overflow, and flood the bathroom and then the living room). When he thinks, "Perhaps I don't really love Valerie," this is a doubt in which he is inferring the possibility that he does not love her and may be making a serious mistake by marrying her.

Our cognitive ability to make inferences or imagine possibilities means that doubt is pervasive and a normal part of human experience. In their international research on normal unwanted intrusive thoughts, Radomsky, Alcolado, and colleagues (2014) found that doubt was, by far, the most common theme of mental intrusions and was selected as individuals' most distressing intrusion over the last 3 months. Unwanted, distressing doubt, then, is a normative experience for most individuals.

Although particularly relevant in compulsive checking, doubt can be seen across many psychological disorders. If doubt is normative and transdiagnostic, what is different about OCD doubt? Table 11.1 summarizes some of the key differences that are discussed more fully below.

Contextual Differences

One of the major differences between normal and abnormal doubt is the context in which it occurs (Julien et al., 2007; O'Connor, Aardema, et al., 2005). OCD doubt occurs in situations that seem more irrational, even absurd, to the nonobsessional person, whereas normal doubt tends to occur in more reasonable, ambiguous situations. For example, the person with OCD might have the doubt "Am I using the right side of my body too much?," whereas a non-OCD person completing a long multiple choice exam might think, "Did I leave any questions blank?" The OCD doubt

TABLE 11.1. Characteristics That Differentiate Pathological and Normative Doubt

Pathological doubt	Normative doubt
• Greater irrationality, even absurdity	• More rationally based
• Presence of inferential confusion	• Greater inferential clarity based on real-world percepts
• More idiosyncratic	• More normative
• Low memory confidence	• Higher memory confidence
• Weaker sense of subjective conviction	• Strong sense of subjective conviction
• Impermeable, absolutistic schemas	• More flexible, adaptable schemas
• Elevated certainty threshold	• Lower certainty threshold
• Strong urge to complete	• Weaker urge to complete
⬇	⬇
—highly persistent —more frequent —more distressing —greater urge to check (neutralize)	—brief episodes —less frequent —slightly distressing —weaker urge to check (neutralize)

is absurd, because who can know what is "too much" and, of course, it doesn't matter whether one side of the body is used more than the other. On the other hand, it is entirely possible to miss a couple of questions on a long multiple-choice test. Pathological doubt, then, occurs in unusual contexts that fall on the more irrational side of imaginative possibilities (e.g., "Did I leave the dryer door open so the cat could jump in and die if the dryer mysteriously started to spin on its own?").

Faulty Reasoning

Pathological doubt is more likely characterized by faulty reasoning or inferential confusion (O'Connor, Aardema, et al., 2005). This occurs because OCD doubt is based on remote hypothetical possibilities rather than on reality-based sensory data. There is a distrust of sensory information in favor of an imagined possibility. So in pathological doubt a person may wonder, "Did I just run over a cyclist?" and become focused on the imagined possibility (i.e., "I am driving in a car that passed close to the cyclist; I could have brushed against the biker or come so close that I knocked him [or her] off the road"). The pathological doubt grows in intensity as the person focuses on this imagined possibility, confusing an imagined possibility as if it were reality. In normal doubt individuals may have the intrusive thought "Did I run over that cyclist?" but then concludes it can't be true because they looked in the rearview mirror and did not see an injured person, and did not feel the car shudder as if running over a body. Normal doubt, then, gets squelched because it is corrected by an appeal to real-life sensory information. Research based on the Inferential Confusion Questionnaire (ICQ; Aardema, O'Connor, & Emmelkamp, 2006) and ICQ—Expanded Version found that individuals with OCD score significantly higher than non-OCD-anxious and nonclinical controls (Aardema, O'Connor, Emmelkamp, Marchand, & Todorov, 2005; Aardema et al., 2010), and that inferential confusion was significantly related to obsessive–compulsive symptoms independent of other OCD belief domains (Aardema et al., 2006).

Idiosyncratic Content

Pathological doubt may involve more idiosyncratic themes than normative doubt. The international study on normal intrusive thoughts found that doubt in the nonclinical population focused on everyday activities like "Did I lock the door?"; "Did I unplug a heating device?"; "Did I turn off the stove?"; and so on (Radomsky, Alcolado, et al., 2014). However, in OCD the primary doubt often focuses on more idiosyncratic issues that are unique to the obsessional concerns of the individual (e.g., "Did I start with the correct foot when walking up the stairs?"). Even when the doubt is about ordinary activities, like locking the door, the person with OCD has a more idiosyncratic way of thinking. There is a tendency to experience (1) even more doubt about an initial conclusion when faced with alternative possibilities generated by others (Pélissier, O'Connor, & Dupuis, 2009) or (2) an overreliance on external proxies or rules because of a reduced sense of subjective conviction or a feeling of knowing (Lazarov, Dar, Oded, & Liberman, 2010). Thus, pathological doubt, even when about mundane affairs, is often experientially more bizarre than normal doubt.

Low Memory Confidence

Numerous studies have shown that OCD is characterized by significant distrust in memory (also referred to as low cognitive confidence), and that repeated checking decreases memory confidence, specifically in vividness and amount of detail recalled (e.g., Radomsky et al., 2001; Radomsky, Dugas, et al., 2014; van den Hout & Kindt, 2003b). Others have found that individuals with OCD also have reduced confidence in attention and that, once again, checking has a deleterious impact (Hermans et al., 2008). Considerable research has focused on the processes responsible for this effect, but it is clear that low memory confidence will intensify doubt in prior actions. Since nonclinical individuals have higher cognitive confidence in their actions and decisions, their doubt is less intense. Low cognitive confidence, then, is an important reason for the intensity one sees in pathological doubt.

Feeling of Knowing

Certainty may be harder to achieve in pathological doubt than in normal doubt because of a greater difficulty in achieving a subjective state of conviction or a "feeling of knowing" (Lazarov et al., 2010; Shapiro, 1965; Szechtman & Woody, 2004). In his discourse on obsessional doubt, Shapiro (1965) stated that a narrowing of attention and preoccupation with detail, along with restricted momentary subjective experience, cause a "loss of the experience of conviction" (p. 50). Pathological doubt and uncertainty are the consequence of this excessive focus on detail and loss of conviction about the world (i.e., a sense of truth), which prevents the person with OCD from seeing the real world in all its richness and changing variations of experience. This pathological doubt is accompanied by a need for some form of ritualistic behavior that is external, detailed, and mechanical; it's an attempt to compensate for "impairment of the sense of substantial reality" (Shapiro, 1965, p. 52).

Shapiro's formulation converges nicely with more recent evidence that individuals with OCD have a deficit in a "feeling of knowing" and so use external proxies or indicators as a compensation to infer their internal state (see also Szechtman & Woody, 2004). In their virtual checking experiments, van den Hout and Kindt (2003a, 2003b) found that repeated checking erodes memory confidence in the outcome of one's checking behavior because it inhibits bottom-up perceptual processing so that the recollections are rooted in "knowing" but not "remembering." That is, recollections after repeated checking are less vivid and detailed, so memory confidence is lower. The repeated checking induces a sense of ambivalence in which the individual has a memory of checking but it is indefinite and unclear (van den Hout & Kindt, 2003a). The "not just right" experience is a related phenomenon that can motivate checking (Summerfeldt, 2004). In sum, doubt will build in the person with OCD in part because the termination criteria—the conviction of remembering, yedasentience, or rightness—are so much more elusive than for the person who experiences normal doubt.

Maladaptive Beliefs

The core beliefs in pathological doubt will be more rigid and impermeable to contradictory evidence than the beliefs underlying normal doubt. However, there is mixed evidence of a relationship between dysfunctional beliefs and doubting or checking. Studies have failed to find a significant relationship between the OBQ belief subscales and the OCI-R Checking subscale in student and OCD samples (Tolin et al., 2008; Woods et al.,

2004). However, OBQ beliefs about inflated responsibility and threat overestimation were significantly related to the DOCS Responsibility for Harm and Mistakes subscale (Wheaton et al., 2010). Others have reported significant associations between OBQ Perfectionism and Importance/Control of Thoughts and OCI Checking in a student sample (Myers et al., 2008). Based on an OCD sample, Julien and associates found that OBQ perfectionism and certainty beliefs predicted the Padua Checking subscale (Julien et al., 2006). From these findings it would appear that threat, responsibility, and certainty beliefs play a role in pathological doubt and checking, although the results are not always consistent.

Intolerance of Uncertainty

Individuals exhibiting pathological doubt likely demand a higher level of certainty because of a preexisting IU (van den Hout & Kindt, 2003b). For example, if asked whether you are certain that you completely turned off a water faucet before leaving for work, you might be 97% certain and able to accept the other 3% of uncertainty. The individual with pathological doubt cannot accept 97% certainty, but strives for absolute certainty. This drive for total certainty forces the doubter to check or to excessively seek reassurance that the water faucet is completely off, because even a miniscule amount of uncertainty is intolerable. There is evidence that individuals with OCD involving checking and repeating had higher intolerance of uncertainty than noncheckers with OCD (Tolin et al., 2003). The authors note that IU may represent an emotional aspect of doubt in which a person feels heightened distress when confronting a number of possibilities.

Incompleteness/NJRE

Individuals with pathological doubt may experience a stronger drive to achieve a feeling of completeness or "just right" compared to normal doubters. There is evidence that the incompleteness sensory experience is significantly related to checking compulsions (Ecker & Gönner, 2008; Ecker, Kupfer, & Gönner, 2014b; Taylor et al., 2014). Thus, pathological doubters may have a stronger felt need to achieve an internal feeling of completeness in their struggle to resolve doubt. To the extent that normal doubters are less driven to achieve this feeling state, their efforts to resolve doubt will be less dire.

From this comparison of pathological and normal doubt, it is evident how the person with OCD can become "stuck in doubt." A tendency to base inferences on harm-related possibilities, a distrust in memory, a weak sense of subjective conviction, an unrealistic threshold of acceptable certainty, and a strong desire for completeness will together conspire toward more intense, persistent, and unresolved doubt.

RACHMAN'S COGNITIVE THEORY OF COMPULSIVE CHECKING

Rachman (2002) proposed a specific application of cognitive theory to explain the persistence of compulsive checking. Its central proposition is that compulsive checking occurs when individuals perceive a heightened responsibility to prevent harm but feel unsure whether they have adequately reduced or removed harm. To be certain that the harmful event will not occur, they repeatedly check for safety. Although checking may provide a temporary reduction in anxiety/distress, it is also associated with a number of other adverse effects that will paradoxically ensure continued repetition of the checking behavior. Rachman referred to these "adverse effects" as self-perpetuating mechanisms that ensure a compulsive repetition of checking.

The first mechanism is the search for certainty. Checking for safety can never provide the desired level of certainty that the likelihood of future harm to self or others has been eliminated because certainty for future events is elusive at best. This elusiveness ensures that the compulsive checking will continue indefinitely. Second, repeated checking clouds individuals' memory of their checking behavior because of the interfering effects of anxious arousal. They are so intently focused on the threat and their emotional reactions that they fail to recall specific details of their checking. Low memory confidence in their checking behavior reduces certainty that safety is established and so increases the likelihood that checking is repeated. Furthermore, negative or catastrophic misinterpretations about the importance of "not remembering" will contribute to an escalation in the checking behavior (e.g., "I must be really stupid or irresponsible because I'm not sure if I completely locked the door").

Third, for individuals with inflated responsibility, checking will increase the perceived probability of the harmful consequence. Checking will increase an individual's sense of personal responsibility after a check for safety is completed. Because of the adverse effects of checking for safety, a self-perpetuating cycle is established that ensures that "one check is never enough."

According to Rachman (2002), there are three cognitive processes that "multiply" checking behavior. The first multiplier is a belief that one has special responsibility to protect self or others from harm. Second, an inflated judgment of the perceived probability of the feared event will also increase the likelihood of checking behavior. The third multiplier is a heightened evaluation of the perceived severity or cost associated with the feared event. Rachman calls these "multipliers" because the presence or absence of each of these cognitive processes will increase or decrease the likelihood of compulsive checking. Thus, Rachman considers inflated responsibility and overestimated threat the two most critical faulty appraisals in compulsive checking. In addition, increased checking impairs memory accuracy of check details, thereby lowering memory confidence and strengthening a belief that one has an abnormally poor memory. Because the CBT model of compulsive checking proposed in this chapter draws heavily on Rachman's theory, a review of the empirical support for the CBT model depicted in Figure 11.1 (p. 296) also is applicable to Rachman's model.

Treatment Considerations

On the basis of this cognitive formulation, Rachman (2002) proposed that cognitive-behavioral treatment of compulsive checking must include three critical components.

- The modification of beliefs that one has a special responsibility to protect self or others from harm.
- Correction of the misinterpretation that one's checking behavior is preventing a possible threat or harm and improving memory confidence.
- Use of response prevention to challenge beliefs about the need to ensure safety.

The actual therapeutic elements of Rachman's (2002) approach focus on a strong didactic component in which the model is explained to clients as a rationale for treatment. Cognitive and experiential exercises are employed to counter inflated responsibility beliefs, although Rachman considered our ability to modify responsibility beliefs rather weak at best. Standard cognitive interventions, but especially behavioral experiments, are recommended to modify overestimated threat appraisals. Rachman considered response prevention of checking a key therapeutic strategy that must be emphasized throughout treatment.

THE INFERENCE-BASED MODEL

O'Connor and associates propose an inference-based theory (IBT) of OCD that is presented as an alternative to the current cognitive appraisal model (O'Connor, Aardema, et al., 2005; see also O'Connor, 2002). O'Connor (2002) argues that obsessions begin with an internal or external percept that is associated with a primary inference about a related state of affairs rather than unwanted intrusive thoughts. An inference is "a plausible proposition about a possible state of affairs, itself arrived at by reasoning but which forms the premise for further deductive/inductive reasoning" (O'Connor, Aardema, et al., 2005, p. 115). In obsessional thinking, the person makes an initial inference about an internal or external percept that relies on erroneous inductive reasoning processes. (These processes are presented in Table 11.2.) This erroneous reasoning leads to the construction of an idio-

TABLE 11.2. **Reasoning Processes Involved in the Inferential Confusion Evident in the Idiosyncratic Obsession Narrative**

Reasoning error	Definition
Category errors	Confusing two logical or ontically distinct properties or objects (e.g., "If this white table is dirty, it means the other white table could need cleaning").
Apparently comparable events	Confusing two distinct events separated by time, place, and/or causal agency (e.g., "My friend often drives off and leaves his garage door open, so mine could be left open")
Selective use of out-of-context facts or misplaced concreteness	Abstract facts are inappropriately applied to specific personal contexts (e.g., "Microbes do exist, so therefore there might be microbes infecting my hand").
Purely imaginary sequences	Making up convincing stories and living them (e.g., "I can imagine waves entering my head, so they could be affecting my brain").
Inverse inference	Inferences about reality precede rather than follow observation of reality (e.g., "A lot of people must have walked on this floor, therefore it could be dirty").
Distrust of normal perception	Disregarding the senses in favor of going deeper into reality (e.g., "Even though my senses tell me there's nothing there, I know by my intelligence that there might be more than I can see").

Note. From Clark and O'Connor (2005). Copyright © 2005 The Guilford Press. Adapted by permission.

syncratic doubting narrative in which imagined possibilities are confused with reality. This is termed *inferential confusion* in IBT and is seen as the primary cognitive process in obsessional doubt. Inferential confusion arises from the obsession-prone individual's distrust of the senses and a preference for possibilities that negate reality (O'Connor, Aardema, et al. 2005; O'Connor & Robillard, 1995). The obsessional inference or doubt is "generated as the result of purely subjective reasoning" (O'Connor, Aardema, et al., 2005, p. 118) in which the person confuses "a remote probability with a completely fictional narrative" (O'Connor & Robillard, 1995, p. 890). The end result is that the pathological doubter rejects sensory information in favor of hypothetical possibilities.

How might IBT explain Mateo's incessant doubt about marrying Valerie? It might start with a conversation in which Valerie is talking about wedding plans. Mateo notices he is not interested in the conversation, but then makes an erroneous inference.

"Why am I so disconnected from this conversation? Maybe this means I'm not serious about marrying Valerie [category error]. If I'm so disinterested in the wedding, it means that I don't really love Valerie and that my commitment to our relationship is weak [inverse inference]. If I marry Valerie without complete certainty that I love her, then I could be trapped in a loveless, tormented marriage [distrust of normal perception]. My life would be ruined forever [purely imaginary sequences]."

One can see from this primary inference or narrative of obsessional doubt that Mateo is building his doubt on an imaginary scenario. He is uninterested in the conversation about bridesmaid's dresses but then erroneously infers the possibility that his momentary disinterest is caused by a lack of love and commitment to the relationship. He then experiences a persistent and recurring doubt about the relationship that causes an increase in anxiety or distress. To relieve the discomfort, he compulsively seeks reassurance about the relationship and his commitment to it (O'Connor & Aardema, 2012).

According to IBT, inferential confusion is a cognitive variable that is evident in all forms of OCD, is disorder-specific, and is distinct from other obsessive–compulsive cognitive constructs such as obsessional beliefs (O'Connor, Aardema, et al., 2005). IBT intervention focuses on the correction of inferential confusion and resolution of doubt to achieve obsessive–compulsive symptom improvement (Aardema & O'Connor, 2012). A tendency to engage in faulty inductive reasoning, especially in relation to obsessive–compulsive-relevant concerns, might be a vulnerability factor for OCD (Clark & O'Connor, 2005), which would make inferential confusion a causal factor in obsessional doubt.

Since first proposing the IBT approach in the mid-1990s, O'Connor, Aardema, and others have carried out an ambitious research program to demonstrate the importance of faulty inductive reasoning or inferential confusion in obsessional doubt. Most of the research has relied on the ICQ to investigate the role of inferential confusion in OCD (Aardema et al., 2006). The 15-item ICQ consists of statements that depict inverse reasoning and distrust of the senses related to unpleasantness, harm, and safety. A later 30-item expanded version of the ICQ (ICQ-EV) was developed to assess a broader range of reasoning errors, such as category errors, reliance on remote or irrelevant associations, absorption into imaginary sequences, and the like (Aardema et al., 2010). Both instruments have good psychometric properties and are significantly correlated with OCD symptom measures (Aardema et al., 2006, 2010). Moreover, inferential confusion (i.e., ICQ Total Scores) is significantly higher in OCD than in non-OCD-anxious and nonclinical controls (Aardema et al., 2006) and is related, but distinct, from other obsessive–compulsive beliefs and continues to predict obsessive–compulsive symptoms when other beliefs are controlled (Aardema et al., 2006). As well, change in inferential confusion was a better predictor of obsessive–compulsive symptom change after a trial of IBT treatment than change in OBQ beliefs (Del Borrello & O'Connor, 2014).

Several studies have shown that inferential confusion increases pathological doubt. For example, when making inferences, the type of inductive reasoning strategy used by people with OCD is associated with more doubt than that of nonobsessional controls (Pélissier et al., 2009). As well, belief in the real probability of the obsessional doubt was inversely related to perceived ability to resist a compulsive act (Grenier, O'Connor, & Bélanger, 2010). Finally, ability to resolve obsessional doubt may be an important change mechanism in IBT (Aardema & O'Connor, 2012). Together, these findings indicate that inferential confusion is an important factor in pathological doubt (see also Nikodijevic, Moulding, Anglim, Aardema, & Nedeljkovic, 2015).

Treatment Considerations

O'Connor and Aardema (2012) developed a cognitive treatment for OCD that focuses on correction of the primary inference or doubt. Change in doubt occurs by resolving inferential confusion, which consists of distrust of the senses or self, and overinvestment in remote possibilities. The goal of IBT, then, is to modify obsessional doubt rather than actual behavior. In IBT behavioral change is a consequence of a reduction in inferential confusion, so behavioral experiments, exposure, and reality testing are not needed to eliminate compulsions. As stated by O'Connor and Aardema in the introduction of their treatment manual, "In IBT the aim is to reorient the client to reality through cognitive education and insight, so that the client relates to reality as reality by performing what we term 'reality sensing' which entails relating to reality in a normal non-effortful way" (p. xv).

IBT usually consists of 12–20 individual sessions that are divided into three parts: (1) education and foundation, (2) intervention, and (3) consolidation. The education component introduces the client to the IBT model and the importance of doubt in the obsessive–compulsive cycle. A unique aspect IBT education is the use of exercises and worksheets to help clients discover their doubt sequence, reasoning errors, and obsessional story or narrative. The *narrative unit* is a story or explanation that convinces individuals of some shred of logic to the obsessional doubt (O'Connor & Aardema, 2012). It contains both reasoning and rhetoric, "interposing associations, bridging, assumptions, generalizations and hearsay and according all equal legitimacy to arrive at the inference that what is not there is, in fact, there" (O'Connor & Aardema, 2012, p. 58). The following is a possible narrative unit Mateo could have used to justify repeatedly walking up and down stairs because he doubts it was done correctly.

THERAPIST: Mateo, you've told me that sometimes you get stuck and find yourself walking up and down stairs several times until you feel that you've done it correctly.

MATEO: Yes, it's so frustrating and embarrassing. I'm afraid someone will catch me doing this.

THERAPIST: I understand that you doubt that you walked up the stairs correctly, but why do you think it's so important to ascend the stairs correctly? [question that probes for the narrative unit]

MATEO: Well, I get halfway up the stairs and I can't remember whether I started the stairs with my left or right foot. I immediately start to feel uncomfortable and realize that I am creating bad *karma* for myself. I need to neutralize bad *karma* by having good, positive thoughts while I go up the stairs. If I don't, the bad *karma* will follow me throughout the day. I'll end up feeling anxious and unable to concentrate at work because I'll be expecting something bad to happen to me or to Valerie. The best way to deal with this situation is to repeat my actions, pay close attention to ensure that I start to ascend the stairs with my right foot and try to keep good positive thoughts in my head throughout the ascension, so I'm creating good *karma*. [Mateo's narrative unit]

The IBT therapist helps clients discover their vulnerable self-theme within the narrative unit. This is the self the person fears becoming and is another important contributor to the individual's obsessions and compulsions. For example, one of Mateo's vulnerability themes was hurting self or others. He feared being the type of person who is callous, uncaring, insensitive; a person who is responsible for causing bad things to happen to others and is completely unconcerned about his ill effect on friends and loved ones.

The second phase of IBT, *intervention,* directly changes the obsessional doubt by first convincing the client that obsessional doubt is constructed without any direct evidence; that it is 100% imaginary (O'Connor & Aardema, 2012). Much of the work at this point is quite similar to the cognitive restructuring seen in CBT for obsessions, although it differs by focusing on the narrative unit and the client's use of reasoning errors. One intervention unique to IBT is called *reality sensing*. Here exercises and worksheets are introduced that guide clients away from the doubt and toward greater trust and reliance on their senses. An alternative narrative is created that is based on external reality—that is, the senses—rather than on imagined possibilities. For example, the alternative narrative for Mateo's "stair compulsion" might be:

"Karma or fate is determined more by actions than by feelings. I am wrong to think that creating a good or right feeling has a direct effect on karma. For example, I could feel great, reading a text message from Valerie that leaves me filled with hope and excitement for the future. I am reading this text as I walk, and I don't see the 'Don't walk' pedestrian sign. I step into the intersection still reading Valerie's wonderful text. I don't see the speeding car and am suddenly hit, causing serious harm that results in a long hospitalization and permanent injuries. My fate was determined by my actions at that moment, not by how I felt or what I did earlier in the day. In fact, we often have little control in guaranteeing the good or bad that happens in our lives. Who can cause good things, like winning the lottery, simply by generating a positive feeling or intuition? In the end much of our fate, or karma, is unpredictable and unknowable. Life is full of surprises; it's an important part of the human experience."

The final phase of IBT is *consolidation*. Its aim is to further weaken the obsessional doubt and strengthen the alternative narrative. The interventions involved at this stage include (1) elaborating the alternative narrative, (2) highlighting reasoning errors that can pull the client back into the obsessional doubt, (3) pinpointing the selectivity of the pathological doubt, (4) implementing action that is based on the alternative narrative, and (5) providing relapse prevention strategies that help maintain gains and deal with any problems that could undermine the client's ability to use the IBT approach (O'Connor & Aardema, 2012).

COGNITIVE-BEHAVIORAL MODEL OF COMPULSIVE CHECKING

Figure 11.1 presents a cognitive-behavioral model of compulsive checking that draws heavily on Rachman's (2002) cognitive theory and some of the key constructs from IBT.

Vulnerability Factors

Based on the IBT research, we might expect that people predisposed to obsessional doubt and checking would have a tendency to commit inductive reasoning errors, especially when dealing with issues that threaten valued self-domains (Clark & O'Connor, 2005; Doron & Kyrios, 2005). However, Simpson, Cove, Fineberg, Msetfi, and Ball (2007) found that an OCD sample differed from nonclinical controls on only one out of four inductive reasoning parameters.

Another potential vulnerability factor is the feared self. In pathological doubt and compulsive checking, the individual might have a self-representation that is overly concerned with avoiding characteristics such as irresponsibility, carelessness, recklessness, or superficiality. This self-

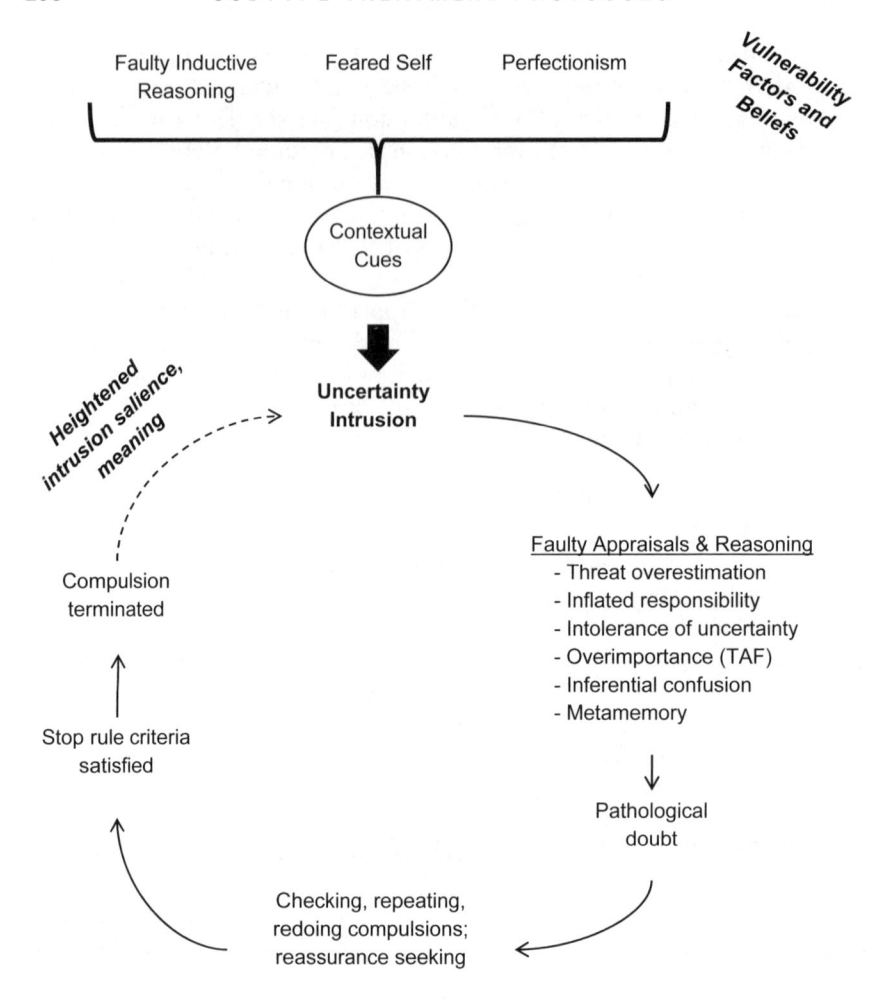

FIGURE 11.1. Cognitive-behavioral model of checking compulsions.

representation is the "feared me" that the compulsive checker is most concerned to avoid, and so processes thoughts and feelings of uncertainty more deeply. Research on the feared self is based on a self-report measure called the Fear of Self Questionnaire (FSQ; Aardema et al., 2013). Most of the FSQ items deal with fear of moral violation, inadequacy, and unworthiness. In the original study the FSQ was a significant predictor of obsessive–compulsive symptoms and beliefs, but there was no specific relationship with checking compulsions. The convergent validity of the FSQ was confirmed in a second study conducted on OCD and nonclinical samples, although the instrument appeared to have particular relevance for repugnant obsessions (Melli, Aardema, & Moulding, 2016). It is likely that selfhood issues play a role in vulnerability to compulsive checking, but whether other self-representational constructs like self-ambivalence or self-domain sensitivities are more relevant than feared self remain to be seen.

Perfectionism is another possible vulnerability factor for doubting and compulsive checking. Perfectionism has long been implicated as a key etiological factor in psychoanalytic theories of OCD and especially obsessive–compulsive personality disorder (OCPD; see Frost et al., 2002). Empirical research indicates that perfectionism is highly relevant for OCD (see Frost et al., 2002; Summerfeldt et al., 1998) and that it correlates with checking symptoms (OCCWQ, 2005; Wu & Cortesi, 2009). Frost and colleagues (2002) concluded in their review that perfectionism plays a specific role in checking compulsions by making people especially concerned about exerting control over certain events in their lives. Unfortunately, the necessary prospective and experimental research is not available, so the vulnerability constructs depicted in Figure 11.1 are merely speculative at the present time.

Context and Uncertainty Intrusions

The precipitates of pathological doubt often involve an external object or situation that requires some action or decision by the individual that involves taking personal responsibility to exert control over an outcome. Common examples are locking a door, turning off water faucets or light switches, driving, filling in forms, etc. The importance of contextual cues was recognized in some of the earliest behavioral research on compulsive checking (e.g., Beech & Perigault, 1974; Rachman & Hodgson, 1980). It is possible that an internal cue, like a feeling or sensation, could also trigger a sense of uncertainty, but this is much less common than external cues that involve some requirement of control by the individual.

A sense of uncertainty or incompleteness in knowledge coupled with a distrust of sensory information is an essential feature of doubt (O'Connor & Aardema, 2012). Thus, in the proposed CBT model, contextual cues trigger an initial intrusive thought or image of uncertainty. That first thought, "Did I lock the door?," represents an initial conscious experience of uncertainty. From that first uncertainty intrusion, a cascade of cognitive processes occurs that leads to a more sustained mental experience of doubt and then checking behavior (see Figure 11.1).

Faulty Appraisals and Reasoning

In the CBT model faulty appraisals of the uncertainty intrusion are the most critical element in the pathogenesis of pathological doubt and checking. We would expect that all of the appraisals discussed in Chapter 5 play a role in checking compulsions. Figure 11.1 highlights four appraisal processes that are especially important in the checking subtype. In their review, Radomsky and colleagues (2008) concluded that correlational and experimental research indicates that inflated responsibility and threat overestimation have a specific relationship with checking behavior. Much of the correlational research is based on the OBQ, which measures responsibility and threat beliefs. However, there is such a close relationship between appraisals and beliefs that we can consider the OBQ a proxy measure of appraisals (i.e., Clark, 2002).

Not all of the empirical research supports a specific relationship between inflated responsibility/threat overestimation and checking compulsions. Julien and colleagues (2006), for example, did not find that the OCD checking subtype scored significantly higher on the OBQ Responsibility/Threat Overestimation subscale than other OCD subtypes, based on symptom classification derived from the Padua Inventory–Revised Checking subscale (see also Tolin et al., 2008). Nevertheless, others have found a relationship between OBQ Responsibility/Threat Overestimation subscale and doubt (Wheaton et al., 2010), and there are experimental studies indicating that heightened responsibility for threatening outcomes does increase the urge to check (for further discussion, see the Chapter 5 section on the causal status of faulty appraisals and beliefs). So we can conclude that faulty appraisals of personal responsibility for perceived threatening outcomes are probably important in the escalation of pathological doubt and checking.

Overimportance of thought (including TAF–Likelihood) and IU are two other appraisal processes that may play a particularly important role in doubt and checking. Again, Radomsky and colleagues (2008) concluded that IU plays an important role in the genesis of compulsive checking. This is hardly surprising, given that uncertainty lies at the very heart of doubt. As well, the nature of the initial intrusion (i.e., sense of uncertainty) and the vulnerability factors implicated in pathological doubt and checking ensure that faulty uncertainty appraisals will lead to an escalation in doubt. (Chapter 5 reviews the empirical research on appraisals and checking; see pp. 122–126.)

In their review of the overimportance of thoughts, Thordarson and Shafran (2002) concluded that the construct was significantly elevated in OCD more generally, but not checking compulsions specifically. Moreover, beliefs in the importance of thought overlap with TAF bias. A general belief in the importance of unwanted thoughts is implicit in the TAF Scale items. However, in their review of TAF, Berle and Starcevic (2005) concluded that the construct was not necessarily specific to OCD, let alone to a particular OCD subtype. In sum, it is likely that overimportance of thought and TAF are relevant faulty appraisal processes in doubt and compulsive checking, but these constructs are clearly not unique to this OCD subtype.

Finally, inferential confusion and deficiencies in metamemory are cognitive processes known to be important in the pathogenesis of checking behavior. The research of O'Connor and associates on inferential confusion indicates that it is a nonspecific determinant of checking. That is, inferential confusion is a faulty cognitive process that characterizes all OCD subtypes (O'Conner, Aardema, et al., 2005). Deficiencies in metamemory, on the other hand, may be more specific to checking. In their review Radomsky and colleagues (2008) argued that memory accuracy may actually be greater in compulsive checking, but that other characteristics of memory, such as vividness, detail, and confidence (i.e., metamemory), are attenuated. For example, more accurate recall or even enhanced memory accuracy (i.e., memory bias) for threat-related stimuli relevant to checking concerns has been reported in some studies (e.g., Ashbaugh & Radomsky, 2007; Constans, Foa, Franklin, & Mathews, 1995; Radomsky et al., 2001), although negative findings have also been reported (Tuna, Tekan, & Topçuoğlu, 2005). Radomsky and colleagues argue that a positive memory bias for threat will only be evident when individuals with compulsive checking truly feel threatened, such as in high-responsibility situations.

More consistent evidence has been found for reduced memory confidence and subjective conviction of knowing (or feeling of knowing) in compulsive checking (e.g., Dar, Rish, Hermesh, Taub, & Fux, 2000; Radomsky et al., 2001; Tuna et al., 2005). As well, individuals with compulsive checking may have reduced memory vividness and detail (Constans et al., 1995) and reduced confidence in their attentional ability (Hermans et al., 2008). A recent series of experimental studies using virtual or real-life situations have shown that repeated checking will cause a decrease in memory confidence, vividness, and detail because of a greater reliance on conceptual rather than perceptual processing, even though memory accuracy remains unaffected (Coles, Radomsky, & Horng, 2006; Radomsky, Dugas, et al., 2014; Radomsky, Gilchrist, & Dussault, 2006; van den Hout & Kindt, 2003a, 2003b). Overall, there is considerable empirical evidence that compulsive checking causes a decrease in metamemory that will exacerbate doubt and increase the likelihood of further repeated checking.

A number of key research questions remain unanswered about memory effects on compulsive checking. The relationship between decreases in metamemory and pathological doubt has not been addressed specifically, although one would expect increases in doubt and uncertainty with decreased memory confidence. And second, there is a confound between sensory processing and the knowing versus remembering ratings. We would assume that memories with high ratings on vividness, detail, and confidence would be more likely remembered, whereas memories that are less vivid and detailed would elicit a sense of knowing (i.e., be more conceptually recalled). It would be interesting to analyze the knowing versus remembering variable after controlling for vividness, detail, and other metamemory ratings. This would help determine the unique contribution of knowing versus remembering in the persistence of compulsive checking.

Pathological Doubt

The combined effects of faulty appraisals and reasoning will elevate the uncertainty intrusions to a higher level of personal significance and threat. Further elaboration and reflection on the uncertainty will intensify the subjective experience of doubt. The individual will become increasingly convinced that an uncertain state of affairs exists that can be rectified only by checking. At first the doubting may extend over several minutes as the individual attempts to resist the urge to check, trying to reappraise the uncertainty in a more adaptive manner. However, in chronic compulsive checking, the doubt may be elicited so automatically that there is little time between the doubt and the occurrence of checking.

Compulsive Checking

With the emergence of pathological doubt, the continuing trajectory of compulsive checking looks remarkably similar to washing compulsions. Individuals will check, repeat, and redo in response to the doubt. However, compared to washing compulsions and contamination fear, checking is not as effective in resolving doubt, so anxiety or guilt reduction, attainment of certainty, or a sense of safety is not as satisfactory (Rachman & Hodgson, 1980). In fact, repeated checking and redoing can lead to an increase in frustration, anger, or tension (see also Rachman & Shafran, 1998), which could be an impetus to stop checking. In a recent experiment on checking and the security motivation system, Hinds and colleagues found that OCD checkers were less able to reduce activation of the security motivation system after a sufficient opportunity to check, indicating that compulsive checkers have a problem in stopping (Hinds, Woody, Schmidt, Van Ameringen, & Szechtman, 2015). Although these results indicate that compulsive checkers had difficulty achieving a sense of safety or confidence that they had not made a mistake, it is possible that other parameters of knowing when to stop could have contributed, such as the frustration caused by continuing to check.

In summary, there is considerable empirical evidence to support the role of faulty appraisals, erroneous reasoning, and pathological doubt in the pathogenesis of compulsive checking. However, much less is known about the vulnerability factors in OCD checking, which states are most important in determining when checking can stop, and the role of failed mental control in the persistence of doubt and checking. As well, many of the cognitive and emotive variables proposed in the pathogenesis of checking are also important in other OCD subtypes. More comparative research on OCD symptom subtypes and experimental studies that manipulate uncertainty are needed to determine the specific cognitive pathway to compulsive checking.

RELATIONSHIP OCD

Recently an obsessive doubt has been identified that focuses specifically on intimate relationships. Labeled *relationship obsessive–compulsive disorder* (ROCD), it refers to "preoccupations and doubts centered on one's feelings towards a relationship partner, the partner's feelings toward oneself, and the 'rightness' of the relationship experience" (Doron, Derby, & Szepsenwol, 2014, p. 169). Although some degree of ambivalence and doubt about intimate relationships is normal, ROCD is considered pathological because of its ego-dystonic and intrusive features as well as its ability to generate a high level of personal distress and functional impairment (Doron, Derby, Szepsenwol, & Talmor, 2012). To assess this clinical phenomenon, Doron and colleagues developed the 12-item Relationship Obsessive Compulsive Inventory (ROCI). Confirmatory factor analysis based on a nonclinical sample revealed three dimensions that reflect doubts about one's love for his or her partner, doubts about the relationship itself, and doubts about whether one is loved by his or her partner (Doron, Derby, et al., 2012). The ROCI subscales evidenced small to moderate correlations with symptom measures of anxiety, depression, OCD, and obsessive–compulsive beliefs, as well as relationship distress and dissatisfaction (Doron, Derby, et al., 2012; Doron, Mizrahi, Szepsenwol, & Derby, 2014). In another nonclinical study, individuals with anxious attachment and a tendency to derive self-worth from their intimate relationships reported the highest ROCI scores, and negative feedback of their relationship competence increased their ROCI responses (Doron, Szepensenwol, Karp, & Gal, 2012). Another study found a positive association between ROCI scores and increased breakup distress in a sample of individuals who experienced a significant romantic breakup in the past 3 months (Clark, O'Sullivan, & Fuller, 2015).

In their conceptual paper on ROCD, Doron, Derby, and Szepsenwol (2014) noted that individuals with obsessive doubts about their intimate relationship will experience unwanted intrusive thoughts and images of doubt about the partner that cause significant personal distress. Attempts to neutralize the distress and doubt can take the form of repeated checking of one's thoughts and feelings about the partner, comparing the partner's characteristics to others in order to rationalize and convince oneself about true feelings toward the partner, reassurance seeking from the partner, or attempts to visualize or recall positive experiences with the partner. Like other forms of obsessive doubt, these neutralizing efforts offer only temporary relief and increase the salience of the doubt. Intense fear of relationship breakup may be evident in some cases of ROCD.

Unfortunately, all of the ROCD research is based on nonclinical samples. Individual case studies of pathological ROCD can be found, but systematic research with clinical samples is missing. Certain fundamental questions about the prevalence of ROCD, its differentiation from other OCD subtypes, and vulnerability/maintenance factors remain unanswered. At this point a conceptual formulation of ROCD has been extrapolated from findings based on normative samples, but caution must be exercised when generalizing to clinical samples. Doron, Derby, and Szepsenwol (2014) provide some treatment insights and indicate that a treatment manual is currently under development. Until published, the practitioner must adapt current CBT interventions for doubt to the specific exigencies of ROCD.

SPECIAL TREATMENT CONSIDERATIONS

Inflated Responsibility

Previous chapters presented cognitive and behavioral strategies for correcting inflated responsibility beliefs and appraisals. Rachman (2002) noted that responsibility beliefs need to be addressed when treating compulsive checking. Cognitive restructuring was the recommended approach, along with transfer and delay of responsibility strategies, but these approaches can be particularly challenging with OCD checkers because the compulsion is intended to prevent an imagined catastrophe.

One option is to use IBT strategies to correct faulty responsibility appraisals. Another is to employ imagery rescripting (see Arntz, Tiesema, & Kindt, 2007; Holmes, Arntz, & Smucker, 2007). To explain how this approach might work, Mateo's email problem provides an example. First, a high-responsibility imagery scenario is developed in which Mateo repeatedly checks an email before sending it. A coworker receives the email, but its impact is uncertain The scenario should be based on a realistic doubting and checking experience. As Mateo imagines the scenario, the therapist offers questions that challenge his faulty responsibility beliefs:

> "How did the repeated checking prevent a misinterpretation? How would you know if your coworker did or did not misinterpret the email?"
>
> "If she did misinterpret the message, how could you have prevented this? How much of the misinterpretation is the fault of the coworker's lack of knowledge?"
>
> "Are you overestimating your responsibility for ensuring the correct interpretation by your coworker?"

"Did you feel more or less responsible by checking repeatedly?"
"What is it costing you personally to keep checking your emails repeatedly?"

Once the therapist has thoroughly explored the high-responsibility scenario, a low-responsibility script is constructed. In this case, Mateo reads over the email once and then sends it. The coworker receives it, but its impact is uncertain. In this scenario, the therapist and Mateo work out how he would deal with the potential misinterpretation and his sense of responsibility for not sending a better email. Several probing questions can be asked:

"How responsible would you feel for sending the misinterpreted email? How much would others hold you responsible? How upset would you feel? Would it last for days? Would it be so intense you could not get out of bed?"
"How much damage would your irresponsibility cause? Would your coworker ever speak to you again?"
"Given your anxiety about the email, could you ask your coworker if she had any concerns about your message? Would this be a better way to deal with your anxiety and uncertainty? Could you imagine yourself using this strategy—if only sparingly?"
"What is the personal cost or benefit to you of reading an email once and then sending it?"
"As you reevaluate your responsibility for miscommunication, what's a more realistic estimate for you and your coworker? Is it really 50/50?"

Once the adaptive and maladaptive responsibility scenarios are developed, it would be important for Mateo to practice the adaptive scenario when he sends emails. The imagery work must be followed by actual ERP in order to be effective.

Inferential Confusion and Faulty Reasoning

There are several elements of the IBT approach to pathological doubt that can be helpful in treating inferential confusion and faulty reasoning. For the present purpose, there are two main themes to the IBT approach. The first is to educate clients that their doubt is the product of faulty reasoning. And the second is to shift the clients' focus from the imaginary world of their doubt to the real world of the senses.

O'Connor and Aardema (2012) describe several homework exercises for increasing awareness of faulty reasoning. This psychoeducational intervention is not unlike teaching individuals to identify their cognitive errors in standard cognitive therapy (Beck et al., 1979). Individuals are provided with this awareness training so that they learn about their doubting narrative of their vulnerable self, and how they interact to create pathological doubt and checking.

O'Connor and Aardema (2012) describe several metaphorical strategies to counter inferential confusion, such as (1) referring to OCD as 100% imaginary and 100% irrelevant, (2) going to the OCD bubble, and (3) practicing reality sensing. Each of these strategies is designed to shift the client from focusing on imaginary possibilities to trusting and acting on the senses. For example, Mateo could be taught to catch himself thinking about the imagined possibility (i.e., "What if my coworker completely misinterprets this email and thinks I am criticizing her?"). It would be important for Mateo to realize that at the moment of sending the email, he is completely (100%) imagining a misinterpretation, and because it is imaginary, it is irrelevant to the task at hand. Mateo would learn to be more aware of when he crosses over into an "OCD bubble," in which he leaves the world of senses for his world of imagined possibilities (O'Connor & Aardema, 2012, p. 3). A series of homework exercises are proposed that encourage obsessional doubters to catch themselves entering the "OCD bubble" and then correct by reentering the real world of the senses. There is a strong element of ERP in these exercises. After correcting their inferential confusion, clients are instructed to "act upon the information from your senses by dismissing the obsession and not engaging in any compulsive rituals" (O'Connor & Aardema, 2012, p. 153). For further explanation of IBT interventions, see O'Connor and Aardema's *Clinician's Handbook for Obsessive Compulsive Disorder* (2012).

Feared Self-Domain

The construct of the feared self is derived from IBT and its emphasis on the *vulnerable self-theme*. According to O'Connor, Aardema, and colleagues (2005), a person's obsessional doubt focuses on a specific self-referential theme that represents a particular concern or sensitivity. Mateo's doubt, for example, often concerned whether he might cause some adverse event to self or others by a careless action. Thus, one of Mateo's vulnerable self-themes was being a careless or thoughtless individual. Consequently, his doubt often focused on making mistakes or being incomplete in his communication. More recently, the notion of a vulnerable self-theme has led to the stronger concept of the "feared" self, although this construct may have more relevance for repugnant obsessions than checking compulsions (Aardema, Moulding, et al., 2018; Nikodijevic et al., 2015). This idea goes beyond the notion of certain selfhood sensitivities and suggests that obsessional doubters might actually experience fear or anxiety at the thought of being careless, thoughtless, inadequate, or the like.

The concept of a feared self could be incorporated into cognitive interventions for compulsive checking. The FSQ could be administered, with the possibility that items concerning inadequacy are more relevant to OCD checkers (Aardema et al., 2013). The therapist could use endorsement of these items to explore with the client a possible feared self that contributes to doubt and excessive checking. As well, IBT offers a more psychoeducational approach for sensitizing individuals to their vulnerable (feared) self-theme and then challenging the veracity of that perceived vulnerability.

As an example of a CBT approach to the feared self, Socratic questioning might reveal that Mateo had a fear of being perceived as a careless, sloppy individual. The therapist could explore the developmental origins and experiences that led to this entrenched selfhood fear. A cost–benefit analysis could be used to determine whether it is advantageous to be driven by this fear of carelessness. A more realistic, balanced perspective on care and meticulousness could be developed by examining how other people deal with the prospect of carelessness. Behavioral experiments could be assigned in which Mateo is exposed to varying levels of "being less thoughtful and observant." He could be taught to use mindful thought labeling in which he practices labeling and then observing the "fear of carelessness thought" in a detached, nonjudgmental manner. We would expect these thoughts to occur in situations that elicit uncertainty, doubt, and checking.

Tolerance of Uncertainty and Distress

Tolerance of uncertainty and distress are not unique to obsessional doubt. They are transdiagnostic constructs evident in most anxiety disorders and subtypes of OCD. Robichaud and Dugas (2006) present three elements in their CBT for GAD that target uncertainty. The first involves increasing clients' awareness of their intolerance of uncertainty, as indicated by "What if . . ." questions. That is, the person learns that thinking "What if _____ happens?" is an indication that uncertainty intolerance has occurred. Second, the client is taught to identify and then reduce avoidance and safety behaviors in order to face the inevitability of uncertainty. And third, "exposure exercises" are assigned in which an action is taken even in the face of uncertainty. In this case individuals are encouraged to process the uncertainty and observe their ability to tolerate the feeling of discomfort.

With compulsive checking, work on uncertainty needs to consider the highly imaginary obsessional fear and the intolerance of even remote possibilities of occurrence. Mateo, for example, "knew" it was extremely unlikely that he had left a stove burner on and the house would catch on fire. And yet, he was drawn back to check by overwhelming doubt. At first, Mateo was convinced he was checking to deal with his intolerance of uncertainty. But multiple checks never left him feeling more certain. He often stopped checking due to mounting frustration, or a vague feeling that "It was all right, he could let it go." The therapist could point out the many occasions, like with the stove, when he eventually stopped checking even with some lingering doubt. From this Mateo could learn that he was tolerating more uncertainty in the obsessional context than he realized.

Strategies to improve distress tolerance in compulsive checking are similar to what are used in other OCD subtypes. Much of this work focuses on correcting maladaptive beliefs about negative emotion and its tolerance through cognitive restructuring. In addition, graduated ERP is critical to training individuals in distress tolerance. The therapist could ensure that the client tests out distress intolerance beliefs through the exposure exercises. For example, Mateo's exposure to sending emails after only one reread would generate considerable distress. When reviewing the exposure homework, the therapist could ask Mateo how well he tolerated the distress, how long it lasted, whether it interfered in his daily functioning, what helped or hindered reduction of the distress, how did the distress compare to other unpleasant states like physical pain, and the like. The goal of these interventions is to strengthen clients' confidence that they can deal with heightened distress in the obsessional context. In their review, Bernstein and colleagues noted that intervention strategies from interoceptive exposure, mindfulness training, dialectical behavior therapy, and acceptance-based emotion regulation might prove helpful with improving distress tolerance (Bernstein, Vujanovic, Leyro, & Zvolensky, 2011).

Response Prevention

Rachman (2002) emphasized that response prevention (RP) is an essential ingredient in CBT for checking compulsions. RP of behavioral checking is relatively straightforward. However, individuals with OCD checking often engage in mental checks, which are much more difficult to control. Trying to do RP with mental checks is tantamount to prescribing thought suppression, which is a notoriously ineffective mental control strategy, especially over a longer time period (i.e., Abramowitz et al., 2001; Najmi et al., 2009; Rassin, 2005). So the challenge is to encourage disengagement from checking, repeating, or redoing without encouraging effortful suppression.

Once again, mindful observation of the mental check might be helpful. Instead of active suppression, the client acknowledges the existence of the mental activity and then gently redirects attention away from the thought. For example, Mateo would often try to form a visual image of the stove dial in the off position as a mental check that it was turned off. When leaving the house and finding himself pulled toward the image of the stove dial, he would acknowledge it, name it as the "dial image," and then focus his attention externally, such as being mindful of his drive to work. Another possibility is to replace the mental check with a fear image.

In this case, Mateo could imagine the stove left on and the red-hot burner left unattended. This would amount to imaginal fear exposure. Of course, it would be important to ensure that the client does not substitute a subtle behavioral check for the mental check, such as looking at the home security app on his smartphone to see that everything is okay at home.

Finally, RP can be more distressing for OCD checkers because the check is intended to prevent some future catastrophe that could be years away. Thus, reducing the checking compulsions through RP means that uncertainty is significantly elevated, which adds to the client's distress. CBT needs to take uncertainty interpretations into account when doing RP for checking compulsions.

TREATMENT EFFICACY

In their review of ERP treatment outcome studies, M. T. Williams and colleagues (2013) concluded that ERP was as effective for doubt and checking compulsions as for other OCD subtypes like contamination fears. Reanalysis of ERP treatment outcome by OCD symptom subtype again revealed no significant difference between compulsive washers and checkers (Abramowitz, Franklin, et al., 2003). Starcevic and Brakoulias (2008) also concluded in their review that checking compulsions respond as well to ERP or CBT as washing compulsions. Reviewers noted that a specialized form of ERP or CBT has not been developed for compulsive checking because checking rituals are so well represented in symptom heterogeneous OCD outcome studies. M. T. Williams and colleagues speculated that CBT may need to be refined when compulsive checking has a strong element of the "not just right" feeling.

CONCLUSION

Doubt and checking compulsions are found in most OCD cases regardless of symptom subtype. Doubt, the primary cognitive symptom in compulsive checking, is rooted in normal inferential states of uncertainty about one's decisions and actions. However, the key distinction in pathological doubt is the presence of inferential confusion, low memory confidence, and a weaker sense of subjective conviction (i.e., the "feeling of knowing").

Two cognitive models were discussed that explain the pathogenesis and treatment of compulsive checking. In Rachman's (2002) cognitive model, checking occurs because individuals are seeking an unrealistic level of certainty that they have achieved safety from possible harm to self or others. However, increased checking causes a reduction in memory confidence along with a heightened sense of responsibility. These factors, combined with exaggerated judgments of the probability and severity of threat, ensure the persistence of checking behavior. A second cognitive model, IBT, focuses on the pathogenesis of doubt, which is considered a central symptom feature in all forms of OCD. O'Connor and associates (O'Connor & Aardema, 2012; O'Connor, Aardema, et al., 2005) argue that the core problem in OCD is the occurrence of inferential confusion and faulty reasoning in which individuals base their inferences (i.e., doubt) on imagined possibilities rather than on sensory information derived from the external world.

A CBT model for compulsive checking was proposed (see Figure 11.1) that recognized the importance of faulty reasoning, inferential confusion, and low memory confidence in the pathogenesis of compulsive checking. Although this model shares similarities with the other cognitive appraisal models of OCD, the greater importance of attentional and memory uncertainty or low confidence, and the increased role played by faulty reasoning and inflated responsibility, are the more distinct features of the model. As well, the initial unwanted intrusion in checking has a strong uncertainty element, with faulty appraisals of threat, responsibility, and TAF salient contributors to the genesis of compulsive checking.

Standard ERP and CBT are as effective for compulsive checking as for other obsessive–compulsive symptoms such as compulsive cleaning. As a result, there is no specific treatment protocol for this OCD subtype. However, the theoretical and empirical research on pathological doubt and checking suggests that our treatments could be enhanced by a greater focus on the more specific cognitive features of this subtype. For example, the cognitive-behavioral therapist could incorporate some of the treatment approaches used in IBT to deal with inferential confusion, offer interventions that strengthen tolerance of uncertainty, refocus the client on reality sensing that improves memory confidence and the "feeling of knowing," identify aspects of the feared or vulnerable self, and challenge inflated responsibility beliefs. Regardless of whether treatment involves a greater emphasis on cognitive or behavioral interventions, RP of checking compulsions must be encouraged over the course of therapy.

CHAPTER 12

Harm, Sex, and Religious Obsessions

CASE ILLUSTRATION

Camilla struggled with disturbing religious, sexual, and harming obsessions that got worse with each passing year. Although not a particularly religious person, daily she experienced fearful thoughts and images that left her wondering if she or her loved ones might suffer eternal damnation. For example, she might be engaged in the most mundane activity, and if she suddenly had a bad thought, such as "I hope my mother has an accident," she would immediately feel anxious and fearful that harm might actually come to her mother, or that God would be so offended by her selfish, unkind thought that she would be condemned to hell. At other times when deciding upon or engaging in an activity, the thought "Have I offended God?" intruded into her mind, and she became overwhelmed with fear. Certain religious symbols like the cross or the number 666 caused intense anxiety because she would think blasphemous thoughts against God, and then ask herself, "Am I Satan's child?" Whenever she engaged in social interaction, she would experience disturbing, intrusive sexual thoughts such as "I'm staring at her breasts." She interpreted such thoughts as a sign of sinful lust and offense against God.

Camilla developed several neutralization strategies to deal with the distressing intrusions. Avoidance was one of her preferred options. She avoided anything religious because it triggered blasphemous thoughts. With the harming obsession, she felt compelled to form a comforting image of God stretching out his hand and offering protection to her family. To be effective, the comforting image had to give Camilla a sense that everything would be all right for her loved ones. When she had the blasphemous thoughts, she imagined Christ on the cross and whispered, "May the blood of Christ cover your sins" seven times. When around people, Camilla tried to control her gaze to prevent a possible glance at a person's genital region. This made her social interactions awkward because she avoided eye contact when talking to people.

This chapter focuses on repugnant obsessions, which include unwanted thoughts, images, and impulses on themes of sex, aggression, harm, and religion. Often the term *pure obsessionals,* or *pure O,* is used for this symptom subtype because overt compulsive rituals are often absent. The chapter begins with a discussion of clinical features and pertinent issues, including the diagnostic validity of pure obsessions, and the role of morality, religiosity, and self-domains in the pathogenesis of repugnant obsessions. These sections are followed by a presentation of the CBT model of repugnant obsessions, its empirical status, and special treatment considerations for the repugnant subtype. The chapter concludes with a brief discussion of treatment efficacy.

CLINICAL FEATURES

Perceived violation of moral principles or standards of personal integrity is a core issue in repugnant obsessions. The most common themes in repugnant obsessions are (1) uncontrolled aggression, harm, or injury toward others; (2) violation of religious or ethical convictions; or (3) forbidden, even disgusting, sexual thoughts or images. One type of sexual obsession that deserves special mention is sexual orientation fears. Labeled *sexual orientation OCD,* individuals fear (1) an unwanted change in sexual orientation, (2) that others might perceive him or her as homosexual, and/or (3) that he or she has latent homosexual desires (Williams, Crozier, et al., 2011). Individuals with sexual orientation OCD experience anxiety and distress rather than pleasure when they have doubtful thoughts about their sexual orientation. Of course, these doubts can include uncertainty over whether they might be experiencing some pleasure or sexual attraction to the same sex. Sexual orientation OCD should not be confused with individuals who are truly conflicted about their sexual orientation or have an authentic sexual attraction to the same sex. When sexual orientation issues arise in therapy, it is critical that the clinician accurately differentiate sexual orientation OCD from sexual orientation conflicts. A misdiagnosis would have adverse effects on the person with genuine sexual orientation conflict and on the person with sexual orientation OCD. Williams and Farris (2011) found that 8% of the participants in the DSM-IV Field Trial for OCD (Foa et al., 1995) had sexual orientation obsessions, which were characterized by greater intensity, interference, and avoidance than other types of obsessions. Despite their severity, there is preliminary evidence that ERP can be effective with sexual orientation obsessions (Williams, Crozier, et al., 2011), although the treatment research is extremely limited at this time.

Repugnant obsessions are found in 20–30% of individuals with OCD (Moulding, Aardema, & O'Connor, 2014). Foa and colleagues (1995) found that 23.6% of their DSM-IV Field Trial sample had a fear of harming self or others as the primary obsession, and 5.9% and 5.5% had primary religious and sexual obsessions, respectively. When lifetime rates of OCD are considered as well as primary and secondary obsessions, the frequency rates of 50–60% have been reported in heterogeneous OCD samples (Pinto et al., 2008). Moreover, there is continuity between the repugnant obsessions in OCD and the unwanted intrusive thoughts of harm, sex, and religion found in nonclinical samples. In the international study of unwanted intrusive thoughts, the percentage of participants within each country who indicated that they had at least one unwanted religious intrusion ranged from 45.5 to 0%, and for sexual intrusions it ranged from 22 to 0% (Clark, Radomsky, et al., 2015). The rates for harm intrusions were even higher (Radomsky, Alcolado, et al., 2014). Repugnant obsessions, then, are quite prevalent in OCD samples, and are experienced even in nonclinical individuals, although less frequently than doubt or contamination intrusions.

Compared to other types of obsessions, those with repugnant content are characterized by greater clinical severity, higher comorbidity, and poorer treatment outcome (see Moulding et al., 2014). For example, individuals with high scores on the YBOCS Symptom Checklist dimension that includes aggression, sex, and religious obsessions have more intense psychopathology, as indicated by greater obsessionality, distress, time spent on obsessions, hostility, prior treatment, male gender, and a past diagnosis of nonalcohol substance dependence (Brakoulias et al., 2013). As well, sexual orientation obsessions are positively correlated with more time spent on obsessions, greater interference, and increased distress (Williams & Farris, 2011). Repugnant obsessions are associated with more comorbidity for anxiety, depression, and alcohol dependence than other OCD symptom subtypes (Hasler et al., 2005). Together these findings indicate that repugnant obsessions represent a more severe form of psychological disturbance that offers particular challenges for the cognitive-behavioral therapist.

Cultural differences are evident in the prevalence and content of repugnant obsessions. In a review of empirical studies on culture and OCD, religious and aggressive obsessions were more prominent in Brazilian and Middle Eastern OCD samples (Fontenelle et al., 2004). There is considerable evidence that religious obsessions are more often seen in countries with strong religious orientation, such as Egypt or Iran (Ghassemzadeh et al., 2002; Okasha et al., 1994). When highly religious individuals who adhere to strict religious beliefs and practices develop OCD, it often takes the form of religious obsessions (Ciarrocchi, 1995). Moreover, devoted Muslims and ultra-orthodox Jews with OCD will be more concerned about contamination and impurity than those of Christian faith (Greenberg & Shefler, 2002; Tek & Ulug, 2001). Even in nonclinical samples, highly religious individuals have more frequent unwanted religious, but not more sexual or harm intrusive thoughts, than the nonreligious (Altin, Clark, & Karanci, 2007).

Life experiences can play an important role in the etiology and form of obsessional symptoms (e.g., Rosso et al., 2012). One of the best examples of environmental risk factors for obsessive–compulsive symptoms is the emergence of harm intrusions in parents of newborn infants. In an early study of obsessional symptoms in the postpartum period, Abramowitz, Schwartz, and colleagues (2003) obtained mail-out survey data from fathers and mothers of newborns. Approximately two-thirds (66%) reported unwanted intrusive thoughts about the baby, with thoughts of intentionally harming the child occurring in one-fifth (21%) of the sample. However, the parents reported only mild distress and were able to control their intrusions. These findings were replicated in other studies, which also showed that dysfunctional beliefs and appraisals mediate the relationship between harm intrusions and obsessive–compulsive symptoms (Abramowitz, Khandker, Nelson, Deacon, & Rygwall, 2006; Abramowitz, Nelson, Rygwall, & Khandker, 2007).

In a subsequent study Fairbrother and Woody (2008) found that all of their new mothers ($N = 91$) reported intrusive thoughts of accidental harm to their newborns, but only 49.5% reported intentional harm cognitions. By 12 weeks postpartum, the percentage of mothers still experiencing intentional harm intrusions had dropped to 27%. However, less than 5% of women experienced intentional harm intrusions that were clinically significant, but these women were no more likely to report harsh parenting behavior. A more recent experiment found that first-time mothers who listened to a 10-minute recording of continuous infant crying experienced more infant-related harm intrusions than mothers listening to 10 minutes of infant cooing (Fairbrother, Barr, Pauwels, Brant, & Green, 2015). This is one of the first studies to find that a specific stressful experience can trigger an increase in unwanted harm intrusions.

In addition to current concerns and stressful life experiences, depressive symptoms can intensify the frequency and severity of harming intrusions (Abramowitz, Schwartz, et al., 2003; Jennings, Ross, Popper, & Elmore, 1999). Together these findings indicate that cognitive-behavioral therapists must be cognizant of the environmental and emotional triggers that contribute to a resurgence of distressing mental intrusions. This domain should be included in the cognitive case formulation and clients should be educated on the reactive nature of their repugnant obsessions. As well, the postpartum research is consistent with the clinical opinion that fears of losing control and acting on one's repugnant obsessions are usually unfounded.

DIAGNOSIS AND THE CASE FOR "PURE O"

As noted in Chapter 1, various structural analyses of the YBOCS Symptom Checklist indicate that harming, sexual, religious, and sometimes somatic obsessions load together with checking compulsions on a single dimension (e.g., Baer, 1994; Summerfeldt et al., 1999). In their meta-analysis, Bloch and colleagues (2008) concluded that a forbidden thoughts dimension consistently emerged as a distinct symptom dimension. This research suggests that harming, religious, and sexual obsessions constitute a distinct symptom subtype of OCD. Others, however, have questioned the differentiation of repugnant obsessions. In their review McKay and colleagues concluded that evidence of a repugnant obsession subtype (sexual/religious, harming, pure obsessions) is mixed at best (McKay et al., 2004). These contradictory conclusions can be traced to methodological limitations of the YBOCS Symptom Checklist. Structural solutions are dependent on the item representation of symptom dimensions (Radomsky & Taylor, 2005). The YOBCS Symptom Checklist contains twice as many items for contamination and harm obsessions, with only two items representing sexual or religious obsessions. The uneven representation of symptom dimensions will constrain the structural solutions that emerge from these datasets. The most parsimonious conclusion is to argue that identifying individuals with primary repugnant obsessions has clinical utility, but the mixed empirical findings remind us that repugnant obsessions can occur as secondary symptoms in all OCD subtypes.

The controversy over repugnant obsessions extends beyond issues of symptom structure and composition to the very label used to identify this obsessional phenomenon. Early psychiatric accounts of OCD recognized that some individuals suffer from obsessions without overt compulsions (e.g., Ingram, 1961a; Lewis, 1936). These "pure obsessions" often presented with themes of repugnant religious, sexual. and, to a lesser extent, aggressive content (see Clark & Guyitt, 2008, for review). However, the word *pure* is a misnomer, because mental (i.e., covert) compulsions are often present in repugnant obsessions (Sibrava et al., 2011; Williams, Farris, et al., 2011). Approximately 25% of individuals with OCD have no overt compulsive rituals (see Clark & Guyitt, 2008; McKay et al., 2004). Absence of overt compulsions is associated with greater clinical severity, chronicity, and lower functioning (Sibrava et al., 2011), and possibly weaker response to ERP (see Clark & Guyitt, 2008). Thus, the absence of overt compulsions has clinical relevance, but the label *pure obsessions* is misleading.

MORALITY, RELIGIOSITY, AND THE SELF

Three phenomena often discussed in the context of OCD are particularly important in the etiology, maintenance, and treatment of repugnant obsessions. They are most aptly considered nonspecific vulnerability factors that act in concert with other risk factors to increase vulnerability for repugnant obsessions.

Morality

It has long been recognized that moral issues play an important role in the pathogenesis of OCD, but this is especially true for repugnant obsessions. Individuals with repugnant obsessions are strongly invested in "a sense of self-as-could-be as opposed to sense of self-as-is" (Aardema & O'Connor, 2007 p. 191). This fear of "what I could be" (i.e., feared self) often involves violations of morality, in which individuals wonder if they are inwardly depraved, violent, perverted, or evil. In such cases, the fear concerns "that which might lie within their own state" (p. 163), rather than a fear focused on factors in the external world, like a dirty or contaminated place (Moulding et al., 2014). Given this internal focus, it is not surprising that morality, religion, and self-discrepancies offer a confluence of possible factors in the pathogenesis of this OCD subtype.

Research into morality and OCD has tended to rely on the TAF–Moral subscale (Rachman & Shafran, 1998; Shafran et al., 1996). Generally, studies find that the TAF–Moral subscale has a less consistent relationship with obsessive–compulsive symptoms than TAF–Likelihood–Self or Others (e.g., Rassin, Merckelbach, et al., 2001; Shafran et al., 1996). Berle and Starcevic (2005) concluded that TAF–Moral may be more closely associated with depressive than obsessive–compulsive symptoms. As well, TAF–Moral may be associated with guilt and a tendency to engage in thought suppression, although the research indicates that its relationship with inflated responsibility beliefs is weaker than it is for TAF–Likelihood (Berle & Starcevic, 2005).

TAF–Moral has a closer association with religiosity than the other TAF subscales (Rassin & Koster, 2003; Siev, Chambless, & Huppert, 2010). Berman, Abramowitz, Pardue, and Wheaton (2010) had highly religious Protestant students and atheist/agnostic participants engage in two variants of a TAF induction (i.e., participants are told to write a statement that they hope to have sex with their sibling, or that they hope their parent or sibling has a car accident today, respectively). The religious group had significantly higher ratings of moral wrongness for the TAF–Moral statement and engaged in more neutralizing behavior but did not differ from the nonreligious in rated likelihood of committing incest. The authors concluded that acceptance of strict religious doctrine about the unacceptability of certain thoughts might foster TAF beliefs.

Morality has also been researched in the context of selfhood processes. Several studies suggest that low moral self-perception may be relevant to OCD in general. For example, there is a specific association between sensitivity in the moral self-domain and obsessive–compulsive symptoms (Doron, Kyrios, & Moulding, 2007; Doron, Moulding, Kyrios, & Nedeljkovic, 2008). Furthermore, induction of a negative moral self-perception increased rated urge to engage in neutralization in response to hypothetical contamination-relevant scenarios (Doron, Sar-El, & Mikulincer, 2012). Similarly, priming of negative morality was associated with significant endorsement of overestimated threat, perfectionism, and importance/control beliefs (Abramovitch, Doron, Sar-El, & Altenburger, 2013). Together these studies suggest that perceived shortcomings in adherence to moral values might have particular relevance to OCD. Individuals with OCD might be especially sensitive to perceived threats to the moral values that contribute to their sense of self.

If threats to moral integrity have any bearing on OCD, one would expect this to be especially true for those who have repugnant obsessions. The obsessional content for this subtype represents the most obvious threat to individuals' moral self-domain. However, no published studies to date have determined whether moral threats have a closer relationship with repugnant obsessions than other obsessive–compulsive symptoms. Nevertheless, clinicians should be cognizant of the probable importance of moral values when treating clients with repugnant obsessions, and that perceived morality conflicts and deficiencies may reach to the very core of individuals' self-view.

Religiosity and Scrupulosity

Given the prominence of sexual and religious themes in repugnant obsessions, we might expect the religiosity–OCD relationship to be especially strong in this symptom subtype. Moreover, it is commonly recognized that religious obsessions, or what has been termed *scrupulosity,* represents a special type of obsessional problem that falls under the umbrella of repugnant obsessions.

Weisner and Riffel (1960) defined *scruple* as "an unhealthy and morbid kind of meticulousness which hampers a person's religious adjustment" (p. 314). Abramowitz (2008) noted that in scrupulosity, religious beliefs and rituals become transformed from comforting spiritual practices to disturbing preoccupations and compulsions that are performed out of a fear of possible punishment. Individuals are frightened of having committed a sin in thought, word, or deed, or of having offended or not pleased God. A wide range of religious obsessions can occur, such as blasphemous thoughts or images against the divine, unwanted and impulsive swearing, doubts of having committed a sin or of not being sufficiently repentant, concerns about offending God or not pleasing Him, fears of inadequate or insincere confession, doubts of having performed a religious ritual correctly or completely, and fears of not praying enough. Greenberg and Witztum (2001) noted two main areas of concern with religious obsessions: ideas of impurity and uncleanliness that can result in compulsive cleaning rituals, and issues of liturgy such as unwanted, forbidden mental intrusions while praying or offering confession. Abramowitz (2008) noted that religious obsessions can also co-occur with sexual, aggressive, and somatic obsessions.

Although religious obsessions are more likely to manifest in people of faith (Ciarrocchi, 1995; Greenberg & Witztum, 2001), agnostics and nonreligious individuals can also have these types of obsessions. Tek and Ulug (2001) found that Turkish patients with religious obsessions were no more likely to be religious than individuals with other obsessive–compulsive symptoms. This point is well illustrated in the case example presented at the beginning of this chapter. The irrationality of Camilla's obsessions was accentuated by the fact that religious devotion was largely absent in her family tradition and personal background.

Even though OCD is not more prevalent in religious populations, the presence of religious devotion can influence the focus and experience of obsessive–compulsive symptoms (Steketee, Quay, & White, 1991). People who are highly religious have a greater fear of God and concern about committing sin (Abramowitz, Huppert, Cohen, Tolin, & Cahill, 2002). In addition, guilt is more pervasive in religious samples (Hale & Clark, 2013; Steketee et al., 1991), and individuals who are religious evidence greater endorsement of beliefs about the importance and control of unwanted thoughts, as well as personal responsibility and overestimated threat (Inozu, Karanci, & Clark, 2012; Sica, Novara, & Sanavio, 2002). Witzif and Pollard (2013) found a positive correlation between the Penn Inventory of Scrupulosity (PIOS; Abramowitz et al., 2002) Total Score and OBQ-44 Total Score in a large sample of Christian fundamentalists. Moreover, scrupulosity was negatively correlated with religious commitment and spiritual well-being. In their CBT model of scrupulosity, Abramowitz and Jacoby (2014) argued that a person's religious beliefs and values can foster maladaptive beliefs, such as TAF–Moral and importance of thought, that increase the probability that unwanted immoral intrusive thoughts will be misinterpreted as a highly significant personal threat. Overall, scrupulosity can be particularly maladaptive in highly religious samples, and its negative effects may be amplified by heightened levels of anxiety and depression.

Subtle differences are evident between religious traditions in the experience of scrupulosity. For example, Turkish Muslim students scored higher on the PIOS Fear of God subscale than did Christian Canadian students (Inozu, Clark, et al., 2012), whereas Abramowitz and colleagues (2002) found that Jews had less fear of God than did Catholics and Protestants. Abramowitz and Jacoby (2014) concluded that religious traditions, values, and doctrine will influence the specific content of religious obsessions and compulsions.

In general, the presence of scrupulosity in highly religious individuals is problematic. Abramowitz and Jacoby (2014) contend that IU is a key process in the pathogenesis of scrupulosity. The scrupulous person strives for certainty that he or she has not sinned or has pleased God. Of course, the highly desired feeling of certainty is impossible to attain, causing the scrupulous person to fall into a religious experience that is "fear-based" rather than "faith-based." When treating scrupulosity, the goal is to help individuals relinquish their fear-based religion for one that is faith-based. This is accomplished by (1) correcting maladaptive fear-based beliefs, (2) increasing tolerance of uncertainty, and (3) relinquishing religious compulsions, safety seeking, and avoidance (Abramowitz & Jacoby, 2014). Table 12.1 presents several important treatment issues when providing CBT for religious obsessions.

Selfhood

Moulding and colleagues (2014) commented that negative self-perception might contribute to a propensity to misinterpret the significance of unwanted intrusive thoughts perceived as relevant to the individual's self-construct. For example, Camilla was compassionate, understanding, and kind toward others. She avoided confrontation and was uncomfortable with anger and irritability in others. Thus, intrusive thoughts of causing harm or offense toward others were considered highly significant because they represented a threat to her self-definition. Recently, various self-representational constructs have been proposed that might be important in the development of repugnant obsessions. Although ego dystonicity is a construct highly relevant to self-construal, in this chapter it is discussed as a faulty appraisal in the CBT model of repugnant obsessions. Below various self-construal constructs are considered that might be especially relevant to harming, sexual, and religious obsessions.

Ambivalent Self

Bhar and Kyrios (2007) proposed that individuals with OCD have a fragile or ambivalent self-view that contributes to a greater likelihood that unwanted ego-dystonic intrusions will be misinterpreted as meaningful threats to valued aspects of the self. Nonobsessional individuals have a stronger self-view, so that self-recriminating or contradictory thinking must be rejected in order to protect their positive self-construction. Because an ambivalent self-view consists of contradictory and opposing elements, an unwanted intrusion becomes evidence for the negative as opposed to the positive self-view. Bhar and Kyrios found that self-worth and moral ambivalence were significantly related to OCD symptoms and beliefs, although both were also elevated in anxious controls. In another study self-ambivalence correlated significantly with self-reported obsessive–compulsive symptoms, trait anxiety, and rumination (Tisher, Allen, & Crouch, 2014). Although empirical research on this construct is scant, self-ambivalence has particular relevance for repugnant obsessions. The heightened frequency and intensity of unwanted mental intrusions that contradict cherished values might be

TABLE 12.1. Pertinent Issues in CBT for Religious Obsessions

Treatment issue	Guidance
Be able to differentiate scrupulosity from normal religious practice.	Therapists must be knowledgeable about the normative beliefs and practices of the client's religion. Scrupulosity can be distinguished as being excessively time-consuming and involving a preoccupation with a single, usually minor area of religious concern, often to the detriment of the main tenets of the individual's faith (Greenberg & Huppert, 2010). As well, negative emotions such as anxiety and guilt dominate the religious focus in scrupulosity.
Spend time strengthening the therapeutic alliance.	Demonstrating sensitivity, knowledge, and respect of the client's religious values, beliefs, and experiences will foster trust, therapist respect, and a willingness to collaborate in the therapy process.
Maintain the therapeutic focus on reducing obsessive–compulsive symptoms and associated emotional disturbance.	Consistently redirect treatment focus to reducing clinical distress caused by unwanted, disturbing thoughts and repetitive behavior. Avoid intervention that could be construed as a direct threat to the client's personal religious beliefs or practices.
Adopt a cognitive conceptualization of scrupulosity.	Redefine religious doubts in terms of unwanted mental intrusions and repetitive religious rites, prayers, and confessions as neutralization responses (Abramowitz, 2008). Treat scrupulosity as an expression of OCD and not an aberrant form of religious devotion (Greenberg & Witztum, 2001).
Expect an elevated level of treatment ambivalence (Greenberg & Huppert, 2010).	Individuals may enter therapy to obtain relief from their distress but be reluctant to consider alternative perspectives on their scrupulosity for fear that it threatens their faith.
Focus on beliefs about the importance and control of thoughts.	In CBT for religious obsessions the client's erroneous belief that more mental control is needed must be changed to a realization that acceptance of unwanted repugnant thoughts is the most adaptive approach.
Conduct an "exposure tolerance test" prior to assigning *in vivo* exercises.	Given the importance of morality and religious conviction in scrupulosity, therapists should determine the moral and ethical acceptability of any exposure task prior to its assignment (e.g., urging Christian fundamentalists to practice imaginal exposure to blasphemous swear words might be entirely reprehensible to these clients).

more likely to contribute to obsessive thinking in those with an ambivalent or fragile self-view.

Sensitive Self-Domains

Doron and Kyrios (2005) contend that individuals with OCD have a self-view that consists of relatively few highly sensitive domains of competence. Intrusive thoughts representing a failure in these sensitive domains would threaten the individual's self-worth and so attain processing priority in terms of heightened attention, evaluation, and associated distress (Moulding et al., 2014). The presence of these sensitive domains of self-competence, together with beliefs that the world is dangerous but controllable, creates a vulnerability to misinterpret mental intrusions and their control in a manner that leads to the development of obsessions. Experimental studies by Doron and colleagues have shown that threats to the moral self-domain, in particular, can influence obsessive–compulsive symptoms and beliefs (e.g., Abramovitch et al., 2013; Doron, Sar-El, & Mikulincer, 2012). In addition, sensitivity in the moral self-domain was significantly greater in an OCD sample than in a sample of other anxiety disorders (Doron et al., 2008).

Research based on perceived success or failure to achieve self-worth in various obsessive–compulsive-specific domains failed to find a relation between obsessive–compulsive symptoms and low moral self-worth attainment (García-Soriano & Belloch, 2012; García-Soriano, Clark, Belloch, del Palacio, & Castanñeiras, 2012). Of course, all of these studies were performed on heterogeneous OCD or nonclinical samples, so the specific relationship between selfhood sensitivities in the moral domain and repugnant obsessions remains unknown.

Feared Self

Aardema and O'Connor (2007) contend that discordant self-representations form a critical component of self-representation in obsessional states. This occurs because individuals with OCD commit a number of reasoning errors that causes them to treat thoughts of a possible self as representing the real self (i.e., inferential confusion; see Chapter 11). A negative self-representation that involves a possibility (e.g., "Am I having a sexual feeling when around minors?") becomes confused with a reality (e.g., "Because I am thinking this way, I could become a child molester"). In this way individuals with OCD act as if the possible were a real probability. Obsession-prone individuals then become immersed in "a fear of who they could be or might become" (Aardema & O'Connor, 2007, p. 191). This causes a strong sense of self-doubt and a distrust of the self-as-is because of their heavy investment in the "self-as-could-be." Fear develops of a nonexistent self (Aardema & O'Connor, 2007); that is, of the qualities that represent "the 'me' that the person does not want to become" (Aardema et al., 2013, p. 307), leading to the misinterpretation of mental intrusions relevant to the "feared self."

As noted in Chapter 11, there is emerging empirical evidence to support a role for the feared self in OCD: for instance, elevated fear of self predicted scores on the DOCS Unacceptable Thoughts subscale in an OCD sample, after controlling for OBQ beliefs (Melli, Aardema, & Moulding, 2016). Also, the feared self may have more relevance for repugnant obsessions than other obsessive-compulsive symptom subtypes (Aardema, Moulding, et al., 2018). Together, ambivalence, heightened self-domain sensitivities, and the feared self may all play a role in elevating the importance of incongruent thinking to high-risk individuals. It is likely that perceived threats to the moral self-domain and their relevance to the feared self are particularly crucial to susceptibility to repugnant obsessions. Clearly, selfhood issues should be incorporated in the cognitive-behavioral treatment plan for repugnant obsessions.

A COGNITIVE-BEHAVIORAL MODEL OF REPUGNANT OBSESSIONS

Figure 12.1 presents a CBT model of repugnant obsessions that has several unique features compared to the conceptualization of contamination and checking symptom subtypes. External triggers play a less prominent role in the occurrence of repugnant intrusions. Thus, the label *autogenous intrusions* is used to denote the cognitive experience that initiates the vicious cycle of obsessive thinking (i.e., Lee & Kwon, 2003). Repugnant obsessions often do not involve overt compulsions, and so the term *mental control strategies* is used to denote a broader array of neutralization strategies utilized in response to the obsession. Unlike overt compulsions, individuals with repugnant obsessions may be less focused on stopping their control efforts and more concerned with thought suppression. Therefore, stop rules may be less relevant in repugnant obsessions. As well, the attainment of comfort or safety will be less important than preventing recurrence of the offensive intrusion.

Cognitive Vulnerability

It is expected that repetitive unwanted thoughts or images of harm, offensive sex, and/or blasphemy are more closely linked to discrepancies in individuals' self-perceptions than are other types of obsessions. Discrepancies between the real and feared self would be experienced most acutely by individuals with a fragile sense of self. The emergence of unacceptable mental intrusions of relevance to the feared self, or a valued self-domain perceived as deficient, would promote a tendency to misinterpret the intrusion as a

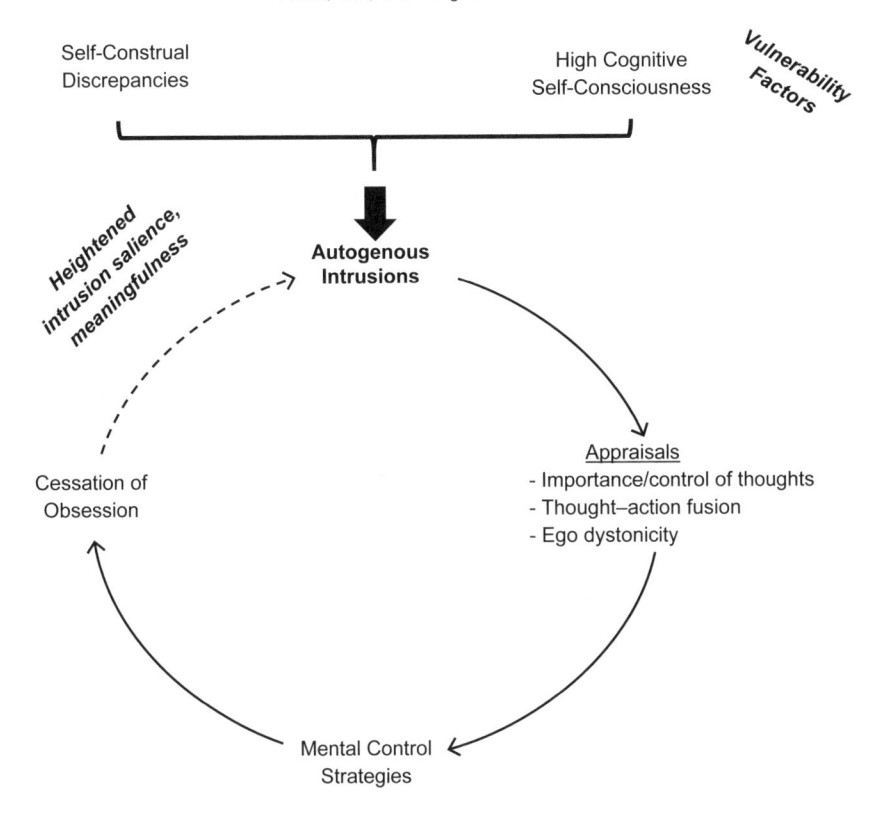

FIGURE 12.1. Cognitive-behavioral model of repugnant obsessions.

highly significant threat (Rachman, 2003). Moreover, it is likely that these self-construal deficiencies stem from developmental issues and so constitute predisposing factors for obsessionality. However, the longitudinal research needed to investigate these assertions is not available, and so the cognitive vulnerability for repugnant obsessions remains speculative at this time.

Cognitive self-consciousness is another construct that could play an etiological role in repugnant obsessions. Emerging as a distinct factor of the Metacognitions Questionnaire (MCQ; Cartwright-Hatton & Wells, 1997), *cognitive self-consciousness* (CSC) refers to a tendency to be aware of and monitor thinking. In the original psychometric study, the CSC subscale of the MCQ showed some relationship with self-reported obsessive–compulsive symptoms, although the relationship was mediated by other meta-cognitive constructs. Using an expanded self-report measure of CSC, Janeck, Calamari, Riemann, and Heffelfinger (2003) found that an OCD group scored significantly higher than other anxiety-disordered groups on the CSC measure, and elevated CSC continued to differentiate the OCD group after controlling for OBQ beliefs. Moreover, elevated CSC in obsessional states is associated with impairments in implicit learning (Marker, Calamari, Woodward, & Riemann, 2006), selective attention to neutral stimuli (Koch & Exner, 2015), and verbal memory performance (Kikul, van Allen, & Exner, 2012; Weber et al., 2014). However, in some studies CSC did not have a more negative effect on cognitive performance than major depression or other anxiety disorders.

Research on CSC indicates that the construct is relevant to OCD and that increased attention to one's thoughts does have the expected deleterious effect on information processing. However, many critical questions remain, such as whether CSC is a cause or consequence of OCD, and whether it is a specific cognitive characteristic of obsessional states. Furthermore, it is unknown whether the construct might have more relevance for repugnant obsessions. Together with a fragile or discrepant self-view, a tendency for inner reflection could provide the seeds for misguided evaluation and control of discordant and offensive cognitions.

Autogenous Intrusions

In their original article Lee and Kwon (2003) contend that obsessions can be categorized into *autogenous* and *reactive* subtypes based on how the obsessions are provoked and experienced. Their description of the autogenous subtype is almost identical to a description of repugnant obsessions, and so the two terms can be considered synonymous. Autogenous obsessions enter conscious awareness abruptly, without external evoking stimuli, are ego-dystonic and highly unacceptable, and usually focus on repugnant themes. Reactive obsessions tend to be triggered by external stimuli, are more likely considered realistic given the provoking stimuli, and involve concerns about dirt, contamination, mistakes, symmetry, and the like. In a series of studies involving clinical and nonclinical samples, Lee, Kwon, and associates (Lee & Kwon, 2003; Lee, Kwon, Kwon, & Telch, 2005; Lee, Lee, Kim, Kwon, & Telch, 2005) were able to demonstrate that autogenous and reactive obsessions are dimensional constructs found in both clinical and nonclinical samples, and that the two subtypes are distinct in phenomenological and cognitive features.

In the first study utilizing Korean undergraduates as participants, Lee and Kwon (2003) found that autogenous intrusions were rated as more unacceptable, guilt-inducing, and important to control. Students who selected an autogenous thought as their most distressing intrusion attached greater importance to the thought, felt more pressure to control the intrusion, and preferred maladaptive avoidant control strategies (e.g., thought stopping, self-blame, praying, avoiding anxious triggers, and counterimaging) compared to students who selected a reactive thought as their most distressing intrusion. A subsequent study of an American student sample found that autogenous intrusions were more distinct from worry than reactive intrusions, and were rated as more bizarre, unrealistic, unacceptable, and less likely to come true (i.e., more ego-dystonic) than worry (Lee, Lee, et al., 2005). A more recent Australian study confirmed the autogenous–reactive distinction, although reactive obsessions had a stronger relation with obsessive–compulsive symptoms and beliefs than did autogenous obsessions (Moulding et al., 2007). As well, there is some evidence that amygdala–hippocampal abnormalities were more evident in OCD participants with autogenous obsessions, suggesting possible biological differences between autogenous and reactive obsessions (Besiroglu et al., 2011).

There is some evidence that the autogenous–reactive distinction might have a differential relationship with selfhood constructs. Moulding and colleagues (2007) found that both intrusion subtypes exhibited a significant correlation with self-ambivalence but not global self-esteem. However, Seo and Kwon (2013) found that students whose primary intrusion was autogenous were more likely to make negative self-inferences because of the intrusion than individuals whose primary intrusion was reactive. As well, the autogenous students experienced more feelings of guilt and were more likely to employ neutralizations that protected their self-worth than the reactive students. Fergus (2013) reported that the relationship between autogenous but not reactive intrusions and obsessive–compulsive symptoms was moderated by thought controllability, such that a significant association between symptom severity and autogenous intrusions occurred only in those reporting high-thought controllability. Although Fergus concludes that thought control may have more relevance for autogenous intrusions, the findings are counterintuitive: We would expect that low-thought controllability would be associated with obsessive–compulsive symptom severity.

Lee, Kwon, and colleagues (2005) replicated their findings in a small OCD sample, finding that autogenous obsessions were more guilt-inducing, more important to control, more threatening, and more likely associated with avoidant coping. Furthermore, individuals with OCD whose primary obsession was autogenous had more severe obsessions and greater concerns about losing control, although the autogenous and reactive groups did not differ on OBQ Importance and Control of Thoughts. The authors concluded that individuals with autogenous obsessions struggle with the thoughts themselves, whereas those with primarily reactive obsessions struggle with the thought triggers (Lee, Kwon, et al., 2005).

It might be assumed that ERP would be more effective for reactive obsessions (i.e., dirt, contamination, checking related to doubts), whereas cognitive therapy would be more appropriate for autogenous obsessions. This prediction was supported in the only treatment study to test this subtype distinction. Belloch, Cabedo, Carrió, and Larsson (2010) found a comparatively better treatment outcome for individuals with autogenous as opposed to reactive obsessions after 18 sessions of cognitive therapy without formal exposure and response prevention.

In the CBT model represented in Figure 12.1, it is proposed that autogenous unwanted thoughts provoke the escalating cycle of repugnant obsessions. Lee and Kwon's research suggests that the very nature of these abrupt, spontaneously occurring autogenous intrusions causes them to be experienced as more distressing, unacceptable, guilt-inducing, and difficult to control. As well, these intrusions might provoke more negative self-inferences and thought controllability issues. Given these experiential features, it is little wonder that autogenous intrusions may be especially primed to elicit faulty beliefs and appraisals that will ensure escalation of the intrusion into a truly troubling repugnant obsession.

Faulty Appraisals and Beliefs

There are three categories of faulty appraisals and beliefs that may be particularly important in the pathogenesis of repugnant obsessions: importance/control of thoughts, TAF bias, and ego dystonicity. Given the cognitive vulnerability factors proposed in the CBT model (see Figure 12.1) and the nature of autogenous intrusions, it is not difficult to see why these three appraisal processes may be especially important in repugnant obsessions. What follows is a brief review of the empirical support for each appraisal/belief category.

Importance/Control of Thoughts

Several studies indicate that beliefs and appraisals about *importance/control* are prominent processes in the presence of repugnant obsessions. M. T. Williams and colleagues (2013) concluded that unacceptable obsessions are often evaluated as overly important and dangerous, and so considerable mental effort is directed at suppressing them. Brakoulias and associates (2013) found that higher scores on the YBOCS Unacceptable/Taboo dimension were associated with stronger beliefs in the importance of controlling unwanted thoughts. In a small OCD study, religious obsessions correlated with a broad range of dysfunctional beliefs (e.g., overimportance of thought, need to control, inflated responsibility, and threat estimation), whereas sexual obsessions were associated only with overimportance and control of thoughts (Siev, Steketee, Fama, & Wilhelm, 2011). An online study of the distinct and shared characteristics of worry and obsessions found that the DOCS Unacceptable Thoughts subscale was significantly associated with low attentional control, high negative affect, and greater negative urgency (which is the propensity to engage in rash action in order to feel better; Macatee et al., 2016). Both low attentional control and heightened negative urgency are consistent with a concern about control of repugnant obsessions.

TAF Bias

Although no studies have determined whether TAF is more prominent in repugnant obsessions than in other OCD subtypes, there is indirect evidence that TAF appraisals might be especially important in this subtype. For example, the TAF Scale correlates with the Obsessions subscale of the OCI-R, which could be considered a proxy for unacceptable obsessions. Meyer and Brown (2012) found that TAF Total Score and TAF–Likelihood subscale correlated with the OCI-R Obsessions subscale, whereas Abramowitz and Deacon (2006) found that only TAF–Moral correlated with the subscale. Other studies have found that TAF is associated with religious obsessions and intrusions, which, of course, are included within the repugnant obsessions subtype. TAF–Moral, in particular, is significantly correlated with religiosity (Rassin & Koster, 2003) and mediates the effects of religiosity on obsessive–compulsive symptoms in Christians only (A. D. Williams et al., 2013). In other studies TAF–Moral was associated with obsessive–compulsive symptoms in Jews but not in Christians (Siev et al., 2010). In a recent study of Muslim students, TAF Total and disgust sensitivity mediated the relationship between religiosity and obsessive–compulsive symptoms (Inozu, Ulukut, Ergun, & Alcolado, 2014). Together these findings indicate that TAF–Moral, in particular, might be a crucial faulty appraisal in repugnant obsessions.

Ego Dystonicity

A third appraisal and belief construct implicated in the escalation of repugnant obsessions is *ego dystonicity* (Moulding et al., 2014; Purdon, 2004a). This construct refers to the extent that the theme of an obsession is inconsistent or in conflict with a person's self-view, as reflected in his or her core values, ideals, or moral tenets (Clark, 2004). Camilla, for example, had distressing sexual obsessions such as "I am staring at his crotch." This was interpreted as a highly significant threatening intrusive thought because Camilla considered it a sign of some underlying sexual deviance. Morality and high ethical standards were valued self-construal domains for Camilla, so the unwanted sexual intrusion represented a tendency that was completely contrary to her self-view. In this sense it was appraised as highly ego-dystonic, causing Camilla's attention to be drawn to it with each intrusion into consciousness.

Research indicates that moral-based obsessions and unwanted intrusive thoughts are rated as more ego-dystonic (Belloch, Roncero, & Perpiná, 2012; Purdon, Cripps, Faull, Joseph, & Rowa, 2007) than other obsessional phenomena. As well, there is evidence that obsessions, in general, are considered more upsetting when appraised as contradicting valued aspects of the self (Rowa & Purdon, 2003; Rowa et al., 2005). Consequently, ego dystonicity has been implicated in self-construct models of repugnant obsessions. Aardema and colleagues (2013), for example, found a positive correlation between the FSQ Total Score and the Ego-Dystonicity Questionnaire (EDQ) developed by Purdon, Cripps, and colleagues (2007). A more recent nonclinical study found that individuals whose intrusions occurred without direct evidence for their relevance in the real world had more obsessive–compulsive symptoms, higher endorsement of OCD-related beliefs, greater ego dystonicity, and higher probability that the intrusions were repugnant (Audet et al., 2016). Moreover, 95% of the ego-dystonic intrusions were classified as occurring without direct evidence. Overall, there is some evidence that ego-dystonic appraisals may play a critical role in producing the faulty appraisal of significance associated with the repugnant intrusion.

Mental Control Strategies

Mental rituals rather than overt compulsions are more often seen in repugnant obsessions than in other OCD subtypes. In this regard, Williams and colleagues (2011) found that mental compulsions and reassurance seeking loaded on the same dimension with repugnant obsessions in a reanalysis of the DSM-IV Field Trial data. Moulding and colleagues (2014) note that individuals with repugnant obsessions may engage in "testing behaviors or compulsions" in an attempt to reduce pathological doubt caused by the obsession. An example of this would be someone with a sexual obsession who intentionally glances at the genital region of strangers to test whether he or she is inappropriately aroused. As well, repugnant obsessions can be associated with safety behaviors, such as wearing sunglasses, so people can't tell where the individual is looking.

It is likely that individuals with repugnant obsessions rely on a broader range of mental control strategies such as reassurance seeking, rationalization, thought stopping, self-punishment, and distraction because the purpose of neutralization is to resolve the ego-dystonic nature of the intrusion. In the case of harming and sexual obsessions, the neutralization is an attempt to convince oneself that the repugnant obsession is irrelevant to one's self-definition and to reassure oneself that one would never act on the intrusion. For a religious obsession, the neutralization may be focused more on the prevention of some abstruse dreaded outcome, such as eternal damnation or offending God.

Termination Rules

Little is known about the stop rules that pertain to repugnant obsessions. OCD researchers have only recently begun this line of research with more common washing and checking rituals, so it is understandable why there has been no exploration of termination criteria for repugnant obsessions. However, because of its more intense internal orientation and ego-dystonic nature, we would expect different stop criteria for repugnant obsessions.

For instance, individuals might be more concerned with achieving cessation of the intrusion rather than a desired emotional state, like reduction of distress or attainment of safety. As well, neutralization may continue until individuals perceive some temporary resolution of their ego-dystonic state. Individuals with repugnant obsessions might continue with their mental control strategies until they achieve a sense of certainty that the obsession is not representative of their feared self (C. L. Purdon, personal communication, April 15, 2016). One can only speculate whether the more severe psychopathology found with repugnant obsessions might be due, in part, to reliance on more nebulous termination criteria.

COGNITIVE-BEHAVIORAL CASE FORMULATION

Figure 12.1 provides the basis for the cognitive-behavioral case formulation of repugnant obsessions. A copy of the figure is made, and examples of the client's specific autogenous intrusions, appraisals, and mental control strategies are noted on the diagram. A copy of the completed case formulation is given to the client, and this becomes the basis for psychoeducation. Table 12.2 summarizes several aspects of the case formulation that must be considered.

TABLE 12.2. Special Considerations in the Case Conceptualization of Repugnant Obsessions

Construct	Explanation
Concealment	Given the overimportance and self-representational significance of the repugnant thoughts and images, individuals will be reluctant to admit to their occurrence.
Ego dystonicity	The extent to which the obsession contradicts, or is at least inconsistent with, valued selfhood domains and therefore represents a threat to self-representation (Purdon, Cripps, et al., 2007).
TAF–Moral	The extent to which the mere occurrence of the obsession is as morally reprehensible as acting on the obsession (Shafran & Rachman, 2004).
Importance/ control of thoughts	The belief that the mere occurrence of the obsession confers it with personal significance that necessitates heightened mental control effort.
Feared self	The extent to which self-representation involves self-relevant qualities that the person does not want to possess and that pose a threat or danger to personal integrity.

Note. From Clark and Hilchey (2017). Adapted with permission from John Wiley & Sons, Inc.

Concealment

Given the ego-dystonic nature of repugnant obsessions, clients often find it difficult to talk about their obsessions (Newth & Rachman, 2001; Purdon, 2004a). Also, resistance to self-disclosure could be influenced by the "natural stigma" associated with repugnant obsessions. When presented with OCD symptom vignettes, nonclinical individuals were less likely to label the harm and taboo symptom vignettes as OCD but endorsed significantly higher stigma ratings for taboo vignettes compared to the other symptom vignettes (McCarty, Guzick, Swan, & McNamara, 2017). Not only is talking about the repugnant thoughts highly distressing, but individuals may also fear that the therapist will confirm their worst fears about the significance of the intrusion as a measure of their true personality and their capacity to act on the disturbing thoughts. In this way, concealment functions as an avoidance response and strategy to maintain a sense of safety and security. There are several steps the therapist can take to help overcome concealment.

- Offer validation to the client, recognizing that disclosure of repugnant obsessions is highly distressing. It is important to build trust into the therapeutic relationship and to take a professional, detached approach to the obsession (i.e., no matter how repugnant, "A thought is a thought").

- Ensure that the repugnant obsessions are truly ego-dystonic and conduct a risk assessment for committing harmful or inappropriate acts to self or others. This is especially true of unlawful sexual or aggressive acts, which involve physical, sexual, or emotional harm to children or unsuspected adults. Moreover, it is important to discuss ethical and legal confidentiality issues and mandatory reporting laws at the outset of the intake interview. This needs to be done in a highly sensitive and therapeutic manner so the client is not frightened by the confidentiality discussion.

- Utilize a graduated approach to disclosure in which the client first talks about the obsession in general terms. I often use a label when working with a repugnant obsession (e.g., the "sexual thought" or the "blasphemous image"). Later more detailed, specific descriptions of obsessional content should be encouraged, which will be a therapeutic experience because just talking about the obsession will be an exposure experience.

- The cognitive therapist may also need to deal with dysfunctional beliefs involved in the concealment or reluctance to talk about obsessional content. For example, the client might believe that "Talking about the obsession makes it more likely to happen" (TAF–Likelihood), "It is immoral to verbalize such thoughts" (TAF–Moral), "You [therapist] will judge me as immoral, perverted, or dangerous," or "It's too embarrassing."

- Rachman (2003) describes a therapeutic strategy to concealment that challenges beliefs that self-disclosure will result in negative consequences. Clients are asked if they told anyone about the obsession. If answered in the affirmative, clients are questioned on whether the person's subsequent behavior changed toward them. Clients are then asked whether their behavior would change toward a friend who disclosed the same obsession to them. It is expected that clients will deny any behavioral change toward the friend upon disclosure, which provides disconfirming evidence of the perceived negative consequences associated with disclosure.

Ego Dystonicity

There are two key features that need to be addressed with ego dystonicity. First, to what extent is the repugnant obsession a deviation from the individual's realistic self-view? And second, how is the repugnant obsession a violation of cherished goals and values that comprise the client's self-definition? Both of these questions can be addressed within the cognitive clinical interview.

The therapist begins by identifying the goals, principles, and moral attributes valued by the individual, as well as the behaviors that are consistent with the person's moral tenets. This requires an in-depth exploration of the client's principles and values in various life domains, such as relationships, work, community, health, spirituality, physical appearance, leisure/recreation, and the like. A narrative can be written that could be labeled "My Ideal Self" or "The Person I Strive to Be." The following is an example of Camilla's ideal self-narrative:

> "Relationships are most important to me. I strive to be in harmony with everyone I meet. It's important that I treat people with understanding, sensitivity, and compassion. I want people to feel comfortable around me and to desire my company. I strive to be a conscientious, reliable, and efficient employee. I want people to feel confident in my skills and professional in my conduct. I maintain close and loving relationships with my family. As my parents age, I want them to feel they can rely on me to look after them. Although I'm not a religious person, I want to be infused with meaning and purpose; I don't want to be shallow or materialistic but rather to have a true sense of the transcendence of human nature. It's important that I take care of my health and physical well-being, but beauty is not important to me. Most of all I want to be a person of balance, integrity, and self-assurance."

After constructing the ideal self-narrative, the repugnant obsession is referred to as a "threat to the ideal self." The threat, of course, represents the extent that the obsession is ego-dystonic to the ideal. This is illustrated by noting the client's values on a series of continuums. Each end of the continuum represents the extreme opposite of the value. The client then labels on the continuums where the obsession lies and where the client's nature/character realistically lies. The difference between these two points represents the extent of ego dystonicity or threat associated with the obsession. Figure 12.2 illustrates this exercise with reference to two important values derived from Camilla's ideal self-narrative.

The therapist can also use the ideal self-narrative and ego-dystonic continuums to educate the client on the role of ego dystonicity in the persistence of repugnant obsessions. As well, this information is useful for cognitive restructuring of faulty beliefs about the obsession's significance. For example, the therapist might ask whether there is any evidence that the obsession will pull clients toward the negative end of their "value con-

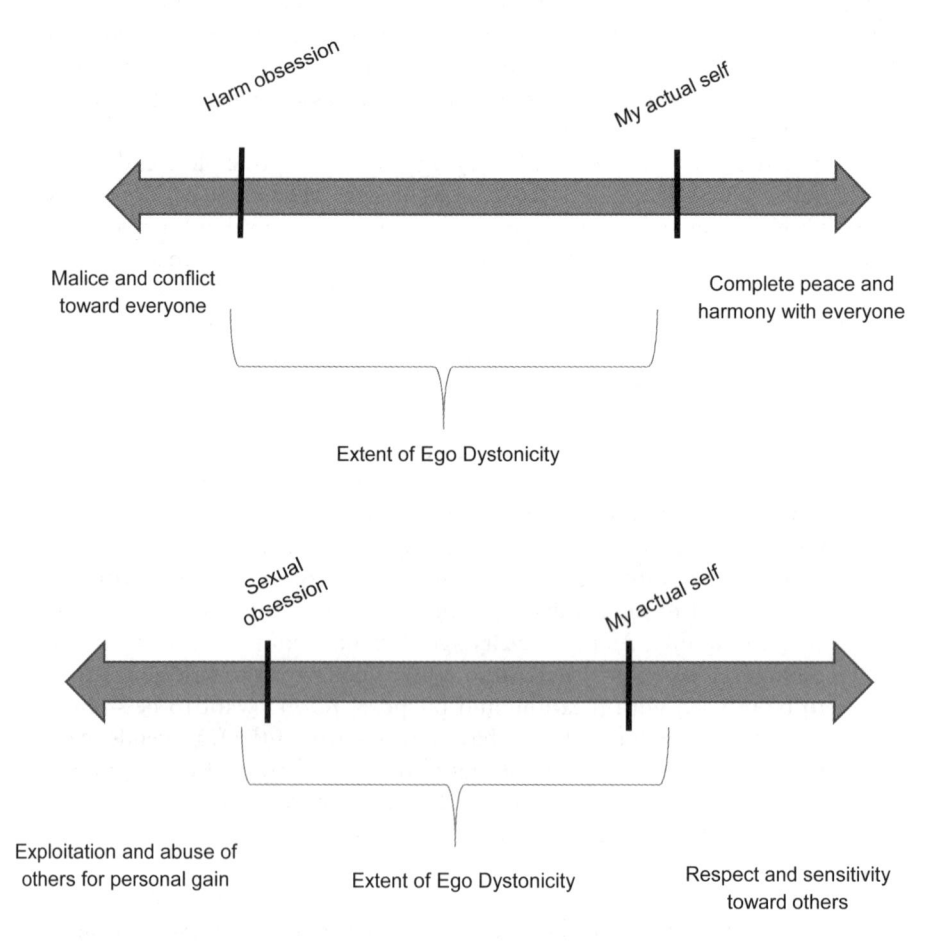

FIGURE 12.2. Camilla's ego-dystonicity continuum.

tinuum." Has the presence of the repugnant obsession had any effect on their commitment to the stated ideals, values, or principles?

TAF–Morality Bias

Intense guilt, ritualistic confession, and self-punishment are often associated with TAF–Moral. The TAF Scale (Shafran et al., 1996) can be administered with scores in the mid to upper 20s, indicating a heightened sense of moral TAF (Shafran & Rachman, 2004). However, a cognitive clinical interview will offer more insight into the client's perspective on morality. The key issue is the extent to which an individual believes the repugnant obsession is highly immoral. Are bad thoughts really considered equivalent to bad deeds? What is the feared consequence of these thoughts? Is there an intense feeling of guilt and, if so, what is the meaning of this guilt; that is, how is it interpreted or understood? To what extent do clients believe that their private mental state is a true reflection of their moral character?

A series of comparative questions can be asked to determine the perceived equivalence of the immoral thought to its expression as an immoral deed. For example, assume that the client has repugnant sexual obsessions of molesting a child. The following questions could be asked:

> "How bad is the thought of shoplifting compared to actually stealing an item from a store?"
> "How bad is the thought of lying to your boss versus actually lying to your boss?"
> "How bad is the thought of falsely taking credit for something you did not achieve, versus actually taking false credit for an undeserved achievement?"
> "How bad is the thought of punching someone versus actually punching that person ?"
> "How bad is the thought of touching a child inappropriately versus actually touching the child?"

The therapist can continue with this line of comparative questioning to determine the extent of moral TAF. Does the client exhibit a generalized moral TAF in which many different "bad thoughts" are considered nearly as bad as their corresponding misconduct, or is the focus solely on the repugnant obsession? In the previous example, the client might agree that deeds are worse than thoughts until the therapist gets to the final comparison, whereupon the client admits that the thought of molesting a child seems as bad as the actual deed. This analysis will be very useful for the psychoeducational phase of treatment as well as for introducing the adverse impact of importance and the need to control appraisals/beliefs on the frequency and intensity of the repugnant intrusion.

Importance/Control of Thoughts

It is important to identify the client's beliefs about the importance and control of the obsession, magnitude of thought control effort, and the anticipated consequences resulting from failures in mental control. Of course, it is also critical to make note of the mental control strategies used to suppress or terminate the repugnant obsession.

The OBQ-44 is one of the best standardized self-report questionnaires for assessing overimportance/need to control beliefs (OCCWG, 2005). In addition, the therapist can use the following questions to more fully understand the clients' beliefs and appraisals of overimportance and need to control in relation to their repugnant obsessions (see also the semistructured interview by Rachman, 2003).

- "When the repugnant obsession pops into your mind, are you able to distract yourself, or is your attention fully drawn to the thought? How good is your mental control over the obsession?"
- "What makes this obsessive thought so important that it grabs your attention? Are you concerned that just having the thought will cause harm to you or others, or are you more concerned about what you are thinking about; that is, its content? Is there any evidence in the real world that the obsession represents a significant personal threat?"
- "How important is it to inhibit the repugnant obsession or to stop thinking about it? What are you afraid will happen if the obsession doesn't go away?"
- "For you, what's so bad when you fail to control the obsession? Is there anything that prevents you from accepting the obsession; that is, just carrying on with your life regardless of whether the obsession is in your mind or not? Have you tried ignoring the thought? What happened?"
- "Do you blame yourself for having lost control over the obsession? What do you think is wrong that you seem to have so little mental control? What have you done to improve your mental control over the obsession?"

Feared Self

A final construct in the case conceptualization is the feared self. Although the FSQ (Aardema et al., 2013) could be administered, it is not clear what would be considered an abnormal score. Once again, the clinical interview will be more helpful in providing a wealth of idiographic information for the case formulation and treatment plan. Specific questions can be asked about the most feared aspects of the obsessional content and how these dreaded characteristics relate to a sense of self. In fact, a feared self-narrative could be constructed in juxtaposition to the ideal narrative discussed earlier. To develop the feared self-narrative, the therapist needs to explore what clients would not want to become; that is, what self-attributes they dread the most that represent a threat to the ideal self. The following is an example of Camilla's feared self-narrative:

> "I would never want to be known as a selfish and inconsiderate person. To go around manipulating and exploiting others simply to satisfy my own desires and pleasures would threaten my basic values of human decency and understanding. To be careless, egocentric, and impulsive, living only for immediate gratification of my momentary wants and desires, is not the type of person I want to be. As well, losing self-control and failing to live a disciplined, well-organized life can only lead to misery and the scorn of others."

Once the clinician has obtained a clear description of the "ideal and feared selves," the emergence of the repugnant obsession can be evaluated from these perspectives. To what extent is the obsession highly distressing because it threatens the "ideal self" and its values, as opposed to confirming elements of the feared self? Knowledge of the client's "self-narratives" provides key information for understanding the etiology and persistence of the repugnant obsession.

SPECIAL TREATMENT CONSIDERATIONS

CBT for repugnant obsessions employs the same treatment strategies as discussed in Chapters 8 and 9. However, the absence of overt rituals and the importance of self-construal processes require some refinements in the treatment protocol.

Imaginal Exposure

Imaginal exposure is an important ingredient in the treatment of repugnant obsessions because of its heightened internal focus. In many cases the mere occurrence of the obsession elicits significant anxiety and guilt. Sustained directed attention on the repugnant obsession through imaginal exposure homework provides a critical empirical hypothesis-testing experience that challenges the individual's belief in the significance of the obsession and the fear of losing control. To begin, the therapist collaborates with the client in construction of an exposure narrative. Clients are encouraged to write a detailed script of the obsessional content in their own words. A gradual approach to construction of the script is necessary if there is considerable anxiousness and reluctance to talk about the obsessional content.

Once a vivid account of the repugnant obsession is available, several in-session imaginal exposures are provided to deal with any avoidance or neutralization responses. Moulding and colleagues (2014) discuss several approaches to imaginal exposure that can be used when assigning homework, such as audio recording, intentionally verbalizing the obsession while preventing neutralization, and exposure to avoided real-life obsession triggers. As well, smartphone apps are available, so the obsession can be confronted frequently. Whatever the methodology employed, imaginal exposure is a critical element of CBT for repugnant obsessions.

Neutralization Prevention

Another important treatment component involves the reduction and eventual elimination of all neutralization responses (Moulding et al., 2014; M. T. Williams et al., 2013). Mental compulsions, reassurance seeking, rationalization, thought suppression, and avoidance are the most common mental control strategies associated with repugnant obsessions. The therapist first identifies the client's most common neutralization responses and then, during provocation of the obsession in the session, helps the client learn healthier, acceptance- and distraction-based responses to replace maladaptive neutralization. For example, reassurance seeking is a common response to religious obsessions. When Camilla, for example, had the intrusive thought "Have I offended God?," she would search the Internet for theological information on the nature of offense against God. She was seeking information that would reassure her that her intrusive thoughts were not offending God. Others who are more religiously inclined might seek out ministers, priests, rabbis, or imams to obtain reassurance that they have not sinned against God. Cessation of all reassurance activities is an important goal in CBT for repugnant obsessions.

To help with response prevention of neutralization, individuals are taught acceptance and distraction strategies that include cognitive and behavioral activities of daily living that replace the neutralization responses. For example, when the urge to seek reassurance arises, the client could engage in physical exercise, read a novel, answer email, cook, work on a puzzle, and so on. The objective is to shift attentional resources to a response that competes with the urge to neutralize. Often a gradual approach to response prevention is required (Clark, 2004; Moulding et al., 2014). This can be done by encouraging the client to delay neutralization, at first for a brief time, and then gradually increasing the delay period so that eventually the neutralization response is completely discontinued. This might also require expansion of the alternate response options and problem-solving any difficulties that might arise with neutralization prevention.

Cognitive Restructuring

An important aspect of CBT is normalizing the repugnant obsession by correcting the dysfunctional beliefs of its overimportance and personal significance. Clients are taught that the occurrence of even repugnant thoughts is normal, but it's the appraisal or interpretation of the intrusion that causes an escalation in its frequency, intensity, and emotional distress. This point can be demonstrated by comparing clients' interpretation of a nondistressing "normal" intrusion with their faulty interpretation of the repugnant obsession (see Chapter 8 for details).

Cognitive structuring can be used to weaken the link between the repugnant obsession and the client's self-definition. The groundwork for this intervention is laid in the psychoeducational phase that highlights the link between the obsession and feared self. The repugnant obsession is considered significant because of its ego dystonicity and its relevance to the feared self.

The therapist begins by asking the client to choose a value or characteristic that is threatened by the presence of repugnant obsessions. The value or characteristic could be obtained from the ideal self-narrative discussed previously. As an example, Camilla might state that she desires to be a person with high moral standards. The therapist then asks, "What is the evidence that you are a moral person?," and Camilla identifies several reality-based indicators of her morality, such as honesty in her dealings with customers, generosity with her time and money, efforts to put the interests of others before herself, etc. Then Camilla could be asked for evidence that she is a selfish, immoral, and inconsiderate person—characteristics articulated in her feared self-narrative. When asked for evidence of immorality, no doubt having repugnant obsessions is Camilla's main proof. The therapist then contrasts the "imagined, inferred evidence for an immoral self" against the realistic, external real-life evidence for the ideal, moralistic self. Once the faulty nature of her self-construal process is identified, the therapist could then work with Camilla to help her shift the source of her self-definition from a "possibility bias" (i.e., "I have repugnant thoughts that mean that I'm immoral") to an external evidence basis (e.g., "My actions are more consistent with morality than immorality"). It is important to spend time elaborating on this cognitive work, helping the client search for more external evidence and practice basing her self-evaluation on external, sensory-based criteria rather than inferred, imagined criteria (Audet et al., 2016; O'Connor & Aardema, 2012).

It is also important to assign empirical hypothesis-testing homework to consolidate the externally based self-construal. Camilla could be assigned homework that involves collecting information from family and close friends on what indicators they use to make judgments of other people's moral character. This information could be used to gauge Camilla's level of moral standing relative to others. Over several weeks Camilla could self-monitor daily activities that are congruent or incongruent with high moral value (e.g., "Today I spent extra time explaining a prescription to an elderly person, even though it made me rushed the rest of the morning"; "I actually defended a coworker whom I felt was being unfairly criticized by our supervisor"). Over time Camilla would be able to shift the basis of her moral self-evaluation from "what I am thinking" to "what I am doing." This would weaken the link between repugnant obsessions and the self-construal process.

Treatment Efficacy and Other Modalities

The most consistent conclusion about treatment effectiveness of OCD symptom subtypes is that pharmacotherapy and ERP are less effective for obsessions without overt compulsions (e.g., Starcevric & Brakoulias, 2008; M. T. Williams et al., 2013). In an early meta-analysis of pharmacotherapy and/or ERP, "pure obsessionals" had smaller than average effect sizes compared to other OCD subtypes, although the difference was not statistically significant (Christensen, Hadzi-Pavlovic, Andrews, & Mattick, 1987). In another study individuals with sexual/religious obsessions had a poorer long-term outcome at 1- to 5-year follow-up when treated with SSRIs and/or ERP (Alonso et al., 2001). A large multicenter treatment study of computer- versus clinician-assisted ERP found that those with sexual/religious obsessions had a poorer treatment response (Mataix-Cols et al., 2002). Likewise, Abramowitz and colleagues found that individuals with OCD, who fell in their Unacceptable/Taboo obsessions cluster, had one of the lowest rates of clinically significant improvement, although not a statistically significant difference from the other symptom clusters (Abramowitz, Franklin, et al., 2003). A more recent study involving regression analysis based on two combined treatment outcome studies found that OCD participants with Unacceptable/Taboo obsessions had significantly smaller YBOCS score reductions at posttreatment than individuals with other primary symptom dimensions (Williams et al., 2014). However, another treatment outcome review concluded that the findings of a worse outcome for sexual/religious obsessions cannot be considered reliable (Knopp et al., 2013).

There are several reasons for the less encouraging outcomes for repugnant obsessions (see also review by McKay et al., 2015). ERP tends to focus on overt compulsions, which are often absent in repugnant obsessions. It is also more challenging to use exposure with autogenous, internally precipitated intrusions (Moulding et al., 2014). Core self-definitional processes are often linked to repugnant obsessions, and so individuals may have more difficulty taking a detached approach to their obsessions. Thus, cognitive interventions may play a more critical role in the treatment of repugnant obsessions (Lee, Kwon, et al., 2005; Rachman, 2003; Williams, Crozier, et al., 2011).

One of the first treatment outcome studies of CBT specially tailored for obsessions without overt compulsions was conducted by Freeston and colleagues (1997). After receiving approximately 25 sessions of CBT, 67% of the sample showed clinically significant improvement at posttreatment, but this dropped to 53% at 6-month follow-up. Likewise, O'Connor, Freeston, and colleagues (2005) randomly assigned 26 individuals with obsessions and no overt compulsions to 12 sessions of either individual or group CBT. Posttreatment analysis revealed that 68% of the individual CBT condition achieved significant symptom improvement, compared to 38% who received the group format. Both treatment conditions maintained their gains at 6-month follow-up. The researchers noted that there was a fairly high refusal rate (38%) for assignment to the group format.

Whittal, Woody, McLean, Rachman, and Robichaud (2010) conducted one of the most rigorous outcome trials on obsessions without overt compulsions. Seventy-three individuals were randomly assigned to 12 individual sessions of cognitive therapy without ERP, stress management training (SMT), or wait-list control. Posttreatment analysis revealed some advantage of cognitive therapy over SMT, but this disappeared at the 6- and 12-month follow-ups. Both treatments were more effective than a wait-list control. In terms of clinical significance, 59% achieved this criterion in the cognitive therapy group and 43% in the SMT condition. This difference was not statistically significant. A subsequent mediational analysis indicated that change in dysfunctional appraisals was a mediator of change in obsessional symptoms, although further analysis of temporal precedence suggested that obsessional symptoms may have had a greater impact on appraisals of personal significance than the reverse (Woody et al., 2011). Finally, Belloch and colleagues (2010) found that cognitive therapy with no ERP was significantly more effective for autogenous than reactive obsessions, with 73% of the completers in the autogenous group reaching recovery criteria at posttreatment.

Findings from more recent outcome studies indicate that treatment efficacy for obsessions without overt compulsions may be more nuanced than previously thought. It may be that contemporary treatment approaches that specifically target dysfunctional appraisals, beliefs, and mental control strategies are more effective than treatments that focus exclusively on ERP. And yet, these more cognitive interventions have reported significant improvement in only 40–65% of individuals who complete therapy. Obviously, there is considerable room for improvement in CBT treatment of repugnant obsessions.

CONCLUSION

Although fewer individuals with OCD have repugnant obsessions as their primary symptom presentation, the 25% of OCD samples with this symptomatology represent a considerable challenge for CBT therapists. Most often people with primary repugnant obsessions do not engage in overt rituals but instead rely on a broader range of mental control strategies to inhibit their distressing intrusions. Moreover, threats to morality and self-definition are central features of the obsession, which then results in appraisals of the obsession as highly ego-dystonic. TAF–Likelihood and –Moral beliefs are elevated, which lead to the conclusion that control or inhibition of the obsession is of utmost importance. Less emphasis is placed on anxiety reduction or prevention of some dreaded outcome than on cessation of the repugnant intrusions. Moreover, certain types of repugnant obsessions, such as religious obsessions or scrupulosity, present even greater challenges for conceptualization and treatment.

CBT for repugnant obsessions requires a greater focus on schemas related to the self as well as beliefs in the necessity of mental control. Practically all the treatment process research that has investigated the treatment efficacy for repugnant obsessions has focused on pharmacotherapy or ERP. The general finding is that medication and behavioral treatment are less effective for repugnant obsessions than they are for washing or checking symptom dimensions. A new generation of outcome studies derived from the CBT appraisal model has reported promising findings, but it is unclear whether these treatments are much better than more conventional behavior therapy. What is needed are comparative outcome studies in which individuals with primary repugnant obsessions are randomly assigned to CBT versus ERP. However, it is unlikely we will see this type of research for years to come. Given the low base rate of repugnant obsessions, samples of sufficient size to allow random assignment are difficult to generate. As well, debate continues on whether it is feasible or even desirable to pit cognitive against behavioral interventions, since most treatment in the clinical setting incorporates both cognitive and exposure-based strategies.

Many conceptual and methodological challenges face researchers interested in the phenomenology and treatment of repugnant mental intrusions. Despite this reality, the need for evidence-based knowledge and treatment could not be greater for those who suffer from this tormenting type of OCD.

CHAPTER 13

Symmetry, Ordering, and Arranging

CASE ILLUSTRATION

Elaine considered herself a perfectionist. She recalls having a strong preference for order, balance, and neatness since childhood. Everything in her room had its place and when something was not right, she felt upset until it was rearranged properly. Her parents worked hard to ensure that they did not upset Elaine by accidentally misplacing her toys, clothing, and other possessions. She refused to have friends over in case they messed up her room during play.

In her early teens Elaine became even more preoccupied with symmetry and balance. She developed a concern about using the right side of her body more than the left and would try to correct this perceived imbalance by using her left hand more or focusing her attention more to the left side of her visual field. In university she eventually had to live on her own because roommates would invade her private space and misplace her stuff. In many ways her meticulousness, organization, and attention to detail served her well academically and as an accountant. She was so well organized that others came to rely on her to find needed information.

The negative effects of Elaine's order and rearranging were felt most acutely at home. The mess and chaos caused by her children troubled her greatly. Her husband tried to share in housecleaning chores, but it was never good enough for Elaine. She would follow after him, "correcting" his tidying efforts. For example, when he loaded the dishwasher with dirty dishes, Elaine would rearrange everything, so the plates, glasses, and utensils were facing the right way. She was constantly rearranging the cupboards because he didn't put things back in their rightful place. She was continually picking up after the children, even when they were not finished playing. Elaine was spending several hours each evening and most of the weekends tidying up. This incessant ordering and rearranging were putting strain on the marriage. At work, Elaine had been passed over for promotion because she was considered too rigid, uncompromising, and so preoccupied with orderliness that her actual work productivity suffered. Elaine tried repeatedly to curb her ordering and rearranging behavior, but each time her efforts ended in failure. The feeling that "things were not right" was so overpowering that she could not simply ignore the disorder and relax. Whatever was out of order *had to be corrected.*

Elaine is the prototypical case of a subtype of OCD that is distinct from all the other obsessive–compulsive presentations discussed in this volume. Referred to as symmetry, order, and arranging (SOA), this subtype of OCD has a different affective–motivational characteristic than do contamination, doubt/checking, and repugnant obsessions (Summerfeldt, 2004). Whereas the latter symptom presentations are motivated by harm avoidance, SOA is driven by a profound sense of imperfection, incompletenesss, or "not just right" experiences (NJRE; e.g., Coles et al., 2003; Radomsky & Rachman, 2004; Rasmussen & Eisen, 1992; Summerfeldt, 2004; Summerfeldt, Kloosterman, Antony, & Swinson, 2014). This chapter discusses the cognitive-behavioral approach to SOA, beginning with the clinical features that are unique to this obsessive state. Next, research is reviewed that supports the symptom distinctiveness of the SOA subtype. This is followed by a discussion of the core cognitive construct in SOA: the sense of incompleteness. The cognitive-behavioral model of SOA is presented, along with a discussion of the CBT case formulation. The chapter concludes by delineating modifications in CBT needed to address the unique features of this OCD subtype.

CLINICAL FEATURES

The symptom heterogeneity of OCD is most apparent in those cases where symptoms of SOA predominate. Numerous OCD researchers, dating back to Pierre Janet in 1903, have noted that the core motivational process that underlies ordering and arranging may be very different from other obsessive–compulsive compulsions like washing and checking. Whereas most OCD presentations are like other anxiety disorders, in which reduction or avoidance of harm is the primary motive, Rasmussen and Eisen (1992) noted that individuals with SOA do not experience elevated anxiety but rather are motivated by a feeling that something is "not just right," imperfect, or incomplete. Summerfeldt (2004) proposed that harm avoidance and incompleteness are two continuous orthogonal dimensions that cut across different types of OCD and are associated with different clinical features, vulnerabilities, and causal factors. Coles and Pietrefesa (2008) argue that SOA symptoms constitute a distinct and very different OCD subtype because they are motivated by a desire to get things "just right," rather than to reduce anxiety or achieve a sense of safety. More recently, Bragdon and Coles (2017) found that individuals with OCD could be differentiated on whether they were high or low on harm avoidance and incompleteness. This fundamental motivational difference for SOA suggests that the causal models and treatment of these symptoms differs substantially from other OCD subtypes. In fact, some have questioned whether CBT models are applicable to OCD symptom presentations that are dominated by concerns with incompleteness or NJREs, rather than anxiety reduction (Cougle, Fitch, Jaconson, & Lee, 2013; Summerfeldt et al., 2014).

Symmetry obsessions are experienced as frequent, intrusive perceptions of imbalance, disorder, or unevenness in personal thought, action, or environment that are associated with an urge to rearrange to achieve a more perfect, even, or ordered state of affairs. Ordering, rearranging, and often checking are the compulsions most often associated with symmetry obsessions. Summerfeldt (2004) noted that the "not just right" feeling evident in symmetry obsessions can involve any sensory modality, including the visual, auditory, tactile, and proprioceptive modes. The sense of incompleteness, or asymmetry, is most often expressed as a visual perception, but the possibility that "not just right" may be evident in other sensory modalities should not be overlooked.

Symmetry, ordering and rearranging are among the most commonly endorsed symptoms in OCD samples. Rasmussen and Eisen (1992, 1998) found that 32% of their OCD treatment sample reported symmetry obsessions and 28% had compulsions focused on achieving precision. In the DSM-IV Field Trial, 10% had predominant symmetry obsessions and 5.7% ordering compulsions (Foa et al., 1995). Moreover, ordering (9.1%) was the third most common compulsion reported by respondents in the NCS-R who met diagnostic criteria for OCD (Ruscio et al., 2010). Given such high prevalence in OCD samples, clinicians should always assess for SOA symptoms even when other types of obsessions and compulsions are more prominent.

SOA symptoms can be found in nonclinical populations, although at lower frequency, intensity, and interference in daily functioning. A community survey of 2,261 Canadians found that orderliness (10.9%) was the second most common obsession, whereas less than 3% of the sample reported the compulsion to do things in a particular order (Stein et al., 1997). A community longitudinal study in New Zealand reported that 10% of their 32-year-old age group met symmetry/ordering criteria, making it the second most common obsessive–compulsive symptom dimension (Fullana et al., 2009). Although symmetry/ordering symptoms showed considerable temporal stability, they had the lowest risk for major depression and were not associated with elevated interference or help seeking. Self-report measures of SOA, such as the Symmetry, Ordering and Arranging Questionnaire, indicate that nonclinical individuals endorse many of the questionnaire items, and their scores correlate strongly with other OCD symptom measures (Radomsky & Rachman, 2004; Radomsky et al., 2006).

Coles and Pietrefesa (2008) noted that SOA symptoms may represent an exaggerated form of culturally prescribed rituals. They state that ordering or arranging is a common cultural ritual that serves a useful social function with value or meaning. However, when taken to the extremes seen in OCD, ordering and arranging lose their social usefulness, are driven more by internal motives such as a sense of incompleteness, and end up isolating the individual from wider society (Coles & Pietrefesa, 2008). Although SOA symptoms are common across culturally diverse OCD samples, the frequencies vary, suggesting some cultural influence on their OCD symptom presentation. SOA prevalence was similar to North American rates in Turkish (Karadağ et al., 2006) and Indian (Girishchandra & Khanna, 2001) samples, but ostensibly more prevalent in Egyptian (Okasha et al., 1994), Iranian (Ghassemzadeh et al., 2002), and Chinese (Li, Marques, Hinton, Wang, & Xiao, 2009) OCD groups. In these latter studies, men had a higher rate of SOA symptoms than women, although others suggest there are no significant sex differences across the obsessive–compulsive symptom dimensions (Raines et al., 2018). Nevertheless, the SOA symptom pattern has cross-cultural consistency, with Arab, Persian, and Chinese cultures showing a higher preponderance of SOA concerns in their OCD populations.

There is evidence that SOA symptoms are associated with early-onset OCD (Taylor, 2011). In a Brazilian OCD study, the SOA symptom dimension had an earlier age of onset and a more stable clinical course (Kichuk et al., 2013). A study of Chinese patients with OCD also found that SOA symptoms were more frequent in the early-onset group (Zhang, Liu, Cui, & Liu, 2013). Other studies indicate that SOA is associated with higher rates of OCD in first-degree relatives and greater comorbidity with tic disorders (for a review, see Leckman et al., 2010). These findings have not always been supported. A more recent OCD study did not find higher rates of family history for individuals with elevated SOA symptoms or a significant association with tic disorders, and age of onset was actually later, rather than earlier, as previously reported (Brakoulias et al., 2016).

Like other OCD symptoms, the presence of stressful life events may exacerbate SOA symptoms. A study of 200 individuals with OCD who reported at least one stressful life event in the year before onset of their OCD found that SOA symptoms had one of the highest associations with severe life events (Rosso et al., 2012). This finding suggests a strong environmental influence on the course of SOA symptoms.

Several conclusions can be drawn from research on the clinical features of individuals with prominent SOA symptoms. Clearly, concerns about symmetry and order are common in the general population and may serve some adaptive value. In some ways clinical SOA is an exaggeration of its nonclinical counterpart, but it has become so extreme and so driven by unique intrapersonal processes that its connection to normal expressions of order and symmetry become strained. SOA is a cross-cultural phenomenon, although cultural differences appear to influence its preponderance in OCD samples. Finally, differences in age of onset, higher familial rates in first-degree relatives, comorbidity with tic disorders, and responsiveness to environmental influences support the contention that SOA forms a distinct symptom subtype that may not conform to standard CBT formulations and treatment protocols for OCD.

THE DISTINCTIVENESS OF SOA

Most of the OCD subtype research assumes a continuity perspective with individuals differing in terms of the prominence of various symptoms in their obsessive–compulsive experience. This assumption raises the question of whether SOA symptoms are distinct from other OCD symptoms such as contamination fears, checking, doubt, and the like. As noted in Chapter 1, numerous studies have researched this issue. Despite some inconsistency in the findings, a distinct SOA symptom dimension is one of the most robust findings in numerous cluster and factor-analyses of the YBOCS Symptom Checklist (see Bloch et al., 2008; Mataix-Cols et al., 2005). This distinctive symptom dimension has been replicated in OCD samples drawn from different countries (e.g., Kashyap, Kumar, Kandavel, & Reddy, 2017; Matsunaga, Hayashida, Kiriike, Maebayashi, & Stein, 2010; Zhang et al., 2013). Bayesian structural equation modeling of the YBOCS Symptom Checklist revealed a broad second-order factor labeled *Incompleteness* that included most of the miscellaneous items in the YBOCS Symptom Checklist (e.g., keeping order, counting, repeating, hoarding, creating symmetry, list making; Schulze, Kathmann, & Reuter, 2018). Moreover, the SOA symptom dimension may have different comorbidity (Hasler et al., 2005), genetic correlates (López-Solà et al., 2016), and less neurophysiological abnormality (Lázaro et al., 2014) compared to other symptom subtypes.

A broad range of research indicates that SOA symptoms are distinct from other obsessive–compulsive symptom dimensions. The clinical implication is that SOA symptoms should be included in any assessment of OCD, and CBT therapists can expect to find order and symmetry concerns in varying degrees across a broad spectrum of OCD patients. Although there may be some disagreement on the specific symptom items that comprise this dimension, the structural equation modeling study of Schulze and colleagues (2018) indicates that the central feature of this dimension is incompleteness, which is the core construct in the CBT formulation for SOA.

Incompleteness

Summerfeldt (2004) describes incompleteness as a troubling sense or dissatisfaction that one's actions or current state is "not just right." In a further elaboration, Coles and Pietrefesa (2008) note that incompleteness is "a tormenting sensation arising from the perception that one's actions or experiences are insufficient or incomplete" (p. 37). Most researchers consider incompleteness synonymous with the NJRE that was discussed in Chapter 3. Although not confined to the SOA symptom subtype, incompleteness is considered the primary affective–motivational process in SOA (Coles & Pietrefesa, 2008; Rasmussen & Eisen, 1992; Summerfeldt, 2004). In the case illustration at the beginning of this chapter, Elaine's urge to rearrange dishes that her husband had loaded into the dishwasher was an irresistible sensation driven by a sense that it was not done correctly. Even though she knew that rearranging the dishes would precipitate an argument, she nonetheless continued with the compulsion because the sense of dissatisfaction was greater than having to endure a tense marital argument.

Summerfeldt (2004) states that incompleteness is primarily a sensory–affective disturbance, with cognitive beliefs and appraisals playing a secondary role. Thus, it is argued that OCD motivated by incompleteness or NJRE may not be as amenable to CBT. However, the definitive features of incompleteness are not well understood, and its relation to harm avoidance is still under investigation. This latter issue has considerable theoretical and clinical importance. If incompleteness and harm avoidance are distinct constructs, this finding would support the contention that CBT may be applicable only to anxiety-related presentations of OCD. On the other hand, if the two constructs are related, then CBT approaches developed for harm avoidance may have application to forms of OCD dominated by incompleteness (i.e., SOA).

In three studies Summerfeldt and colleagues (2014) found evidence of structural integrity for an incompleteness dimension that was distinct but coexistent with the harm avoidance dimension, with the Harm Avoidance and Incompleteness subscales of the Obsessive–Compulsive Core Dimensions Questionnaire (OC-CDQ) well correlated ($r = .70$). An earlier study by Pietrefesa and Coles (2008) also reported a two-factor solution of incompleteness and harm avoidance based on an undergraduate sample, but again the two dimensions were highly correlated ($r = .76$). As well, a meta-analysis and subsequent study based on a large nonclinical sample found evidence that incompleteness and harm avoidance were distinct dimensions with a moderate to high correlation (Taylor et al., 2014). Further analysis of the nonclinical sample revealed that incompleteness, as measured by the OC-CDQ, had an extremely high correlation with harm avoidance ($r = .93$), whereas NJRE had only a moderate correlation ($r = .45$). Finally, a recent study based on 100 individuals with OCD found low to moderate correlations between the Behavioral and Sensory subscales of the Brown Incompleteness Scale and the Harm Avoidance subscale of the

OC-CDQ, with correlations of r = .31 and .47, respectively (Boisseau et al., 2018). Given the moderate to strong correlation between harm avoidance and incompleteness, it is possible that the compulsions of many people with OCD may be driven by both motivational processes, whereas others may be driven solely by incompleteness. This suggests considerable variability in the motivational processes across individuals with OCD. Individual differences in the preponderance of harm avoidance and/or incompleteness was evident in a cluster analysis of 85 individuals with OCD, in which only 26% of the sample had both elevated incompleteness and harm avoidance (Bragdon & Coles, 2017).

Several studies have investigated the nature of incompleteness in order to better understand its functional relation to OCD. Boisseau and colleagues (2018) found that incompleteness is two-dimensional, with a behavioral feature representing difficulty initiating and completing tasks because of the need to have things just right, and a sensory component characterized by a feeling that things need to be a certain way. Both incompleteness dimensions correlated moderately with obsessive–compulsive symptoms, although incompleteness–sensory was more highly correlated with harm avoidance than incompleteness–behavioral. Bragdon and Coles (2017) reported that their incompleteness-only cluster endorsed more beliefs about perfectionism and fewer beliefs of inflated responsibility/threat overestimation (see also Belloch et al., 2016). Pietrefesa and Coles (2009) showed that incompleteness was specifically related to feelings of tension/discomfort and to the need to perform tasks perfectly or "just right," when university students were asked to engage in certain tasks like arranging books on a bookshelf or hanging pictures. In their analysis of incompleteness and NJRE in clinical and nonclinical samples, Belloch and colleagues (2016) concluded that incompleteness might represent a stable predisposition that activates compulsions, whereas NJRE motivates individuals to act compulsively depending on the meaning ascribed to their experience.

Two experimental studies were conducted to tease apart the defining features of incompleteness. Fornés-Romero and Belloch (2017) used an incompleteness/NJRE induction in nonclinical and OCD samples to show that the induction was associated with greater physical discomfort and a need to check repeatedly. As well, incompleteness scores were associated with state NJRE and physical discomfort during the experimental task. In another study in which students engaged in a task that assessed their preference for, and ability to estimate, symmetry and balance, high-trait incompleteness was characterized by greater symmetry-related concerns and behaviors as well as heightened preference for symmetry in images, although there were no differences in aesthetic skill, such as estimating the objective aesthetic value of images (Summerfeldt, Gilbert, & Reynolds, 2015). Together, research on the nature of incompleteness suggests that it may (1) be multidimensional with behavioral and sensory elements, (2) possess more dispositional or traitlike attributes, (3) have a close association with perfectionism and aesthetic preference for balance and symmetry, and (4) elicit feelings of discomfort and urge to check. Although most researchers emphasize the overlap between incompleteness and NJRE, others suggest that NJRE is more relevant for understanding obsessive thinking and incompleteness as a motivator for compulsions (Belloch et al., 2016).

Research indicates that incompleteness is more prominent in OCD than in other disorders. Ecker and Gönner (2008), for example, performed hierarchical regression on a large OCD sample to show that incompleteness was uniquely associated with symmetry/ordering and checking after controlling for depression, anxiety, and symptom severity. Starcevic and colleagues (2011) found that SOA compulsions were more frequently motived by NJRE (see also Ferrão et al., 2012). A group comparison study found that incompleteness was more pronounced in OCD than in anxiety disorders or depression, with regression analysis indicating that a diagnosis of OCD, and to a lesser extent, depression, contributed to incompleteness severity (Ecker, Kupfer, & Gönner, 2014a). Others have found that the associated construct of NJRE may be a better discriminator of OCD than beliefs (Ghisi et al., 2010) and that induced guilt may increase NJREs in high-trait-guilt individuals (Mancini, Gangemi, Peerdighe, & Marini, 2008).

Research on the symptom specificity of incompleteness has produced mixed results. Several studies have reported a significant relationship between incompleteness and SOA symptoms (e.g., Ecker & Gönner, 2008; Ecker et al., 2014a; Sibrava, Boisseau, Eisen, Mancebo, & Rasmussen, 2016; Starcevic at al., 2011). However, incompleteness also promotes checking compulsions (Cougle et al., 2013) and is associated with obsessive–compulsive personality traits (Ecker, Kupfer, & Gönner, 2014b).

Table 13.1 presents a summary of the key findings on incompleteness.

TABLE 13.1. Key Findings on Incompleteness

- Incompleteness and the "not just right" experience (NJRE) are aspects of a sensory–perceptual motivational construct that plays a key role in the pathogenesis of OCD.
- Most often, compulsions like washing, checking, repeating, mental rituals, and the like are motivated by harm avoidance, whereas other compulsions involving ordering, rearranging, and checking are motivated by incompleteness/NJRE.
- Although incompleteness and harm avoidance are distinct affective–motivational constructs, they are highly correlated and can coexist in the same individual.
- Incompleteness is a key process in the SOA subtype of OCD, although its relevance is not confined to this symptom subtype.
- Incompleteness is a stable dispositional characteristic that is associated with perfectionism, obsessive–compulsive personality traits, and preference for balance and symmetry. However, it is also sensitive to the presence of depressive mood, guilt, and symptom severity.
- Incompleteness may be a vulnerability factor for the SOA symptom presentation of OCD, although research is needed to support this assertion.

Clearly, any model of SOA must include incompleteness as a critical process that motivates compulsive behavior. Although some have questioned whether CBT models are relevant to obsessive–compulsive symptom presentations motivated by incompleteness/NJRE (i.e., Cougle et al., 2013; Summerfeldt et al., 2014), there is no reason to assume that the affective–motivational construct is incompatible with the notion of faulty beliefs and appraisals. As evident in the following section, a cognitive-behavioral formulation of SOA can be proposed that assigns a prominent role to incompleteness and NJRE phenomena.

A COGNITIVE-BEHAVIORAL MODEL OF SOA

From the previous discussion, it is evident that some modification is needed to the generic model (see Figure 5.1) to provide an adequate cognitive-behavioral formulation of SOA. Figure 13.1 presents a possible CBT account of this symptom subtype.

This section highlights key changes needed in the CBT formulation of SOA. As well, research supporting the cognitive-behavioral conceptualization of SOA is reviewed. As will be seen, a CBT conceptualization is plausible, evidence-based, and informative of treatment for this type of obsessive–compulsive symptom presentation.

Vulnerability Factors

Research on the etiology of SOA is practically nonexistent. Coles and Pietrefesa (2008) propose that clinical levels of SOA may represent "a failure to extinguish normal childhood habits or an exacerbation of culturally prescribed patterns of behavior" (p. 39). It is well known that repetitive behaviors like ordering and rearranging, as well as "just right" feelings, are common in early childhood (Evans et al., 1997). It has been speculated that OCD might lie on a continuum with childhood rituals (Leonard, Goldberger, Rapoport, Cheslow, & Swedo, 1990). As children grow older and eventually enter adulthood, the frequency of compulsive-like repetitive rituals decreases but does not disappear entirely. In fact, preference for order remains strong even into adulthood (Radomsky & Rachman, 2004). Reuven, Kahn, and Carmeli (2012) reported that childhood oral and tactile hypersensitivity is related to increased childhood ritualistic behavior and obsessive–compulsive symptoms in adults. This research raises the possibility that clinical levels of SOA might represent a specific type of "arrested development" in which individuals continue to show the heightened concern for order and symmetry found in early childhood (Coles & Pietrefesa, 2008). Individual differences are evident in preference for order and symmetry, so it is entirely possible that an

348   SUBTYPE TREATMENT PROTOCOLS

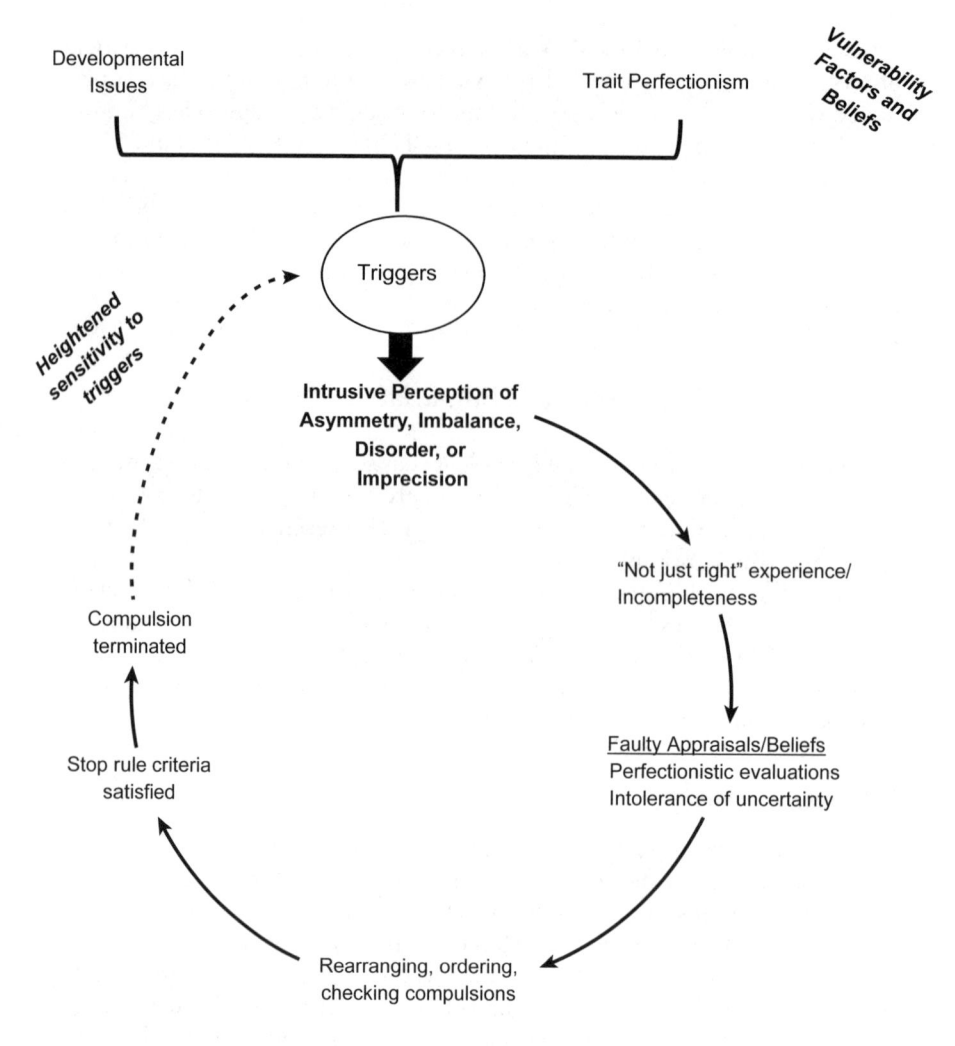

FIGURE 13.1. Cognitive-behavioral model for symmetry, ordering, and rearranging OCD.

elevated concern for order, symmetry, and completeness might be a vulnerability factor for clinical SOA (Belloch et al., 2016; Radomsky & Rachman, 2004; Summerfeldt et al., 2015). At the very least, researchers should consider whether developmental influences might contribute to the etiology of SOA.

There is considerable evidence of an association between perfectionism and SOA. Although CBT research in OCD has tended to focus on perfectionism as a set of faulty appraisals/beliefs that are proximal contributors to obsessive–compulsive symptoms, most consider perfectionism a core personality vulnerability that can predispose an individual to emotional disturbance more generally (Egan et al., 2014; Hewitt, Flett, & Mikail, 2017). Thus, it is reasonable to consider whether perfectionism might play a particularly important role in the etiology of the SOA symptom dimension.

Research has consistently shown a relationship between perfectionism and OCD (e.g., Frost & Steketee, 1997; Rhéaume, Freeston, Dugas, Letartte, & Ladouceur, 1995; for a review, see Frost et al., 2002). Furthermore, perfectionism is related to specific OCD features that are prominent in SOA, such as NJRE, precision, order, and incompleteness (Aardema et al., 2018; Coles et al., 2003, 2005; Martinelli, Chasson, Wetterneck, Hart, & Björgvinsson, 2014). However, a mediational study by Moretz and McKay (2009) indicates that trait anxiety may mediate the relationship between perfectionism and obsessive–compulsive symptoms. As noted in Chapter 1, a significant number of individuals with OCD have comorbid OCPD, which includes perfectionism as a core diagnostic feature. This finding suggests that perfectionism is a significant feature of OCD more generally.

Unfortunately, there are no longitudinal studies to indicate whether childhood ritualistic behavior or a perfectionistic personality predispose individuals to SOA symptoms in adulthood. The research available indicates significant associations but scant evidence for causality or predisposing influence. It is not even clear whether perfectionism, for example, is more relevant for SOA than for other obsessive–compulsive symptom dimensions. Thus, the vulnerability constructs proposed in Figure 13.1 are speculative at the present time.

Intrusive Perception

The CBT formulation of other OCD subtypes posited unwanted intrusive thoughts, images, or impulses as the primary obsessive phenomena. However, with SOA the obsession is a perception of asymmetry, imbalance, or imprecision. Often this perception is triggered by some stimulus or situation in the external environment, such as seeing magazines strewn on a table or a picture not hung straight. In this sense the intrusion takes the form of a *perception* of asymmetry or imbalance rather than a distinct *thought* that things are disorganized. Even if, for example, individuals with SOA symptoms think they are using one side of their body more than the other, the intrusion has a more sensory, intuitive quality to it than seen in other types of obsessions. The more sensory-based, experiential nature of the symmetry obsession may be one reason why NJRE and incompleteness play a more critical role in SOA than in other obsessive–compulsive symptom dimensions.

NJRE/Incompleteness

Another distinctive feature of the model is the juxtaposition of NJRE and incompleteness between the symmetry obsession and faulty appraisals/beliefs. The empirical research on SOA makes a compelling argument for the importance of NJRE and incompleteness in the pathogenesis of this symptom subtype. Summerfeldt (2004) has contributed the most to recognizing the importance of incompleteness in SOA. She contends that it is the interpretation of the NJRE/incompleteness experience that is critical in the pathogenesis of obsessive–compulsive symptoms. Thus, the sensory–affective disturbance, rather than an unwanted intrusive thought or obsession, is the primary source of the faulty misinterpretations in SOA.

In a further elaboration, Summerfeldt and colleagues (2014) concluded that faulty appraisals of intrusions characterize obsessive–compulsive symptoms dominated by anxiety or harm avoidance, whereas intrusion appraisals and beliefs are unrelated to incompleteness and NJRE. However, the empirical support for this assertion is mixed. For example, individuals with OCD were divided into high- and low-scoring groups based on their OBQ-44 scores. Although the high-belief group scored significantly higher on most NJRE indices than the low-belief group, the relation between obsessive–compulsive symptoms and NJRE was greater in the low-belief group (Chik, Calamari, Rector, & Riemann, 2010). Unfortunately, the critical research on whether individuals with SOA symptoms misinterpret incompleteness/NJRE disturbance or unwanted intrusive thoughts has not been conducted.

Faulty Appraisals and Beliefs

Faulty appraisals and beliefs continue to play an important role even in Summerfeldt's (2004) perspective on incompleteness and SOA. Given that these appraisals may be focused on the sense of incompleteness or NJRE, it is plausible that the appraisals in SOA may be different from those prominent in harm avoidant obsessive–compulsive symptoms. As seen in Figure 13.1, it is suggested that perfectionism, IU, and inflated responsibility may be most important, whereas faulty appraisals of threat and importance/control of thoughts would be more important in the anxious obsessions associated with contamination, doubt, or repugnant intrusions.

The empirical research suggests that a different belief pattern may characterize SOA. Tolin and colleagues (2008) found that only OBQ-44 Perfectionism/Uncertainty subscale predicted OCI-R ordering scores in an OCD sample. Likewise, Fergus (2014) found that OBQ-20 Perfectionism/Uncertainty subscale significantly predicted NJRE in a nonclinical sample. Furthermore, Belloch and colleagues (2016) found that the OC-CDQ

Incompleteness subscale was strongly associated with OBQ-44 Perfectionism/Uncertainty in the nonclinical sample, but this association was much weaker in the OCD sample. Cluster analysis of an OCD sample revealed that OBQ-44 Responsibility/Threat was significantly lower, but Perfectionism/Uncertainty was higher in the high-incompleteness cluster (Bragdon & Coles, 2017). These preliminary findings indicate that perfectionism and IU beliefs may be especially relevant to SOA and its motivational construct of incompleteness/NJRE. The other maladaptive appraisals and beliefs proposed in the generic model—such as inflated responsibility, threat estimation, and importance/control of thoughts—do not appear to have a significant role in SOA. As well, mental control effort may not be a relevant factor in the pathogenesis of SOA. However, experimental studies are needed to determine whether the induction of incompleteness/NJRE elicits only faulty appraisals of perfectionism and uncertainty in vulnerable individuals.

Ordering Compulsions and Stop Criteria

Several studies indicate that the induction of incompleteness or NJRE in vulnerable individuals will cause an increase in discomfort and an urge to engage in ordering and rearranging behaviors (Coles et al., 2005; Fornés-Romero & Belloch, 2017; Pietrefesa & Coles, 2009; Summerfeldt et al., 2015). As well, an urge to check can be elicited by an incompleteness induction (Cougle et al., 2013). What is less clear from this research is whether an urge to order/rearrange is elicited only in vulnerable individuals high in trait incompleteness or perfectionism, or whether incompleteness inductions have broader effects in the nonclinical population as well.

As noted in Chapter 3, some resolution of incompleteness and NJRE sensations is often a criterion used to terminate a compulsive ritual. More research is needed on the stop criteria utilized in the context of SOA symptoms, but it would be parsimonious to assume that individuals will continue with their ordering and rearranging behaviors until a sense of completeness, balance, and precision has been achieved. At the same time, we can assume that the entire cognitive–sensory process depicted in Figure 13.1 will cause greater attentional sensitivity to external stimuli that are perceived to be incomplete or disorderly. This heightened environmental sensitivity may be another factor that differentiates SOA from other obsessive–compulsive symptom dimensions. In these latter symptom dimensions, individuals exhibit heightened sensitivity to unwanted cognitive intrusions, although, admittedly, the intrusions may or may not be triggered by certain external stimuli. Nevertheless, the environment may have a greater direct pull on SOA than it does for the other symptom subtypes.

COGNITIVE ASSESSMENT AND CASE FORMULATION OF SOA

CBT case formulation for primary SOA should include a thorough assessment of (1) external and internal triggers, (2) incompleteness and NJRE disturbance, (3) appraisals and beliefs of perfectionism and uncertainty, and (4) stop criteria. A brief review of several self-report measures of SOA symptoms and incompleteness/NJRE is provided as informative resources in developing the case formulation.

Normative Assessment

Symmetry, Ordering and Arranging Questionnaire

The Symmetry, Ordering and Arranging Questionnaire (SOAQ; Radomsky & Rachman, 2004) is a 20-item questionnaire that assesses strength of belief in statements that pertain to thoughts and beliefs about symmetry as well as ordering and arranging compulsions. The SOAQ is unidimensional, so only the total score is utilized. It has strong convergent validity with other self-report measures of obsessive–compulsive symptoms, such as the VOCI and the Padua Inventory—Washington State University Revision, and these correlations are higher than for other symptoms like depression or anxiety (Radomsky & Rachman, 2004; Radomsky, Ouimet, et al., 2006). The SOAQ Total Score correlates with constructs relevant to SOA, such as VOCI Just Right and the Padua Grooming/Dressing subscales. In addition, moderate correlations were reported between the SOAQ and a computer-based measure of symmetry and arranging symptoms (Roh, Kim, Chang, Kim, & Kim, 2013). Although the SOAQ is probably the best self-report measure of SOA symptoms, it lacks strong clinical validation and it may be that only a subset of items is specific to SOA (Gönner et al., 2010). Nevertheless, clinicians should administer the SOAQ when this symptom dimension is part of the case formulation.

Revised NJRE Questionnaire

The Not Just Right Experiences Questionnaire—Revised (NJRE-QR; Coles et al., 2003) is a 19-item questionnaire that evaluates the extent to which individuals have had NJRE experiences in the past month. After providing a definition and examples of NJREs, respondents rate the frequency of having an NJRE in 10 everyday situations (e.g., getting dressed, locking the door, folding clothes, hanging a picture). Next, individuals select the NJRE item that occurred most recently and, based on that experience, complete seven ratings that assess frequency, intensity, immediate distress, delayed distress, rumination, urge to respond, and responsibility. A sum of the first 10 items produces an NJRE–number score, whereas a sum of the seven ratings constitutes an NJRE–severity score (see Fornés-Romero & Belloch, 2017). Alternatively, the seven NJRE ratings can be treated separately to produce a more idiographic assessment of NJRE. Various studies have shown that the NJRE–number score is more highly correlated with obsessive–compulsive symptoms, especially order and symmetry, than non-obsessive–compulsive constructs like anxiety or depression (Coles et al., 2003, 2005; Coles & Ravid, 2016; Sica et al., 2015). Fornés-Romero and Belloch (2017) found that NJRE–number had a significant relationship with response to a free-recall NJRE/Incompleteness induction in both nonclinical and OCD samples. At present, the NJRE-QR is the best validated measure of the NJRE construct.

Obsessive–Compulsive Core Dimensions Questionnaire

The Obsessive–Compulsive Core Dimensions Questionnaire (OC-CDQ; Summerfeldt et al., 2014) is a 20-item questionnaire administered in a state or trait format. Ten items assess harm avoidance and 10 items assess incompleteness, with responses rated on a 5-point Likert scale from 1 ("never applied to me") to 5 ("always applied to me"). Exploratory and confirmatory factor analysis supported the two-factor structure of the OC-CDQ (Summerfeldt et al., 2014). Most of the studies reviewed previously in this chapter used the OC-CDQ, or a condensed version of the instrument, to assess incompleteness. Overall, the research has supported the convergent and discriminant validity of the OC-CDQ, especially the trait version. For example, Ecker and colleagues (2014b) reported that an OCD sample scored significantly higher on a shortened OC-CDQ Incompleteness subscale than depressive or anxious clinical groups. In sum, the OC-CDQ is the best measure of incompleteness, although the state version of the questionnaire may be more informative for clinical purposes. Also, Summerfeldt and colleagues (2014) developed a more detailed interview assessment of incompleteness—the Obsessive–Compulsive Core Dimensions Interview (OC-CDI)—but it has been rarely used in the research literature.

Other Measures

There are several measures that clinicians might find helpful in the assessment of SOA and its related constructs. The Brown Incompleteness Scale (BINGS) is a 21-item clinician-rated measure that assesses two dimensions of incompleteness: behavioral and sensory (Boisseau et al., 2018). The measure is highly correlated with the OC-CDQ Incompleteness subscale and is more strongly associated with obsessive–compulsive symptoms than general distress. The Dimensional Obsessive–Compulsive Scale (DOCS; Abramowitz et al., 2010) has a symmetry subscale that has strong psychometric properties in OCD and nonclinical samples, and the Vancouver Obsessive Compulsive Inventory (VOCI) has Just Right and Indecision subscales that are helpful in the assessment of SOA (Thordarson et al., 2004). For the assessment of perfectionism, the 35-item Frost Multidimensional Perfectionism Scale (Frost, Marten, Lahart, & Rosenblate, 1990) has good psychometric properties, although concern about Mistakes and High Personal Standards subscales may be the most sensitive to obsessive–compulsive symptoms (for a review, see Egan et al., 2014). As well, the Perfectionism/Intolerance of Uncertainty subscale of the OBQ-44 (OCCWG, 2005) is available to assess beliefs that are especially germane to SOA.

Idiographic Assessment

Similar to other symptom subtypes, CBT clinicians must include self-monitoring, *in vivo* observation, and symptom induction procedures in their assessment to develop an accurate cognitive case formulation of SOA symptomatology. The following section presents several idiographic measures that are tailored to the distinct features of SOA, with illustrated reference to the case example.

Contextual Analysis

A clear understanding of the external and internal stimuli that trigger symmetry obsessions is critical to the case formulation. This information can be obtained from the clinical interview and by asking clients to self-monitor the triggers of their symmetry obsessions between sessions. Form 13.1 is a modified version of the Situation Record and Rating Scales (see Form 7.2) used for anxiety-based symptom subtypes.

Once 10–20 triggers of SOA symptoms have been identified, a hierarchy of situations can be developed from the least to most difficult. This hierarchy is based on the client's rating of the strength of incompleteness/NJRE and the likelihood of engaging in ordering and rearranging compulsions. For example, Elaine could have listed rearranging clothes hanging in her closet, folding laundry, straightening pictures, reloading the dishwasher, filing documents at work, and reorganizing her email as triggering situations. However, the dishwasher, filing, and folding laundry were associated with much higher ratings (75–100 on both scales) than straightening pictures or reorganizing her email (ratings of 30–50). Clearly, treatment involving some form of response prevention should begin with the latter situations.

Symptom Induction

It is likely that a person's SOA symptoms can be elicited by presenting relevant triggers within session. Not only does *in vivo* exposure provide the therapist with critical observational data, but clients can also be asked to evaluate their incompleteness/NJREs in real time. For example, an individual could be asked to focus on a misaligned picture hanging on the office wall, disorganized papers on the therapist's desk, misaligned books, or a messy table of magazines. It may be necessary to instruct clients to imagine that the disorganization is occurring in their own home or office, since messiness in another person's environment may not elicit SOA symptoms. As well, clients should be instructed to focus intently on the disorganization for several minutes to ensure sufficient opportunity for symptom induction. After 5–10 minutes of concentrated attention, the therapist can ask clients to rate various aspects of their incompleteness/NJREs and the appraisals associated with the provocation using Form 13.2.

The SOA Symptom Induction Ratings can provide detailed information on the incompleteness/NJRE, as well as on misinterpretations of this experience and the stop criteria used to terminate ordering and rearranging compulsions. The rating scales could be used as a homework assignment in which individuals rate their experience when encountering SOA triggers in their naturalistic environment. This may be especially important if the *in vivo* exposure within the session failed to provoke any semblance of SOA symptomatology.

Once the core symptom processes have been assessed, the therapist can write in the client's experience of each process noted in Figure 13.1. This cognitive case formulation will be the basis for developing treatment goals that will guide subsequent CBT sessions.

SPECIAL TREATMENT CONSIDERATIONS

Based on the previous discussion, one might assume that exposure-based interventions and cognitive restructuring of faulty appraisals and beliefs may be less effective when affective–sensory disturbance is the main motivational process that underlies provocation for obsessive–compulsive symptoms. And yet, it is equally tenable to assert that CBT can be effective for SOA symptoms when certain modifications are made to the therapy protocol.

There is reason to believe that CBT can produce significant symptom reduction in SOA. Coles and Ravid (2016) reported that individuals with OCD reported significant reductions in NJREs after at least 14 sessions of individual CBT with a specific emphasis on ERP. Reviews of treatment outcome associated with various symptom dimensions conclude that ERP can be effective for SOA symptoms, although only a few studies have examined this question (Mataix-Cols et al., 2002; Starcevic & Brakoulias, 2008; M. T. Williams et al., 2013). In an early study, Abramowitz, Franklin, and colleagues (2003) found that individuals with OCD who fell in a symmetry symptom cluster had a significant but weaker ERP treatment response than the harming, contamination, and unacceptable thoughts clusters. A recent meta-analysis of CBT outcome studies of OCD found that incompleteness significantly improved with treatment, especially when the treatment was tailored to deal with this construct (Schwartz, 2018).

Treating Incompleteness/NJRE

Coles and Pietrefesa (2008) note that individuals with primary SOA may show a more modest response to conventional CBT due to the presence of OCPD features such as perfectionism and the absence of feared consequences (i.e., harm avoidance). Summerfeldt (2004) argued that the conventional CBT approach to OCD must be modified to focus on the sensory–affective experience of incompleteness or NJRE. In Summerfeldt's treatment approach, ERP can be applied to situations and stimuli that trigger incompleteness/NJRE instead of fear or anxiety. She recommends five changes to the cognitive component of treatment:

1. Consider faulty appraisals and beliefs as consequences rather than as the cause of incompleteness/NJREs.
2. Focus on faulty appraisals or interpretations of incompleteness/NJRE.
3. Alter the individual's subjective value placed on incompleteness/NJRE.
4. Accept intrusive experiences of incompleteness/NJRE as false messages from the brain.
5. Modify maladaptive beliefs about incompleteness/NJRE.

Based on Summerfeldt's (2004) recommendations, the treatment protocol for Elaine's SOA symptoms would differ from the CBT described for contamination, doubt, and repugnant obsessions. For the behavioral component, graded hierarchical ERP could be utilized based on the intensity of incompleteness/NJRE associated with various triggers (see Form 13.1). In Elaine's case, the therapist would start ERP by asking her to tolerate misaligned pictures and resist organizing emails until the end of the day or the week. The exposures would be presented as behavioral experiments designed to test whether feelings of incompleteness or NJRE are more tolerable than expected. Once Elaine has shown that she can deal with these exposures without engaging in ordering or rearranging compulsions, the therapist would assign tasks associated with more intense incompleteness/NJREs, such as loading the dishwasher haphazardly or leaving clean laundry unfolded for several hours.

The cognitive component of treatment focuses on the individual's misinterpretation of incompleteness/NJREs. This would begin with Socratic questioning that seeks to explore the nature of individuals' interpretation of their incompleteness/NJREs. Several questions could be asked, such as:

> "What's it like for you to feel that something is incomplete or not just right?"
> "Do you always try to correct the situation, or sometimes can you ignore, that is, not give into, the feeling of incompleteness/NJRE?"
> "How difficult is it to ignore or sit with the incompleteness/NJREs? Does it depend on the circumstances, such as having other people around?"
> "What are you concerned might happen if you did nothing when you get the feeling of incompleteness/NJRE? If you resisted ordering, rearranging, or correcting whatever is bothering you, would there be any negative consequences?"
> "Was there a time in your life when you didn't think about whether things were just right or complete?"

The purpose of this line of questioning is to help clients confront their belief that incompleteness/NJREs are intolerable and so they must engage in ordering or rearranging compulsions. This intervention can be followed with behavioral homework assignments in which clients collect data on the consequences of accepting their incompleteness/NJREs. Are they better able to tolerate these experiences than predicted? Based on the threat prediction intervention described in Chapter 9, the client can be asked to predict the tolerability of incompleteness/NJRE when doing a specific exposure, and then record their actual tolerability after exposure to the SOA experience.

Another objective of this exercise is to correct any misinterpretations of consequence. For example, Elaine believed that if she didn't give into her feelings and redo or correct a situation, it would bother her all day and her work would suffer. To put belief to the test, behavioral experiments could be designed, such as allowing files and other documents to accumulate on her desk until the end of the day, or letting emails accumulate in her in-folder to see whether reducing her ordering and rearranging behaviors interfered with her ability to work productively. An alternate-days experiment could be implemented in which she compared distractibility and work productivity on high versus low SOA days. In this way evidence is gathered that challenges the client's misinterpretations of adverse consequences associated with incompleteness/NJREs.

Perfectionism

As noted in Figure 13.1, perfectionism plays a critical role in SOA symptoms, both as vulnerability and maintenance factors. Therefore, successful treatment of order and symmetry OCD must include interventions that target perfectionism. Although the presence of perfectionism has been associated with poorer CBT treatment outcomes for other disorders, such as depression (see review by Egan, Wade, & Shafran, 2011), the development of a specific CBT treatment protocol for perfectionism indicates that significant improvements are possible when construct-specific intervention is provided (Egan et al., 2014). The effective treatment of order and symmetry OCD will require that clinicians incorporate elements of CBT for perfectionism into their treatment protocol for SOA. Egan and colleague's (2014) CBT treatment manual offers the best guidance in treating the critical elements of perfectionism.

Excessively high and inflexible standards of achievement as the basis of self-worth are a maladaptive cognitive element in perfectionism that should be included in CBT for SOA. Egan and colleagues (2014) discuss how self-monitoring, identifying cognitive errors, evidence gathering, cost–benefit analysis, inductive reasoning, and behavioral experiments can be used to challenge core beliefs that strengthen commitment to unrealistic performance standards. For individuals with SOA, treatment of unrealistic performance standards may extend beyond the usual perfectionistic themes of work and relationships to more mundane activities like the need to maintain a tidy, well-organized, and systematic living space. For example, Elaine took great pride in her reputation for planning, promptness, and organization. She believed that "competent people are well organized and efficient" and that any deviation from orderliness threatened her personal worth and value. This belief in order and efficiency was so rigid and pervasive that it affected even the most mundane of daily activities. Clearly, CBT for Elaine's OCD needed to address her rigid, unrealistic standards of efficiency and competence.

Although ordering and rearranging compulsions are the most common response to perfectionism in SOA, the therapist should be vigilant for other compensatory responses that are associated with perfectionism, such as reassurance seeking, avoidance, self-denigration, or overwork. Aware of their SOA symptoms, individuals might seek reassurance from others that their performance is good enough, avoid an SOA trigger (e.g., Elaine's husband would do the vacuuming when she was out of the house to reduce the likelihood that she would redo it), or be self-critical of efforts to rearrange or correct something that was out of order or balance (e.g., Elaine would spend hours tidying up, but still criticize herself for letting the house "get out of control"). Often unrealistic performance standards for the most routine daily activities result in an excessive amount of time spent on them, like cleaning, self-care, tidying, and organizing. For example, individuals with order and symmetry OCD might spend so much time organizing and rearranging their tools and tidying up their workshop that it takes them an inordinate amount of time to complete a woodworking project. In this case the slowness is due to SOA processes of incompleteness/NJRE, as well as perfectionistic standards about a neat and efficient workshop. Effective treatment would need to address the perfectionistic and OCD processes responsible for the maladaptive behavior.

Personal Insignificance and Normalization

Often SOA symptoms are not the primary reason that individuals seek treatment. Washing and checking compulsions are much more common than order and precision symptoms (Rasmussen & Eisen, 1992), and individuals with predominant symmetry obsessions and ordering compulsions are fairly uncommon among those seeking treatment for OCD (e.g., Foa et al., 1995). This means that clinicians could miss the presence of SOA symptoms when other obsessive–compulsive symptoms, such as washing or checking compulsions, are more dominant. Also, individuals may downplay the significance of their SOA symptoms, considering the behavior a quirk of their personalities or a habit that does not cause sufficient distress or interference in daily functioning to warrant treatment. In such cases a thorough assessment is needed to determine whether manifestations of SOA meet the personal distress/impaired functioning threshold required to justify treatment. Since order and symmetry concerns are a feature of perfectionism and OCPD, it can be harder to determine whether an individual's SOA is causing significant interference in daily living.

Treatment goals are important in CBT, and one of the challenges in treating clients with OCD is determining what is normal. It is relatively straightforward to define *normal* handwashing as the treatment goal or to agree that an individual do just one check when leaving the house. However, defining *normal* tidying, organizing, or rearranging is more difficult. Most people spend some time engaged in these activities, and the preference for orderliness, balance, and precision is nearly universal. No doubt the treatment goal in SOA will include increased ability to tolerate incompleteness and feeling that things are not just right. But a more behavioral description of the treatment goal, such as leaving pictures misaligned, putting away laundry more haphazardly, and tolerating a disorganized closet, will be more difficult to achieve.

Finally, there may be a greater degree of situational specificity to SOA than to other OCD symptom presentations. The need for symmetry and order may be apparent only in situations that are personally important to the client. The client may be perfectly able to tolerate a messy and disorganized public space or someone else's home or workspace. SOA symptoms may apply only to situations that are personally significant and the responsibility of the client. Thus, CBT therapists must take into account the situational specificity of these obsessive–compulsive symptoms when designing treatment programs.

CONCLUSION

Symmetry obsessions and order/rearranging compulsions are fairly common in OCD samples, although they are less often the primary obsessive–compulsive symptom that motivates treatment seeking. There is considerable evidence that SOA has a distinct symptom presentation with an early onset and stable clinical course. The core psychological process motivating SOA symptoms is the experience of incompleteness or of "not just right." This makes the psychological substratum of SOA much different from other OCD symptom presentations that are based on harm avoidance.

Summerfeldt (2004) and others have proposed a two-factor motivational model of OCD, with some symptoms motivated by a need to complete or attain a feeling of "just right," and other symptoms motivated by anxiety or fear reduction. Research has tended to view incompleteness and NJREs as interchangeable constructs, with studies showing they have a strong association with perfectionism, OCPD, and SOA symptoms. Incompleteness/NJRE has a higher level of specificity to OCD than harm avoidance, and it is considered a critical factor in the pathogenesis of order and symmetry OCD.

Although various researchers have questioned whether the CBT perspective is applicable to SOA symptoms, a modified CBT formulation was proposed in which incompleteness/NJRE is a mediator between perceptions of asymmetry or imbalance and faulty appraisals and beliefs about perfectionism and IU (see Figure 13.1). The key difference in the SOA model is that faulty appraisals involve a misinterpretation of the incompleteness/NJRE sensory–affective disturbance, rather than the misinterpretation of unwanted intrusive thoughts, as depicted in the generic model (see Figure 5.1). As well, excessive mental control has little influence in the pathogenesis of SOA, compared to other OCD symptom subtypes. Finally, it is proposed that ordering, rearranging, and checking compulsions will continue until a threshold of feeling that a task is complete or "just right" has been achieved. When this happens, the compulsions cease, but the entire process heightens the vulnerable person's attentional bias for disorder, asymmetry, and imbalance.

Based on a modified CBT formulation, treatment of SOA focuses on increasing the client's tolerance for incompleteness/NJRE through graded *in vivo* exposure to SOA triggers and response prevention of order, redoing, rearranging, and checking compulsions. Cognitive restructuring and behavioral experiments target the individual's misinterpretations and beliefs about tolerance of incompletenesss/NJRE, the consequences of failing to meet perfectionistic performance standards, and the benefits of practicing a greater degree of insouciance, flexibility, and acceptance of the mundane tasks of daily living.

FORM 13.1. Record of Triggers for Order and Symmetry

Instructions: Use the worksheet below to list the situations, objects, or circumstances that most often trigger your concern about symmetry, balance, order, or precision and then complete the rating scale associated with each situation.

List of Triggering Situations	Rate Feeling of Incompleteness or NJRE (0 = none to 100 = extreme)	Likelihood of Ordering, Rearranging, Redoing, or Checking Compulsion (0 = can easily ignore to 100 = always engage in compulsion)
1.		
2.		
3.		
4.		
5.		
6.		
7.		
8.		
9.		
10.		

Note. NJRE refers to a "not just right" experience.

From *Cognitive-Behavioral Therapy for OCD and Its Subtypes, Second Edition,* by David A. Clark. Copyright © 2020 The Guilford Press. Permission to photocopy this material is granted to purchasers of this book for personal use or use with individual clients (see copyright page for details). Purchasers can download enlarged versions of this material (see the box at the end of the table of contents).

FORM 13.2. SOA Symptom Induction Ratings

Instructions: Present the client with a situation, object, or stimulus that is likely to elicit SOA symptoms. This should be a trigger associated with moderate ratings on Form 13.1 and amenable to manipulation in the office. Clients should be encouraged to imagine that the disorganization occurred in their home or office and to attend closely to the disorganization for several minutes. After the period of focusing on the trigger, clients rate their incompleteness/"not just right" experience on the following dimensions.

Rating Dimensions	Intensity Rating (0 = not present to 100 = extremely intense, irresistible)
1. How much did you feel that [*state provocation stimulus*] was incomplete or not just right? (**intensity**)	
2. To what extent were you thinking about the [*state provocation stimulus*] throughout the exposure session? (**rumination**)	
3. How strong was the urge to do something to correct the disorganization or imbalance? (**urge to respond**)	
4. How distressed did [*state provocation stimulus*] make you feel? (**distress**)	
5. How responsible did you feel to correct this situation? (**inflated responsibility**)	
6. If you had caused this situation [*state provocation here*], to what extent would this feel like a violation of your personal standards? (**perfectionism**)	
7. To what extent would you feel the need to be certain that you had reestablished order or correctness to this situation [*state the provocation here*]? (**intolerance of uncertainty**)	
8. To what extent would you keep working at [*state provocation stimulus here*] until you could leave the situation because you felt it was just right or complete? (**stop criteria**)	

From *Cognitive-Behavioral Therapy for OCD and Its Subtypes, Second Edition*, by David A. Clark. Copyright © 2020 The Guilford Press. Permission to photocopy this material is granted to purchasers of this book for personal use or use with individual clients (see copyright page for details). Purchasers can download enlarged versions of this material (see the box at the end of the table of contents).

References

Aardema, F., Moulding, R., Melli, G., Radomsky, A. S., Doron, G., Audet, J-S., et al. (2018). The role of feared possible selves in obsessive–compulsive and related disorders: A comparative analysis of a core cognitive self-construct in clinical samples. *Clinical Psychology and Psychotherapy, 25*, e19–e29.

Aardema, F., Moulding, R., Radomsky, A. S., Doron, G., Allamby, J., & Sourki, E. (2013). Fear of self and obsessionality: Development and validation of the Fear of Self Questionnaire. *Journal of Obsessive–Compulsive and Related Disorders, 2*, 306–315.

Aardema, F., & O'Connor, K. (2007). The menace within: Obsessions and the self. *Journal of Cognitive Psychotherapy: An International Quarterly, 21*, 182–196.

Aardema, F., & O'Connor, K. (2012). Dissolving the tenacity of obsessional doubt: Implications for treatment outcome. *Journal of Behavior Therapy and Experimental Psychiatry, 43*, 855–861.

Aardema, F., O'Connor, K. P., & Emmelkamp, P. M. G. (2006). Inferential confusion and obsessive beliefs in obsessive–compulsive disorder. *Cognitive Behaviour Therapy, 35*, 138–147.

Aardema, F., O'Connor, K. P., Emmelkamp, P. M. G., Marchand, A., & Todorov, C. (2005). Inferential confusion in obsessive–compulsive disorder: The Inferential Confusion Questionnaire. *Behaviour Research and Therapy, 43*, 293–308.

Aardema, F., Wu, K., Careau, Y., Moulding, R., Audet, J.-S., & Baraby, L.-P. (2018). The relationship of inferential confusion and obsessive beliefs with specific obsessive–compulsive symptoms. *Journal of Obsessive–Compulsive and Related Disorders, 18*, 98–105.

Aardema, F., Wu, K., Careau, Y., O'Connor, K., Julien, D., & Dennie, S. (2010). The expanded version of the Inferential Confusion Questionnaire: Further development and validation in clinical and non-clinical samples. *Journal of Psychopathology and Behavioral Assessment, 32*, 448–462.

Abramovitch, A., Doron, G., Sar-El, D., & Altenburger, E. (2013). Subtle threats to moral self-perceptions trigger obsessive–compulsive related cognitions. *Cognitive Therapy and Research, 37,* 1132–1139.

Abramowitz, J. S. (1998). Does cognitive-behavioral therapy cure obsessive–compulsive disorder?: A meta-analytic evaluation of clinical significance. *Behavior Therapy, 29,* 339–355.

Abramowitz, J. S. (2004). Treatment of obsessive–compulsive disorder in patients who have comorbid depression. *Journal of Clinical Psychology, 60,* 1133–1141.

Abramowitz, J. S. (2008). Scrupulosity. In J. S. Abramowitz, D. McKay, & S. Taylor (Eds.), *Clinical handbook of obsessive–compulsive disorder and related problems* (pp. 156–172). Baltimore: Johns Hopkins University Press.

Abramowitz, J. S. (2018). *Getting over OCD: A 10-step workbook for taking back your life* (2nd ed.). New York: Guilford Press.

Abramowitz, J. S., & Deacon, B. J. (2006). Psychometric properties and construct validity of the Obsessive–Compulsive Inventory—Revised: Replication and extension with a clinical sample. *Journal of Anxiety Disorders, 20,* 1016–1035.

Abramowitz, J. S., Deacon, B. J., Olatunji, B. O., Wheaton, M. G., Berman, N. C., Losardo, D., et al. (2010). Assessment of obsessive–compulsive symptom dimensions: Development of the Dimensional Obsessive–Compulsive Scale. *Psychological Assessment, 22,* 180–198.

Abramowitz, J. S., Deacon, B. J., & Whiteside, S. P. H. (2011). *Exposure therapy for anxiety: Principles and practice.* New York: Guilford Press.

Abramowitz, J. S., Fabricant, L. E., Taylor, S., Deacon, B. J., McKay, D., & Storch, E. A. (2014). The relevance of analogue studies for understanding obsessions and compulsions. *Clinical Psychology Review, 34,* 206–217.

Abramowitz, J. S., & Foa, E. B. (2000). Does comorbid major depression influence outcome of exposure and response prevention for OCD? *Behavior Therapy, 31,* 795–800.

Abramowitz, J. S., Foa, E. B., & Franklin, M. E. (2003). Exposure and ritual prevention for obsessive–compulsive disorder: Effects of intensive versus twice-weekly sessions. *Journal of Consulting and Clinical Psychology, 71,* 394–398.

Abramowitz, J. S., Franklin, M. E., Schwartz, S. A., & Furr, J. M. (2003). Symptom presentation and outcome of cognitive-behavioral therapy for obsessive–compulsive disorder. *Journal of Consulting and Clinical Psychology, 71,* 1049–1057.

Abramowitz, J. S., Franklin, M. E., Street, G. P., Kozak, M. J., & Foa, E. B. (2000). Effects of comorbid depression on response to treatment for obsessive–compulsive disorder. *Behavior Therapy, 31,* 517–528.

Abramowitz, J. S., Huppert, J. D., Cohen, A. B., Tolin, D. F., & Cahill, S. P. (2002). Religious obsessions and compulsions in a non-clinical sample: The Penn Inventory of Scrupulosity (PIOS). *Behaviour Research and Therapy, 40,* 825–838.

Abramowitz, J. S., & Jacoby, R. J. (2014). Obsessive–compulsive disorder in the DSM-5. *Clinical Psychology: Science and Practice, 21,* 221–245.

Abramowitz, J. S., Khandker, M., Nelson, C. A., Deacon, B. J., & Rygwall, R. (2006). The role of cognitive factors in the pathogenesis of obsessive–

compulsive symptoms: A prospective study. *Behaviour Research and Therapy, 44,* 1361–1374.

Abramowitz, J. S., Nelson, C. A., Rygwall, R., & Khandker, M. (2007). The cognitive mediation of obsessive–compulsive symptoms: A longitudinal study. *Journal of Anxiety Disorders, 21,* 91–104.

Abramowitz, J. S., Schwartz, S. A., & Moore, K. A. (2003). Obsessional thoughts in postpartum females and their partners: Content, severity, and relationship with depression. *Journal of Clinical Psychology in Medical Settings, 10,* 157–164.

Abramowitz, J. S., Storch, E. A., Keeley, M., & Cordell, E. (2007). Obsessive–compulsive disorder with comorbid major depression: What is the role of cognitive factors? *Behaviour Research and Therapy, 45,* 2257–2267.

Abramowitz, J. S., Tolin, D. F., & Street, C. P. (2001). Paradoxical effects of thought suppression: A meta-analysis of controlled studies. *Clinical Psychology Review, 21,* 683–703.

Abramowitz, J. S., Whiteside, S., Kalsy, S. A., & Tolin, D. F. (2003). Thought control strategies in obsessive–compulsive disorder: A replication and extension. *Behaviour Research and Therapy, 41,* 529–540.

Abramowitz, J. S., Whiteside, S., Lynam, D., & Kalsy, S. (2003). Is thought–action fusion specific to obsessive–compulsive disorder?: A mediating role of negative affect. *Behaviour Research and Therapy, 41,* 1069–1079.

Adam, Y., Meinlshmidt, G., Gloster, A. T., & Lieb, R. (2012). Obsessive–compulsive disorder in the community: 12-month prevalence, comorbidity and impairment. *Social Psychiatry and Psychiatric Epidemiology, 47,* 339–349.

Ahern, C., & Kyrios, M. (2016). Self-processes in obsessive compulsive disorder. In M. Kyrios, R. Moulding, G. Doron, S. S. Bhar, M. Nedeljkovic, & M. Mikulincer (Eds.), *The self in understanding and treating psychological disorders* (pp. 112–122). Cambridge, UK: Cambridge University Press.

Ahern, C., Kyrios, M., & Meyer, D. (2015). Exposure to unwanted intrusions, neutralizing and their effects on self-worth and obsessive–compulsive phenomena. *Journal of Behavior Therapy and Experimental Psychiatry, 49,* 216–222.

Akhtar, S., Varma, V. K., Pershad, D., & Verma, S. K. (1978). Socio-cultural and clinical determinants in obsessional neurosis. *International Journal of Psychiatry, 24,* 157–162.

Akhtar, S., Wig, N. N., Varma, V. K., Pershad, D., & Verma, S. K. (1975). A phenomenological analysis of symptoms in obsessive–compulsive neurosis. *British Journal of Psychiatry, 127,* 342–348.

Alonso, P., Menchón, J. M., Pifarre, J., Mataix-Cols, D., Torres, L., Salgado, P., et al. (2001). Long-term follow-up and predictors of clinical outcome in obsessive–compulsive patients treated with serotonin reuptake inhibitors and behavioral therapy. *Journal of Clinical Psychiatry, 62,* 535–540.

Alonso, P., Menchón, J. M., Segalàs, C., Jaurrieta, N., Jiménez-Murcia, S., Cardoner, N., et al. (2008). Clinical implications of insight assessment in obsessive–compulsive disorder. *Comprehensive Psychiatry, 49,* 305–312.

Altin, M., Clark, D. A., & Karanci, N. (2007, July). *The impact of religiosity on obsessive–compulsive cognitions and symptoms in Christian and Muslim students.* Paper presented at the World Congress for Behavioural and Cognitive Therapies, Barcelona, Spain.

American Psychiatric Association. (1980). *Diagnostic and statistical manual of mental disorders* (3rd ed.). Washington, DC: Author.

American Psychiatric Association. (2007). Practice guideline for the treatment of patients with obsessive–compulsive disorder. Retrieved from *www.psych.org/psych_pract/treatg/pg/prac_ guide.cfm.*

American Psychiatric Association. (2012). DSM-5: The future of psychiatric diagnosis. Retrieved from *www.dsm5.org.*

American Psychiatric Association. (2013). *Diagnostic and statistical manual of mental disorders* (5th ed.). Arlington, VA: Author.

Amir, N., Cashman, L., & Foa, E. B. (1997). Strategies of thought control in obsessive–compulsive disorder. *Behaviour Research and Therapy, 35,* 775–777.

Amir, N., Foa, E. B., & Coles, M. E. (1997). Factor structure of the Yale–Brown Obsessive–Compulsive Scale. *Psychological Assessment, 9,* 312–316.

Amir, N., Freshman, M., & Foa, E. B. (2000). Family distress and involvement in relatives of obsessive–compulsive patients. *Journal of Anxiety Disorders, 14,* 209–217.

Amir, N., Freshman, M., Ramsey, B., Neary, E., & Brigidi, B. (2001). Thought-action fusion in individuals with OCD symptoms. *Behaviour Research and Therapy, 39,* 765–776.

Andrews, G., Henderson, S., & Hall, W. (2001). Prevalence, comorbidity, disability and service utilization: Overview of the Australian National Mental Health Survey. *British Journal of Psychiatry, 178,* 145–153.

Angelakis, I., Gooding, P., Tarrier, N., & Panagioti, M. (2015). Suicidality in obsessive–compulsive disorder (OCD): A systematic review and meta-analysis. *Clinical Psychology Review, 39,* 1–15.

Anholt, G. A., van Oppen, P., Cath, D. C., Emmelkamp, P. M. G., Smit, J. H., & van Balkom, A. J. L. M. (2010). Sensitivity to change of the Obsessive Beliefs Questionnaire. *Clinical Psychology and Psychotherapy, 17,* 154–159.

Antony, M. M. (2001). Measures for obsessive–compulsive disorder. In M. M. Antony, S. M. Orsillo, & L. Roemer (Eds.), *Practitioner's guide to empirically based measures of anxiety* (pp. 219–243). New York: Kluwer Academic/Plenum.

Antony, M. M., Downie, F., & Swinson, R. P. (1998). Diagnostic issues and epidemiology in obsessive–compulsive disorder. In R. P. Swinson, M. M. Antony, S. Rachman, & M. A. Richter (Eds.), *Obsessive–compulsive disorder: Theory, research, and treatment* (pp. 3–32). New York: Guilford Press.

Arch, J. J., & Abramowitz, J. S. (2015). Exposure therapy for obsessive–compulsive disorder: An optimizing inhibitory learning approach. *Journal of Obsessive–Compulsive and Related Disorders, 6,* 174–182.

Armstrong, T., Tomarken, A. J., & Olatunji, B. O. (2012). The moderating effects of contamination sensitivity on state affect and information processing: Examination of disgust specificity. *Cognition and Emotion, 26,* 136–143.

Arntz, A., Rauner, M., & van den Hout, M. (1995). "If I feel anxious, there must be danger": Ex-consequentia reasoning in inferring danger in anxiety disorders. *Behaviour Research and Therapy, 33,* 917–925.

Arntz, A., Tiesema, M., & Kindt, M. (2007). Treatment of PTSD: A comparison of imaginal exposure with and without imagery rescripting. *Journal of Behavior Therapy and Experimental Psychiatry, 38,* 345–370.

Arntz, A., Voncken, M., & Goosen, A. C. A. (2007). Responsibility and obsessive–compulsive disorder: An experimental test. *Behaviour Research and Therapy, 45,* 425–435.

Ashbaugh, A. R., & Radomsky, A. S. (2007). Attentional focus during repeated checking influences memory but not metamemory. *Cognitive Therapy and Research, 31,* 291–306.

Audet, J.-S., Aardema, F., & Moulding, R. (2016). Contextual determinants of intrusions and obsessions: The role of ego-dystonicity and the reality of obsessional thoughts. *Journal of Obsessive–Compulsive and Related Disorders, 9,* 96–106.

Baer, L. (1994). Factor analysis of symptom subtypes of obsessive compulsive disorder and their relation to personality and tic disorder. *Journal of Clinical Psychology, 55,* 18–23.

Baer, L., Brown-Beasley, W., Sorce, J., & Henriques, A. I. (1993). Computer-assisted telephone administration of a structured interview for obsessive–compulsive disorder. *American Journal of Psychiatry, 150,* 1737–1738.

Bailey, B. E., Wu, K. D., Valentiner, D. P., & McGrath, P. B. (2014). Thought–action fusion: Structure and specificity in OCD. *Journal of Obsessive–Compulsive and Related Disorders, 3,* 39–45.

Baptista, M. N., Magna, L. A., McKay, D., & Del-Porto, J. A. (2011). Assessment of obsessive beliefs: Comparing individuals with obsessive–compulsive disorder to a medical sample. *Journal of Behavior Therapy and Experimental Psychiatry, 42,* 1–5.

Barlow, D. H. (2002). *Anxiety and its disorders: The nature and treatment of anxiety and panic* (2nd ed.). New York: Guilford Press.

Barrera, T. L., & Norton, P. J. (2011). The appraisal of intrusive thoughts in relation to obsessional–compulsive symptoms. *Cognitive Behavior Therapy, 40,* 98–110.

Basoglu, M., Lax, T., Kasvikis, Y., & Marks, I. M. (1988). Predictors of improvement in obsessive–compulsive disorder. *Journal of Anxiety Disorders, 2,* 299–317.

Beck, A. T. (1967). *Depression: Causes and treatment.* Philadelphia: University of Pennsylvania Press.

Beck, A. T. (1976). *Cognitive therapy and the emotional disorders.* New York: New American Library.

Beck, A. T., & Emery, G. (with Greenberg, R. L.). (1985). *Anxiety disorders and phobias: A cognitive perspective.* New York: Basic Books.

Beck, A. T., Freeman, A., & Davis, D. D. (2015). General principles and specialized techniques in cognitive therapy of personality disorders. In A. T. Beck, D. D. Davis, & A. Freeman, (Eds.), *Cognitive therapy of personality disorders* (3rd ed., pp. 97–124). New York: Guilford Press.

Beck, A. T., Rush, A. J., Shaw, B. F., & Emery, G. (1979). *Cognitive therapy of depression.* New York: Guilford Press.

Beck, A. T., Steer, R. A., & Brown, G. (1996). *Beck Depression Inventory manual* (2nd ed.). San Antonio, TX: Psychological Corporation.

Beck, J. S. (1995). *Cognitive therapy: Basics and beyond.* New York: Guilford Press.

Beck, J. S. (2011). *Cognitive behavior therapy: Basics and beyond* (2nd ed.). New York: Guilford Press.

Beech, H. R., & Perigault, J. (1974). Toward a theory of obsessional disorder. In H. R. Beech (Ed.), *Obsessional states* (pp. 113–141). London: Methuen.

Belloch, A., Cabedo, E., Carrió, C., & Larsson, C. (2010). Cognitive therapy for autogenous and reactive obsessions: Clinical and cognitive outcomes at post-treatment and 1-year follow-up. *Journal of Anxiety Disorders, 24,* 573–580.

Belloch, A., Carrió, C., Cabedo, E., & García-Soriano, G. (2015). Discovering what is hidden: The role of non-ritualized covert neutralizing strategies in obsessive–compulsive disorder. *Journal of Behavior Therapy and Experimental Psychiatry, 49,* 180–187.

Belloch, A., Fornés, G., Carrasco, A., López-Solá, C., Alonso, P., & Menchón, J. M. (2016). Incompleteness and not just right experiences in the explanation of obsessive–compulsive disorder. *Psychiatry Research, 236,* 1–8.

Belloch, A., Morillo, C., & García-Soriano, G. (2009). Strategies to control unwanted intrusive thoughts: Which are relevant and specific in obsessive–compulsive disorder? *Cognitive Therapy and Research, 33,* 75–89.

Belloch, A., Morillo, C., Lucero, M., Cabedo, E., & Carrió, C. (2004). Intrusive thoughts in non-clinical subjects: The role of frequency and unpleasantness on appraisal ratings and control strategies. *Clinical Psychology and Psychotherapy, 11,* 100–110.

Belloch, A., Roncero, M., García-Soriano, G., Carrió, C., Cabedo, E., & Frenández-Álvarez, H. (2013). The Spanish version of the Obsessive–Compulsive Inventory—Revised (OCI-R): Reliability, validity, diagnostic accuracy, and sensitivity to treatment effects in clinical samples. *Journal of Obsessive–Compulsive and Related Disorders, 2,* 249–256.

Belloch, A., Roncero, M., & Perpiná, C. (2012). Ego-syntonicity and ego-dystonicity associated with upsetting intrusive cognitions. *Journal of Psychopathology and Behavioral Assessment, 34,* 94–106.

Bellodi, L., Sciuto, G., Diaferia, G., Ronchi, P., & Smeraldi, E. (1992). Psychiatric disorders in the families of patients with obsessive–compulsive disorder. *Psychiatry Research, 42,* 111–120.

Berle, D., & Starcevic, V. (2005). Thought–action fusion: Review of the literature and future direction. *Clinical Psychology Review, 25,* 263–284.

Berlin, G. S., & Hollander, E. (2014). Compulsivity, impulsivity, and the DSM-5 process. *CNS Spectrum, 19,* 62–68.

Berman, N. C., Abramowitz, J. S., Pardue, C. M., & Wheaton, M. C. (2010). The relationship between religion and thought–action fusion: Use of an *in vivo* paradigm. *Behaviour Research and Therapy, 48,* 670–674.

Bernstein, A., Vujanovic, A. A., Leyro, T. M., & Zvolensky, M. J. (2011). Research synthesis and the future. In M. J. Zvolensky, A. Bernstein, & A. A. Vujanovic (Eds.), *Distress tolerance: Theory, research, and clinical applications* (pp. 263–279). New York: Guilford Press.

Bernstein, G. A., Victor, A. M., Nelson, P. M., & Lee, S. S. (2013). Pediatric obsessive–compulsive disorder: Symptom patterns and confirmatory factor analysis. *Journal of Obsessive–Compulsive and Related Disorders, 2,* 299–305.

Besiroglu, L., Sozen, M., Ozbebit, Ö., Avcu, S., Selvi, Y., Bora, A., et al. (2011). The involvement of distinct neural systems in patients with obsessive–compulsive disorder with autogenous and reactive obsessions. *Acta Psychiatrica Scandinavica, 124,* 141–151.

Bhar, S. S., & Kyrios, M. (2007). An investigation of self-ambivalence in obsessive-compulsive disorder. *Behaviour Research and Therapy, 45,* 1845–1857.

Bienvenu, O. J., Samuels, J. F., Wuyek, L. A., Liang, K.-Y., Wang, Y., Grados, M. A., et al. (2012). Is obsessive–compulsive disorder an anxiety disorder, and what, if any, are spectrum conditions?: A family study perspective. *Psychological Medicine, 42,* 1–13.

Birrell, J., Meares, K., Wilkinson, A., & Freeston, M. H. (2011). Toward a definition of intolerance of uncertainty: A review of factor analytical studies of the Intolerance of Uncertainty Scale. *Clinical Psychology Review, 31,* 1198–1208.

Bjornsson, A. S., Didie, E. R., Grant, J. E., Menard, W., Stalker, E., & Phillips, K. A. (2013). Age at onset and clinical outcomes in body dysmorphic disorder. *Comprehensive Psychiatry, 54,* 893–903.

Black, A. (1974). The natural history of obsessional neurosis. In H. R. Beech (Ed.), *Obsessional states* (pp. 19–54). London: Methuen.

Blakey, S. M., & Abramowitz, J. S. (2016). The effects of safety behaviours during exposure therapy for anxiety: Critical analysis from an inhibitory learning perspective. *Clinical Psychology Review, 49,* 1–15.

Blakey, S. M., Jacoby, R. J., Reuman, L., & Abramowitz, J. S. (2016). The relative contributions of experiential avoidance and distress tolerance to OC symptoms. *Behavioural and Cognitive Psychotherapy, 44,* 460–471.

Bloch, M. H., Landeros-Weisenberger, A., Rosario, M. C., Pittenger, C., & Leckman, J. F. (2008). Meta-analysis of the symptom structure of obsessive-compulsive disorder. *American Journal of Psychiatry, 165,* 1532–1542.

Blom, R. H., Koeter, M., van den Brink, W., de Graaf, R., ten Have, M., & Denys, D. (2011). Co-occurrence of obsessive–compulsive disorder and substance use disorder in the general population. *Addiction, 106,* 2178–2185.

Bocci, L., & Gordon, P. K. (2007). Does magical thinking produce neutralizing behavior?: An experimental investigation. *Behaviour Research and Therapy, 45,* 1823–1833.

Boisseau, C. L., Sibrava, N. J., Garnaat, S. L., Mancebo, M. C., Eisen, J. L., & Rasmussen, S. A. (2018). The Brown Incompleteness Scale (BINGS): Measure development and initial evaluation. *Journal of Obsessive–Compulsive and Related Disorders, 16,* 66–71.

Bordin, E. S. (1979). The generalizability of the psychoanalytic concept of the working alliance. *Psychotherapy: Theory, Research and Practice, 16,* 252–260.

Borkovec, T. D. (1994). The nature, functions and origins of worry. In G. C. L. Davey & F. Tallis (Eds.), *Worrying: Perspectives on theory, assessment and treatment* (pp. 5–33). Chichester, UK: Wiley.

Bottesi, G., Ghisi, M., Sica, C., & Freeston, M. H. (2017). Intolerance of uncertainty, not just right experiences, and compulsive checking: Test of a moderated mediation model of a non-clinical sample. *Comprehensive Psychiatry, 73,* 111–119.

Boulougouris, J. C., & Bassiakos, L. (1973). Prolonged flooding in cases with obsessive–compulsive neurosis. *Behaviour Research and Therapy, 11,* 227–231.

Boulougouris, J. C., Rabavilas, A. D., & Stefanis, C. (1977). Psychophysiological responses in obsessive–compulsive patients. *Behaviour Research and Therapy, 15,* 221–230.

Bouvard, M., Fournet, N., Denis, A., Sixdenier, A., & Clark, D. (2017). Intrusive thoughts in patients with obsessive compulsive disorder and non-clinical participants: A comparison using the International Intrusive Thought Interview Schedule. *Cognitive Behaviour Therapy, 46,* 287–299.

Bragdon, L. B., & Coles, M. E. (2017). Examining heterogeneity of obsessive–compulsive disorder: Evidence for subgroups based on motivations. *Journal of Anxiety Disorders, 45,* 64–71.

Brakoulias, V., Starcevic, V., Berle, D., Milicevic, D., Moses, K., Hannan, A., et al. (2013). The characteristics of unacceptable/taboo thoughts in obsessive–compulsive disorder. *Comprehensive Psychiatry, 54,* 750–757.

Brakoulias, V., Starcevic, V., Martin, A., Berle, D., Milicevic, D., & Viswasam, K. (2016). The familiality of specific symptoms of obsessive–compulsive disorder. *Psychiatry Research, 239,* 315–319.

Brander, G., Pérez-Vigil, A., Larrson, H., & Mataix-Cols, D. (2016). Systematic review of environmental risk factors for obsessive–compulsive disorder: A proposed roadmap from association to causation. *Neuroscience and Biobehavioral Reviews, 65,* 36–62.

Braun, J. D., Strunk, D. R., Sasso, K. E., & Cooper, A. A. (2015). Therapist use of Socratic questioning predicts session-to-session symptom change in cognitive therapy for depression. *Behaviour Research and Therapy, 70,* 32–37.

Brewin, C. R., Hunter, E., Carroll, F., & Tata, P. (1996). Intrusive memories in depression: An index of schema activation? *Psychological Medicine, 26,* 1271–1276.

Bronisch, T., & Hecht, H. (1990). Major depression with and without a coexisting anxiety disorder: Social dysfunction, social integration, and personality features. *Journal of Affective Disorders, 20,* 151–157.

Brown, T. A. (1998). The relationship between obsessive–compulsive disorder and other anxiety-based disorders. In R. P. Swinson, M. M. Antony, S. Rachman, & M. A. Richter (Eds.), *Obsessive–compulsive disorder: Theory, research, and treatment* (pp. 207–226). New York: Guilford Press.

Brown, T. A., & Barlow, D. H. (1992). Comorbidity among anxiety disorders: Implications for treatment and DSM-IV. *Journal of Consulting and Clinical Psychology, 60,* 835–844.

Brown, T. A., & Barlow, D. H. (2014). *Anxiety and related disorders: Interview schedule for DSM-5 (ADIS-5)—client interview schedule.* Oxford, UK: Oxford University Press.

Brown, T. A., Campbell, L. A., Lehman, C. L., Grisham, J. R., & Mancill, R. B. (2001). Current and lifetime comorbidity of the DSM-IV anxiety and mood disorders in a large clinical sample. *Journal of Abnormal Psychology, 110,* 585–599.

Brown, T. A., Di Nardo, P. A., & Barlow, D. H. (1994). *Anxiety Disorders Interview Schedule for DSM-IV: Client interview schedule*. San Antonio, TX: Graywind & Psychological Corporation.

Brown, T. A., Dowdall, D. J., Côté, G., & Barlow, D. H. (1994). Worry and obsessions: The distinction between generalized anxiety disorder and obsessive-compulsive disorder. In G. C. L. Davey & F. Tallis (Eds.), *Worrying: Perspectives on theory, assessment and treatment* (pp. 229–246). New York: Wiley.

Brown, T. A., Moras, K., Zinbarg, R. E., & Barlow, D. H. (1993). Diagnostic and symptom distinguishability of generalized anxiety disorder and obsessive-compulsive disorder. *Behavior Therapy, 24*, 227–240.

Bucarelli, B., & Purdon, C. (2015). A diary study of the phenomenology and persistence of compulsions. *Journal of Behavior Therapy and Experimental Psychiatry, 49*, 209–215.

Bucarelli, B., & Purdon, C. (2016). Stove checking behaviour in people with OCD vs. anxious controls. *Journal of Behavior Therapy and Experimental Psychiatry, 53*, 17–24.

Buhr, K., & Dugas, M. J. (2002). The Intolerance of Uncertainty Scale: Psychometric properties of the English version. *Behaviour Research and Therapy, 40*, 931–945.

Bulli, F., Melli, G., Cavalletti, V., Stopani, E., & Carraresi, C. (2016). Comorbid personality disorders in obsessive–compulsive disorder and its symptom dimension. *Psychiatry Quarterly, 87*, 365–376.

Burns, G. L., Keortge, S. G., Formea, G. M., & Sternberger, L. G. (1996). Revision of the Padua Inventory of obsessive compulsive disorder symptoms: Distinctions between worry, obsessions and compulsions. *Behaviour Research and Therapy, 34*, 163–173.

Byers, E. S., Purdon, C., & Clark, D. A. (1998). Sexual intrusive thoughts of college students. *Journal of Sex Research, 35*, 359–369.

Calamari, J. E. (2005). Understanding the heterogeneity of OCD. *American Journal of Psychiatry, 162*, 2193–2194.

Calamari, J. E., Cohen, R. J., Rector, N. A., Szacun-Shimizu, K., Riemann, B. C., & Norberg, M. M. (2006). Dysfunctional belief-based obsessive–compulsive disorder subtypes. *Behaviour Research and Therapy, 44*, 1347–1360.

Calamari, J. E., & Janeck, A. S. (1997, March). *Negative intrusive thoughts in obsessive–compulsive disorder: Appraisal and response differences*. Poster presented at the annual convention of the Anxiety Disorders Association of America, New Orleans, LA.

Calamari, J. E., Wiegartz, P. S., & Janeck, A. S. (1999). Obsessive–compulsive disorder subgroups: A symptom-based clustering approach. *Behaviour Research and Therapy, 37*, 113–125.

Calamari, J. E., Wiegartz, P. S., Riemann, B. C., Cohen, R. J., Greer, A., Jacob, D. M., et al. (2004). Obsessive–compulsive disorder subtypes: An attempted replication and extension of a symptom-based taxonomy. *Behaviour Research and Therapy, 42*, 647–670.

Calleo, J. S., Hart, J., Björgvinsson, T., & Stanley, M. A. (2010). Obsessions and worry beliefs in an inpatient OCD population. *Journal of Anxiety Disorders, 24*, 903–908.

Calvocoressi, L., Lewis, B., Harris, M., Trufan, S. J., Goodman, W. K., McDougle,

C. J., et al. (1995). Family accommodation in obsessive–compulsive disorder. *American Journal of Psychiatry, 152,* 441–443.

Camuri, G., Oldani, L., Dell'Osso, B., Benatti, B., Lietti, L., Palazzo, C., et al. (2014). Prevalence and disability of comorbid social phobia and obsessive–compulsive disorder in patients with panic disorder and generalized anxiety disorder. *International Journal of Psychiatry in Clinical Practice, 18,* 248–254.

Carleton, R. N., Norton, P. J., & Asmundson, G. J. G. (2007). Fearing the unknown: A short version of the Intolerance of Uncertainty Scale. *Journal of Anxiety Disorders, 21,* 105–117.

Carr, A. T. (1974). Compulsive neurosis: A review of the literature. *Psychological Bulletin, 81,* 311–318.

Cartwright-Hatton, S., & Wells, A. (1997). Beliefs about worry and intrusions: The Meta-Cognitions Questionnaire and its correlates. *Journal of Anxiety Disorders, 11,* 279–296.

Catapano, F., Perris, F., Fabrazzo, M., Cioffi, V., Giacco, D., De Santis, V., et al. (2010). Obsessive–compulsive disorder with poor insight: A three-year prospective study. *Progress in Neuro-Psychopharmacology and Biological Psychiatry, 34,* 323–330.

Chakraborty, V., Cherian, A. V., Math, S. B., Venkatasubramanian, G., Thennarasu, K., Mataix-Cols, D., et al. (2012). Clinically significant hoarding in obsessive–compulsive disorder: Results from an Indian study. *Comprehensive Psychiatry, 53,* 1153–1160.

Chamberlain, S. R., Fineberg, N. A., Blackwell, A. D., Robbins, T. W., & Sahakian, B. J. (2006). Motor inhibition and cognitive inflexibility in obsessive–compulsive disorder and trichotillomania. *American Journal of Psychiatry, 163,* 1282–1284.

Chase, T., Wetterneck, C. T., Bartsch, R. A., Leonard, R. C., & Riemann, B. C. (2015). Investigating treatment outcomes across OCD symptom dimensions in a clinical sample of OCD patients. *Cognitive Behaviour Therapy, 44,* 365–376.

Cherian, A. V., Narayanswamy, J. C., Viswanath, B., Guru, N., George, C. M., Math, S. B., et al. (2014). Gender differences in obsessive–compulsive disorder: Findings from a large Indian sample. *Asian Journal of Psychiatry, 9,* 17–21.

Chik, H. M., Calamari, J. E., Rector, N. A., & Riemann, B. C. (2010). What do low-dysfunctional beliefs obsessive–compulsive disorder subgroups believe? *Journal of Anxiety Disorders, 24,* 837–846.

Christensen, H., Hadzi-Pavlovic, D., Andrews, G., & Mattick, R. (1987). Behavior therapy and tricyclic medication in the treatment of obsessive–compulsive disorder: A quantitative review. *Journal of Consulting and Clinical Psychology, 55,* 701–711.

Christoff, K. (2012). Undirected thought: Neural determinants and correlates. *Brain Research, 1428,* 51–59.

Ciarrocchi, J. W. (1995). *The doubting disease: Help for scrupulosity and religious compulsions.* Mahwah, NJ: Paulist Press.

Clark, D. A. (1992). Depressive, anxious and intrusive thoughts in psychiatric inpatients and outpatients. *Behaviour Research and Therapy, 30,* 93–102.

Clark, D. A. (2002). Commentary on cognitive domains section. In R. O. Frost & G. Steketee (Eds.), *Cognitive approaches to obsessions and compulsions: Theory, assessment, and treatment* (pp. 107–113). Amsterdam: Elsevier Science.

Clark, D. A. (2004). *Cognitive-behavioral therapy for OCD.* New York: Guilford Press.

Clark, D. A. (2005). Lumping versus splitting: A commentary on subtyping in OCD. *Behavior Therapy, 36,* 401–404.

Clark, D. A. (2013). Collaborative empiricism: A cognitive response to exposure reluctance and low distress tolerance. *Cognitive and Behavioral Practice, 20,* 445–454.

Clark, D. A. (2018). *The anxious thoughts workbook: Skills to overcome the unwanted intrusive thoughts that drive anxiety, obsessions and depression.* Oakland, CA: New Harbinger.

Clark, D. A., Abramowitz, J., Alcolado, G. M., Pino, A., Belloch, A., Bouvard, M., et al. (2014). Part 3: A question of perspective: The association between intrusive thoughts and obsessionality in 11 countries. *Journal of Obsessive–Compulsive and Related Disorders, 3,* 292–299.

Clark, D. A., Antony, M. M., Beck, A. T., Swinson, R. P., & Steer, R. A. (2003). *ROC analysis of the Clark–Beck Obsessive–Compulsive Inventory.* Unpublished manuscript, Department of Psychology, University of New Brunswick, Canada.

Clark, D. A., Antony, M. M., Beck, A. T., Swinson, R. P., & Steer, R. A. (2005). Screening for obsessive and compulsive symptoms: Validation of the Clark–Beck Obsessive–Compulsive Inventory. *Psychological Assessment, 17,* 132–143.

Clark, D. A., & Beck, A. T. (2002). *Clark–Beck Obsessive–Compulsive Inventory Manual.* San Antonio, TX: Harcourt Assessment.

Clark, D. A., & Beck, A. T. (2010). *Cognitive therapy of anxiety disorders: Science and practice.* New York: Guilford Press.

Clark, D. A., & Brown, G. P. (2015). Cognitive clinical assessment: Contributions and impediments to progress. In G. P. Brown & D. A. Clark (Eds.), *Assessment in cognitive therapy* (pp. 3–26). New York: Guilford Press.

Clark, D. A., & Claybourn, M. (1997). Process characteristics of worry and obsessive intrusive thoughts. *Behaviour Research and Therapy, 35,* 1139–1141.

Clark, D. A., & de Silva, P. (1985). The nature of depressive and anxious, intrusive thoughts: Distinct or uniform phenomena? *Behaviour Research and Therapy, 23,* 383–393.

Clark, D. A., & Guyitt, B. D. (2008). Pure obsessions: Conceptual misnomer or clinical anomaly? In J. S. Abramowitz, D. McKay, & S. Taylor (Eds.), *Obsessive–compulsive disorder: Suptypes and spectrum conditions* (pp. 53–75). Amsterdam: Elsevier.

Clark, D. A., & Hilchey, C. A. (2017). Repugnant obsessions. In J. S. Abramowitz, D. McKay, & E. A. Storch (Eds.), *The Wiley handbook of obsessive compulsive disorders* (Vol. 1, pp. 421–440). New York: Wiley.

Clark, D. A., & O'Connor, K. (2005). Thinking is believing: Ego-dystonic intrusive thoughts in obsessive–compulsive disorder. In D. A. Clark (Ed.), *Intrusive thoughts in clinical disorders: Theory, research, and treatment* (pp. 145–174). New York: Guilford Press.

Clark, D. A., O'Sullivan, L., & Fuller, R. (2015, September). *Obsessing about love: How relationship OCD tendencies affect romantic breakup in young Canadian adults.* Paper presented at the 45th Congress of the European Association for Behavioural and Cognitive Therapies, Jersualem, Israel.

Clark, D. A., & Purdon, C. (1993). New perspectives for a cognitive theory of obsessions. *Australian Psychologist, 28,* 161–167.

Clark, D. A., & Purdon, C. (2016). Still cognitive after all these years?: Perspectives for a cognitive behavioural theory of obsessions and where we are 30 years later—a commentary. *Australian Psychologist, 51,* 14–17.

Clark, D. A., Radomsky, A. S., Alcolado, G. M., Abramowitz, J. S., Alonso, P., Belloch, A., et al. (2015, September). *Repugnant thoughts: An international perspective on distressing sexual and religious intrusions.* Paper presented at the 45th Congress of the European Association for Behavioural and Cognitive Therapies, Jerusalem, Israel.

Clark, D. A., Sugrim, I., & Bolton, D. (1982). Primary obsessional slowness: A nursing treatment programme with a thirteen year old male adolescent. *Behaviour Research and Therapy, 20,* 289–292.

Clark, D. M. (1986). A cognitive approach to panic. *Behaviour Research and Therapy, 24,* 461–470.

Coles, M. E., Frost, R. O., Heimberg, R. G., & Rhéaume, J. (2003). "Not just right experiences": Perfectionism, obsessive–compulsive features and general psychopathology. *Behaviour Research and Therapy, 41,* 681–700.

Coles, M. E., Hart, A. S., & Schofield, C. A. (2012). Initial data characterizing the progression from obsessions and compulsions to full-blown obsessive compulsive disorder. *Cognitive Therapy and Research, 36,* 685–693.

Coles, M. E., Heimberg, R. G., Frost, R. O., & Steketee, G. (2005). Not just right experiences and obsessive–compulsive features: Experimental and self-monitoring perspectives. *Behaviour Research and Therapy, 43,* 153–167.

Coles, M. E., Mennin, D. S., & Heimberg, R. G. (2001). Distinguishing obsessive features and worries: The role of thought–action fusion. *Behaviour Research and Therapy, 39,* 947–959.

Coles, M. E., & Pietrefesa, A. S. (2008). Symmetry, ordering, and arranging. In J. S. Abramowitz, D. McKay, & S. Taylor (Eds.), *Obsessive–compulsive disorder: Subtypes and spectrum conditions* (pp. 36–52). Amsterdam: Elsevier.

Coles, M. E., Pinto, A., Mancebo, M. C., Rasmussen, S. A., & Eisen, J. L. (2008). OCD with comorbid OCPD: A subtype of OCD? *Journal of Psychiatric Research, 42,* 289–296.

Coles, M. E., Radomsky, A. S., & Horng, B. (2006). Exploring the boundaries of memory distrust from repeated checking: Increasing external validity and examining thresholds. *Behaviour Research and Therapy, 44,* 995–1006.

Coles, M. E., & Ravid, A. (2016). Clinical presentation of not-just right experiences (NJREs) in individuals with OCD: Characteristics and response to treatment. *Behaviour Research and Therapy, 87,* 182–187.

Coluccia, A., Fagiolini, A., Ferretti, F., Pozza, A., Costoloni, G., Bolognesi, S., et al. (2016). Adult obsessive–compulsive disorder and quality of life outcomes: A systematic review and meta-analysis. *Asian Journal of Psychiatry, 22,* 41–52.

Constans, J. I., Foa, E. B., Franklin, M. E., & Mathews, A. (1995). Memory for actual and imagined events in OC checkers. *Behaviour Research and Therapy, 33,* 665–671.

Corcoran, K. M., & Woody, S. R. (2008). Appraisals of obsessional thoughts in normal samples. *Behaviour Research and Therapy, 46,* 71–83.

Corcoran, K. M., & Woody, S. R. (2009). Effects of suppression and appraisals on thought frequency and distress. *Behaviour Research and Therapy, 47,* 1024–1031.

Coryell, W. (1981). Obsessive–compulsive disorder and primary unipolar depression: Comparisons of background, family history, course, and mortality. *Journal of Nervous and Mental Disease, 169,* 220–224.

Costa, D. L. C., Assunção, M. C., Ferrão, Y. A., Conrado, L. A., Gonzalez, C. H., Fontenelle, L. F., et al. (2012). Body dysmorphic disorder in patients with obsessive–compulsive disorder: Prevalence and clinical correlates. *Depression and Anxiety, 29,* 966–975.

Coughtrey, A. E., Shafran, R., Knibbs, D., & Rachman, S. J. (2012). Mental contamination in obsessive–compulsive disorder. *Journal of Obsessive–Compulsive and Related Disorders, 1,* 244–250.

Cougle, J. R., Fitch, K. E., Jacobson, S., & Lee, H.-J. (2013). A multi-method examination of the role of incompleteness in compulsive checking. *Journal of Anxiety Disorders, 27,* 231–239.

Cougle, J. R., Goetz, A. R., Fitch, K. E., & Hawkins, K. A. (2011). Terminating of washing compulsions: A problem of internal reference criteria or "not just right" experience? *Journal of Anxiety Disorders, 25,* 801–805.

Cougle, J. R., & Lee, H.-J. (2014). Pathological and non-pathological features of obsessive–compulsive disorder: Revisiting basic assumptions of cognitive models. *Journal of Obsessive–Compulsive and Related Disorders, 3,* 12–20.

Cougle, J. R., Lee, H.-J., Horowitz, J. D., Wolitzky-Taylor, K. B., & Telch, M. J. (2008). An exploration of the relationship between mental pollution and OCD symptoms. *Journal of Behaviour Therapy and Experimental Psychiatry, 39,* 340–353.

Cougle, J. R., Lee, H.-J., & Salkovskis, P. M. (2007). Are responsibility beliefs inflated in non-checking OCD patients? *Journal of Anxiety Disorders, 21,* 153–159.

Cougle, J. R., Timpano, K. R., Fitch, K. E., & Hawkins, K. A. (2011). Distress tolerance and obsessions: An integrative analysis. *Depression and Anxiety, 28,* 906–914.

Coyne, J. C. (1976). Toward an interactional description of depression. *Psychiatry, 39,* 28–40.

Craske, M. G., Kircanski, K., Zelikowsky, M., Mystkowski, J., Chowdhury, N., & Baker, A. (2008). Optimizing inhibitory learning during exposure therapy. *Behaviour Research and Therapy, 46,* 5–27.

Craske, M. G., Treanor, M., Conway, C., Zborinek, T., & Vervliet, B. (2014). Maximizing exposure therapy: An inhibitory learning approach. *Behaviour Research and Therapy, 58,* 10–23.

Crino, R. D., & Andrews, G. (1996). Obsessive–compulsive disorder and Axis I comorbidity. *Journal of Anxiety Disorders, 10,* 37–46.

Cromer, K. R., Schmidt, N. B., & Murphy, D. L. (2007). An investigation of traumatic life events and obsessive–compulsive disorder. *Behaviour Research and Therapy, 45,* 1683–1691.

Cuzen, N. L., Stein, D. J., Lochner, C., & Fineberg, N. A. (2014). Comorbidity of obsessive–compulsive disorder and substance use disorder: A new heuristic. *Human Psychopharmacology, 29,* 89–93.

Dar, R., Rish, S., Hermesh, H., Taub, M., & Fux, M. (2000). Realism of confidence in obsessive–compulsive checkers. *Journal of Abnormal Psychology, 109,* 673–678.

Darwin, C. R. (1965). *The expression of the emotions in man and animals.* Chicago: University of Chicagp Press. (Original work published 1872)

David, B., Olatunji, B. O., Armstrong, T., Ciesielski, B. G., Bondy, C., & Broman-Fulks, J. (2009). Incremental specificity of disgust sensitivity in the prediction of obsessive–compulsive disorder symptoms: Cross-sectional and prospective approaches. *Journal of Behavior Therapy and Experimental Psychiatry, 40,* 533–543.

de Bruin, G. O., Muris, P., & Rassin, E. (2007). Are there specific meta-cognitions associated with vulnerability to symptoms of worry and obsessional thoughts? *Personality and Individuals Differences, 42,* 689–699.

de Haan, E., van Oppen, P., van Balkom, A. J. L. M., Spinhoven, P., Hoogduin, K. A. L., & van Dyck, R. (1997). Prediction of outcome and early vs. late improvement in OCD patients treated with cognitive behaviour therapy and pharmacotherapy. *Acta Psychiatria Scandinavia, 96,* 354–361.

de Jong, P. J., Vorage, I., & van den Hout, M. (2000). Counterconditioning in the treatment of spider phobia: Effects on disgust, fear and valence. *Behaviour Research and Therapy, 38,* 1055–1069.

de Putter, L. M. S., Van Yper, L., & Koster, E. H. W. (2017). Obsessions and compulsions in the lab: A meta-analysis of procedures to induce symptoms of obsessive–compulsive disorder. *Clinical Psychology Review, 52,* 137–147.

de Silva, P. (1986). Obsessional–compulsive imagery. *Behaviour Research and Therapy, 24,* 333–350.

de Silva, P. (2003). Obsessions, ruminations and covert compulsions. In R. G. Menzies & P. de Silva (Eds.), *Obsessive–compulsive disorder: Theory, research and treatment* (pp. 195–208). Chichester, UK: Wiley.

de Silva, P., & Marks, M. (1999). The role of traumatic experiences in the genesis of obsessive–compulsive disorder. *Behaviour Research and Therapy, 37,* 941–951.

de Silva, P., & Rachman, S. (1992). *Obsessive–compulsive disorder: The facts.* Oxford, UK: Oxford University Press.

Deacon, B., & Maack, D. J. (2008). The effects of safety behaviors on the fear of contamination: An experimental investigation. *Behaviour Research and Therapy, 46,* 537–547.

Deacon, B., & Olatunji, B. O. (2007). Specificity of disgust sensitivity in the prediction of behavioral avoidance in contamination fear. *Behaviour Research and Therapy, 45,* 2110–2120.

Del Borrello, L., & O'Connor, K. (2014). The role of obsessive beliefs and inferential confusion in predicting treatment outcomes for different subtypes of obsessive–compulsive disorder. *International Journal of Cognitive Therapy, 7,* 43–66.

References

Del Re, A. C., Flückiger, C., Horvath, A. O., Symonds, D., & Wampold, B. E. (2012). Therapist effects in the therapeutic alliance–outcome relationship: A restricted-maximum likelihood meta-analysis. *Clinical Psychology Review, 32*, 642–649.

Demal, U., Lenz, G., Mayrhofer, A., Zapotoczky, H.-G., & Zitterl, W. (1993). Obsessive–compulsive disorder and depression: A retrospective study on course and interaction. *Psychopathology, 26*, 145–150.

Denys, D. (2011). Obsessionality and compulsivity: A phenomenology of obsessive–compulsive disorder. *Philosophy, Ethics, and Humanities in Medicine, 6*, 1–7.

Denys, D., Tenney, N., van Megen, H. J. G. M., de Geus, F., & Westenberg, H. G. M. (2004). Axis I and II comorbidity in a large sample of patients with obsessive–compulsive disorder. *Journal of Affective Disorders, 80*, 155–162.

Diedrich, A., Sckopke, P., Schwartz, C., Schlegl, S., Osen, B., Stierle, C., et al. (2016). Change in obsessive beliefs as predictor and mediator of symptom change during treatment of obsessive–compulsive disorder: A process-outcome study. *BMC Psychiatry, 16*, 220.

Dixon, M. L., Fox, K. C., & Christoff, K. (2014). A framework for understanding the relationship between externally and internally directed cognition. *Neuropsychologia, 62*, 321–330.

Dobson, D. J. G., & Dobson, K. S. (2013). In-session structure and collaborative empiricism. *Cognitive and Behavioral Practice, 20*, 410–418.

Doron, G., Derby, D. S., & Szepsenwol, O. (2014). Relationship obsessive compulsive disorder (ROCD): A conceptual framework. *Journal of Obsessive-Compulsive and Related Disorders, 3*, 169–180.

Doron, G., Derby, D. S., Szepsenwol, O., & Talmor, D. (2012). Tainted love: Exploring relationship-centered obsessive compulsive symptoms in two non-clinical cohorts. *Journal of Obsessive–Compulsive and Related Disorders, 1*, 16–24.

Doron, G., & Kyrios, M. (2005). Obsessive compulsive disorder: A review of possible specific internal representations within a broader cognitive theory. *Clinical Psychology Review, 25*, 415–432.

Doron, G., Kyrios, M., & Moulding, R. (2007). Sensitive domains of self-concept in obsessive–compulsive disorder (OCD): Further evidence for a multidimensional model of OCD. *Journal of Anxiety Disorders, 21*, 433–444.

Doron, G., Mizrahi, M., Szepsenwol, O., & Derby, D. (2014). Right or flawed: Relationship obsessions and sexual satisfaction. *Journal of Sexual Medicine, 11*, 2218–2224.

Doron, G., Moulding, R., Kyrios, M., & Nedeljkovic, M. (2008). Sensitivity of self-beliefs in obsessive compulsive disorder. *Depression and Anxiety, 25*, 874–884.

Doron, G., Sar-El, D., & Mikulincer, M. (2012). Threats to moral self-perceptions trigger obsessive compulsive contamination-related behavioral tendencies. *Journal of Behavior Therapy and Experimental Psychiatry, 43*, 884–890.

Doron, G., Szepensenwol, O., Karp, E., & Gal, N. (2012). Obsessing about intimate relationships: Testing the double relationship–vulnerability hypothesis. *Journal of Behavior Therapy and Experimental Psychiatry, 44*, 433–440.

Drake, R. E., Mueser, K. T., Brunette, M. F., & McHugo, G. J. (2004). A review of treatment for people with severe mental illnesses and co-occurring substance use disorders. *Psychiatric Rehabilitation Journal, 27,* 360–374.

Dugas, M. J., Gagnon, F., Ladouceur, R., & Freeston, M. H. (1998). Generalized anxiety disorder: A preliminary test of a conceptual model. *Behaviour Research and Therapy, 36,* 215–236.

Dugas, M. J., Gosselin, P., & Ladouceur, R. (2001). Intolerance of uncertainty and worry: Investigating specificity in a nonclinical sample. *Cognitive Therapy and Resarch, 25,* 551–558.

Dugas, M. J., & Robichaud, M. (2006). *Cognitive-behavioral treatment for generalized anxiety disorder: From science to practice.* New York: Routledge.

Dykshoorn, K. L. (2014). Trauma-related obsessive–compulsive disorder: A review. *Health Psychology and Behavioural Medicine, 2,* 517–528.

Ecker, W., & Gönner, S. (2008). Incompleteness and harm avoidance in OCD symptom dimensions. *Behaviour Research and Therapy, 46,* 895–904.

Ecker, W., Kupfer, J., & Gönner, S. (2014a). Incompleteness and harm avoidance in OCD, anxiety and depressive disorders, and non-clinical controls. *Journal of Obsessive–Compulsive and Related Disorders, 3,* 46–51.

Ecker, W., Kupfer, J., & Gönner, S. (2014b). Incompleteness as a link between obsessive–compulsive personality traits and specific symptom dimensions of obsessive–compulsive disorder. *Clinical Psychology and Psychotherapy, 21,* 394–402.

Egan, S. J., Wade, T. D., & Shafran, R. (2011). Perfectionism as a transdiagnostic process: A clinical review. *Clinical Psychology Review, 31,* 203–212.

Egan, S. J., Wade, T. D., Shafran, R., & Antony, M. M. (2014). *Cognitive-behavioral treatment of perfectionism.* New York: Guilford Press.

Ehring, T., & Watkins, E. R. (2008). Repetitive negative thinking as a transdiagnostic process. *International Journal of Cognitive Therapy, 1,* 192–205.

Eisen, J. L., Coles, M. E., Shea, M. T., Pagano, M. E., Stout, R. L., Yen, S., et al. (2006). Clarifying the convergence between obsessive compulsive personality disorder criteria and obsessive compulsive disorder. *Journal of Personality Disorders, 20,* 294–305.

Eisen, J. L., Phillips, K. A., Baer, L., Beer, D. A., Atala, K. D., & Rasmussen, S. A. (1998). The Brown Assessment of Beliefs Scale: Reliability and validity. *American Journal of Psychiatry, 155,* 102–108.

Eisen, J. L., Phillips, K. A., & Rasmussen, S. A. (1999). Obsessions and delusions: The relationship between obsessive–compulsive disorder and the psychotic disorders. *Psychiatric Annals, 29,* 515–522.

Eisen, J. L., Sibrava, N. J., Boisseau, C. L., Mancebo, M. C., Stout, R. L., Pinto, A., et al. (2013). Five-year course of obsessive compulsive disorder: Predictors of remission and relapse. *Journal of Clinical Psychiatry, 74,* 233–239.

Ekman, P., & Friesen, W. V. (1975). *Unmasking the face.* Englewood Cliffs, NJ: Prentice Hall.

Elliott, C. M., & Radomsky, A. S. (2009). Analyses of mental contamination: Part I. Experimental manipulations of morality. *Behaviour Research and Therapy, 47,* 995–1003.

Emmelkamp, P. M. G. (1982). *Phobic and obsessive–compulsive disorders: Theory, research and practice.* New York: Plenum Press.

Emmelkamp, P. M. G., & De Lange, I. (1983). Spouse involvement in the treatment of obsessive–compulsive patients. *Behaviour Research and Therapy, 21,* 341–346.

Emmelkamp, P. M. G., & Kraanen, J. (1977). Therapist controlled exposure in vivo versus self-controlled exposure in vivo: A comparison with obsessive–compulsive patients. *Behaviour Research and Therapy, 15,* 491–495.

Emmelkamp, P. M. G., van Linden van den Heuvell, C., Ruphan, M., & Sanderman, R. (1989). Home-based treatment of obsessive–compulsive patients: Intersession interval and therapist involvement. *Behaviour Research and Therapy, 27,* 89–93.

England, S. L., & Dickerson, M. (1988). Intrusive thoughts: Unpleasantness not the major cause of uncontrollability. *Behaviour Research and Therapy, 26,* 279–282.

Enright, S. J. (1996). Obsessive–compulsive disorder: Anxiety disorder or schizotype? In R. M. Rapee (Ed.), *Current controversies in the anxiety disorders* (pp. 161–190). New York: Guilford Press.

Evans, D. W., Leckman, J. F., Carter, A., Reznick, J. S., Henshaw, D., King, R. A., et al. (1997). Ritual, habit, and perfectionism: The prevalence and development of compulsive rituals in normal young children. *Child Development, 68,* 58–68.

Eysenck, H. J., & Rachman, S. (1965). *The causes and cures of neurosis.* San Diego, CA: Knapp.

Eysenck, M. W. (1992). *Anxiety: The cognitive perspective.* Hove, UK: Erlbaum.

Fairbrother, N., Barr, R. G., Pauwels, J., Brant, R., & Green, J. (2015). Maternal thoughts of harm in response to infant crying: An experimental analysis. *Archives of Women's Mental Health, 18,* 447–455.

Fairbrother, N., Newth, S. J., & Rachman, S. (2005). Mental pollution: Feelings of dirtiness without physical contact. *Behaviour Research and Therapy, 43,* 121–130.

Fairbrother, N., & Rachman, S. (2004). Feelings of mental pollution subsequent to sexual assault. *Behaviour Research and Therapy, 42,* 173–189.

Fairbrother, N., & Woody, S. R. (2008). New mothers' thoughts of harm related to the newborn. *Archives of Women's Mental Health, 11,* 221–229.

Fallon, B. A., Javitch, J. A., Hollander, E., & Liebowitz, M. R. (1991). Hypochondriasis and obsessive compulsive disorder: Overlaps in diagnosis and treatment. *Journal of Clinical Psychiatry, 52,* 457–460.

Fayard, J. V., Bassi, A. K., Bernstein, D. M., & Roberts, B. W. (2009). Is cleanliness next to godliness?: Dispelling old wives' tales: Failure to replicate Zhong and Liljenquist (2006). *Journal of Articles in Support of the Null Hypothesis, 6,* 21–30.

Fear, C., Sharp, H., & Healy, D. (2000). Obsessive compulsive disorder with delusions. *Psychopathology, 33,* 55–61.

Fergus, T. A. (2013). Thought control moderates the relation between autogenous intrusions and the severity of obsessional symptoms: Further support for the autogenous-reactive model of obsessions. *Journal of Obsessive–Compulsive and Related Disorders, 2,* 9–13.

Fergus, T. A. (2014). Are "not just right experiences" (NJREs) specific to obsessive–compulsive symptoms?: Evidence that NJREs span across symptoms of emotional disorders. *Journal of Clinical Psychology, 70,* 353–363.

Fergus, T. A., & Carmin, C. N. (2014). The validity and specificity of the short-form of the Obsessive Beliefs Questionnaire (OBQ). *Journal of Psychopathology and Behavioral Assessment, 36,* 318–328.

Fergus, T. A., & Wu, K. D. (2010). Do symptoms of generalized anxiety and obsessive–compulsive disorder share cognitive processes? *Cognitive Therapy and Research, 34,* 168–176.

Ferrão, Y. A., Shavitt, R. G., Prado, H., Fontenelle, L. F., Malavazzi, D. M., de Mathis, M. A., et al. (2012). Sensory phenomena associated with repetitive behaviors in obsessive–compulsive disorder: An exploratory study of 1001 patients. *Psychiatry Research, 197,* 253–258.

Feske, U., & Chambless, D. L. (2000). A review of assessment measures for obsessive–compulsive disorder. In W. K. Goodman, M. V. Rudorfor, & J. D. Maser (Eds.), *Obsessive–compulsive disorder: Contemporary issues in treatment* (pp. 157–182). Mahwah, NJ: Erlbaum.

Figee, M., Pattij, T., Willuhn, I., Luigjes, J., van den Brink, W., Goudriaan, A., et al. (2015). Compulsivity in obsessive–compulsive disorder and addictions. *European Neuropsychopharmacology, 26,* 856–868.

Fineberg, N. A., Chamberlain, S. R., Goudriaan, A. E., Stein, D. J., Vanderschuren, L. J. M. J., Gillan, C. M., et al. (2014). New developments inhuman neurocognition: Clinical, genetic and brain imaging correlates of impulsivity and compulsivity. *CNS Spectrum, 19,* 69–89.

Fineberg, N. A., Hengartner, M. P., Bergbaum, C., Gale, T., Rössler, W., & Angst, J. (2013). Lifetime comorbidity of obsessive–compulsive disorder and subthreshold obsessive–compulsive symptomatology in the community: Impact, prevalence, socio-demographic and clinical characteristics. *International Journal of Psychiatry and Clinical Practice, 17,* 188–196.

First, M. B., Spitzer, R. L., Gibbon, M., & Williams, J. B. W. (1996). *Structured Clinical Interview for DSM-IV Axis I Disorders—Patient edition (SCID-I/P, version 2.0).* New York: Biometrics Research Department, New York State Psychiatric Institute.

First, M. B., Williams, J. B. W., Karg, R. S., & Spitzer, R. L. (2016). *User's guide for the SCID-5-CV Structured Clinical Interview for DSM-5 Disorders: Clinical version.* Arlington, VA: American Psychiatric Association.

Flückiger, C., Del Re, A. C., Wampold, B. E., Symonds, D., & Horvath, A. O. (2012). How central is the alliance in psychotherapy?: A multilevel longitudinal meta-analysis. *Journal of Counseling Psychology, 59,* 10–17.

Foa, E. B. (1979). Failure in treating obsessive compulsives. *Behaviour Research and Therapy, 17,* 169–176.

Foa, E. B., Abramowitz, J. S., Franklin, M. E., & Kozak, M. J. (1999). Feared consequences, fixity of belief, and treatment outcome in patients with obsessive–compulsive disorder. *Behavior Therapy, 30,* 717–724.

Foa, E. B., Franklin, M. E., & Kozak, M. J. (1998). Psychosocial treatments for obsessive–compulsive disorder: Literature review. In R. P. Swinson, M. M. Antony, S. Rachman, & M. A. Richter (Eds.), *Obsessive–compulsive disorder: Theory, research, and treatment* (pp. 258–276). New York: Guilford Press.

Foa, E. B., Huppert, J. D., Leiberg, S., Langner, R., Kichic, R., Hajcak, G., et al.

(2002). The Obsessive–Compulsive Inventory: Development and validation of a short version. *Psychological Assessment, 14,* 485–496.

Foa, E. B., & Kozak, M. J. (1986). Emotional processing of fear: Exposure to corrective information. *Psychological Bulletin, 99,* 20–35.

Foa, E. B., & Kozak, M. J. (1997). *Mastery of obsessive–compulsive disorder: Client handbook.* San Antonio, TX: Psychological Corporation.

Foa, E. B., & Kozak, M. J. (1996). Psychological treatment for obsessive–compulsive disorder. In M. R. Mavissakalian & R. F. Prien (Eds.), *Long-term treatments of anxiety disorders* (pp. 285–309). Washington, DC: American Psychiatric Press.

Foa, E. B., Kozak, M. J., Goodman, W. K., Hollander, E., Jenike, M. A., & Rasmussen, S. A. (1995). DSM-IV Field Trial: Obsessive–compulsive disorder. *American Journal of Psychiatry, 152,* 90–96.

Foa, E. B., Kozak, M. J., Salkovskis, P. M., Coles, M. E., & Amir, N. (1998). The validation of a new obsessive–compulsive disorder scale: The Obsessive–Compulsive Inventory. *Psychological Assessment, 10,* 206–214.

Foa, E. B., Sacks, M. B., Tolin, D. F., Przeworski, A., & Amir, N. (2002). Inflated perception of responsibility for harm in OCD patients with and without checking compulsions: A replication and extension. *Journal of Anxiety Disorders, 16,* 443–453.

Foa, E. B., Steketee, G. S., & Ozarow, B. J. (1985). Behavior therapy with obsessive–compulsives: From theory to treatment. In M. Mavissakalian, S. M. Turner, & L. Michelson (Eds.), *Obsessive–compulsive disorder: Psychological and pharmacological treatment* (pp. 49–129). New York: Plenum Press.

Fontenelle, L. F., & Hasler, G. (2008). The analytical epidemiology of obsessive–compulsive disorder: Risk factors and correlates. *Progress in Neuro-Psychopharmacology and Biological Psychiatry, 32,* 1–15.

Fontenelle, L. F., Mendlowicz, M. V., Marques, C., & Versiani, M. (2004). Transcultural aspects of obsessive–compulsive disorder: A description of a Brazilian sample and a systematic review of international clinical studies. *Journal of Psychiatric Research, 38,* 403–411.

Fontenelle, L. F., Mendlowicz, M. V., & Versiani, M. (2006). The descriptive epidemiology of obsessive–compulsive disorder. *Progress in Neuro-Psychopharmacology and Biological Psychiatry, 30,* 327–337.

Fornés-Romero, G., & Belloch, A. (2017). Induced not just right and incompleteness experiences in OCD patients and non-clinical individuals: An in vivo study. *Journal of Behavior Therapy and Experimental Psychiatry, 57,* 103–112.

Forrester, E., Wilson, C., & Salkovskis, P. M. (2002). The occurrence of intrusive thoughts transforms meaning in ambiguous situations: An experimental study. *Behavioural and Cognitive Psychotherapy, 30,* 143–152.

Fourtounas, A., & Thomas, S. J. (2016). Cognitive factors predicting checking, procrastination and other maladaptive behaviours: Prospective versus inhibitory intolerance of uncertainty. *Journal of Obsessive–Compulsive and Related Disorders, 9,* 30–35.

Franz, A. P., Rateke, L., Hartmann, T., McLaughlin, N., Torres, A. R., do Rosaário, M. C., et al. (2015). Separation anxiety in adult patients with obsessive–compulsive disorder: Prevalence and clinical correlates. *European Psychiatry, 30,* 145–151.

Freeston, M. H., & Ladouceur, R. (1993). Appraisal of cognitive intrusions and response style: Replications and extension. *Behaviour Research and Therapy, 31,* 185–191.

Freeston, M. H., & Ladouceur, R. (1997a). *The cognitive behavioral treatment of obsessions: A treatment manual.* Unpublished manuscript, École de Psychologie, Université Laval, Québec, Canada.

Freeston, M. H., & Ladouceur, R. (1997b). What do patients do with their obsessive thoughts? *Behaviour Research and Therapy, 35,* 335–348.

Freeston, M. H., & Ladouceur, R. (1999). Exposure and response prevention for obsessional thoughts. *Cognitive and Behavioral Practice, 6,* 362–383.

Freeston, M. H., Ladouceur, R., Gagnon, F., Thibodeau, N., Rhéaume, J., Letarte, H., et al. (1997). Cognitive-behavioral treatment of obsessive thoughts: A controlled study. *Journal of Consulting and Clinical Psychology, 65,* 405–413.

Freeston, M. H., Ladouceur, R., Provencher, M., & Blais, F. (1995). Strategies used with intrusive thoughts: Context, appraisal, mood, and efficacy. *Journal of Anxiety Disorders, 9,* 201–215.

Freeston, M. H., Ladouceur, R., Rhéaume, J., Letarte, H., Gagnon, F., & Thibodeau, N. (1994). Self-report of obsessions and worry. *Behaviour Research and Therapy, 32,* 29–36.

Freeston, M. H., Ladouceur, R., Thibodeau, N., & Gagnon, F. (1991). Cognitive intrusions in a non-clinical population: I. Response style, subjective experience, and appraisal. *Behaviour Research and Therapy, 29,* 585–597.

Freeston, M. H., Ladouceur, R., Thibodeau, N., & Gagnon, F. (1992). Cognitive intrusions in a non-clinical population: II. Associations with depressive, anxious, and compulsive symptoms. *Behaviour Research and Therapy, 30,* 263–271.

Freeston, M. H., Rhéaume, J., & Ladouceur, R. (1996). Correcting faulty appraisals of obsessional thoughts. *Behaviour Research and Therapy, 34,* 433–446.

Freeston, M. H., Rhéaume, J., Letarte, H., Dugas, M. J., & Ladouceur, R. (1994). Why do people worry? *Personality and Individual Differences, 17,* 791–802.

Freud, S. (1959). Character and eroticism. In J. Strachey (Ed. & Trans.), *The standard edition of the complete psychological works of Sigmund Freud* (Vol. 9, pp. 167–175). London: Hogarth Press. (Original work published 1908)

Freund, B., & Steketee, G. (1989). Sexual history, attitudes and functioning of obsessive–compulsive patients. *Journal of Sex and Marital Therapy, 15,* 31–41.

Freund, B., Steketee, G. S., & Foa, E. B. (1987). Compulsive Activity Checklist (CAC): Psychometric analysis with obsessive–compulsive disorder. *Behavioral Assessment, 9,* 67–79.

Friborg, O., Martinussen, M., Kaiser, S., Øvergård, K. T., & Rosenvinge, J. H. (2013). Comorbidity of personality disorders in anxiety disorders: A meta-analysis of 30 years of research. *Journal of Affective Disorders, 145,* 143–155.

Frost, R. O., Marten, P., Lahart, C., & Rosenblate, R. (1990). The dimensions of perfectionism. *Cognitive Therapy and Research, 14,* 449–468.

Frost, R. O., Novara, C., & Rhéaume, J. (2002). Perfectionism in obsessive compulsive disorder. In R. O. Frost & G. Steketee (Eds.), *Cognitive approaches to obsessions and compulsions: Theory, assessment, and treatment* (pp. 91–105). Amsterdam: Elsevier Science.

Frost, R. O., & Steketee, G. (1997). Perfectionism in obsessive–compulsive disorder patients. *Behaviour Research and Therapy, 35,* 291–296.

Frost, R. O., Steketee, G., Krause, M. S., & Trepanier, K. L. (1995). The relationship of the Yale–Brown Obsessive–Compulsive Scale (YBOCS) to other measures of obsessive compulsive symptoms in a nonclinical population. *Journal of Personality Assessment, 65,* 158–168.

Fryman, I., do Brasil, P. E., Torres, A. R., Shavitt, R. G., Ferrão, Y. A., Rosário, M. C., et al. (2014). Late-onset obsessive–compulsive disorder: Risk factors and correlates. *Journal of Psychiatric Research, 49,* 68–74.

Fullana, M. A., Mataix-Cols, D., Caspi, A., Harrington, H., Grisham, J. R., Moffitt, T. E., et al. (2009). Obsessions and compulsions in the community: Prevalence, interference, help-seeking, developmental stability, and co-occurring psychiatric conditions. *American Journal of Psychiatry, 166,* 329–336.

Fullana, M. A., Vilagut, G., Rojas-Farreras, S., Mataix-Cols, D., de Graaf, R., Demyttenaere, K., et al. (2010). Obsessive–compulsive symptom dimensions in the general population: Results from an epidemiological study in six European countries. *Journal of Affective Disorders, 124,* 291–299.

García-Soriano, G., & Belloch, A. (2012). Exploring the role of obsessive–compulsive relevant self-worth contingencies in obsessive–compulsive patients. *Psychiatry Research, 198,* 94–99.

García-Soriano, G., & Belloch, A. (2013). Symptom dimensions in obsessive–compulsive disorder: Differences in distress, interference, appraisals and neutralizing strategies. *Journal of Behavior Therapy and Experimental Psychiatry, 44,* 441–448.

García-Soriano, G., Belloch, A., Morillo, C., & Clark, D. A. (2011). Symptom dimensions in obsessive–compulsive disorder: From normal cognitive intrusions to clinical obsessions. *Journal of Anxiety Disorders, 25,* 474–482.

García-Soriano, G., Clark, D. A., Belloch, A., del Palacio, A., & Castanñeiras, C. (2012). Self-worth contingencies and obsessionality: A promising approach to vulnerability? *Journal of Obsessive–Compulsive and Related Disorders, 1,* 196–202.

García-Soriano, G., Roncero, M., Perpiña, C., & Belloch, A. (2014). Intrusive thoughts in obsessive–compulsive disorder and eating disorder patients: A differential analysis. *European Eating Disorders Review, 22,* 191–199.

Gentes, E. L., & Ruscio, A. M. (2011). A meta-analysis of the relation of intolerance of uncertainty to symptoms of generalized anxiety disorder, major depressive disorder, and obsessive–compulsive disorder. *Clinical Psychology Review, 31,* 923–933.

Gentes, E., & Ruscio, A. M. (2015). Do negative appraisals of unwanted thoughts predict negative outcome?: A test of the effect of negative appraisals across thought types. *Journal of Experimental Psychopathology, 6,* 82–99.

Gershuny, B. S., Baer, L., Radomsky, A. S., Wilson, K. A., & Jenike, M. A. (2003). Connections among symptoms of obsessive–compulsive disorder and posttraumatic stress disorder: A case series. *Behaviour Research and Therapy, 41,* 1029–1041.

Ghassemzadeh, H., Mojtabai, R., Khamseh, A., Ebrahimkhani, N., Issazadegan,

A.-A., & Saif-Nobakht, Z. (2002). Symptoms of obsessive–compulsive disorder in a sample of Iranian patients. *International Journal of Social Psychiatry, 48,* 20–28.

Ghisi, M., Chiri, L. R., Marchetti, I., Sanavio, E., & Sica, C. (2010). In search of specificity: "Not just right experiences" and obsessive–compulsive symptoms in nonclinical and clinical Italian individuals. *Journal of Anxiety Disorders, 24,* 879–886.

Gibbs, N. A. (1996). Nonclinical populations in research on obsessive–compulsive disorder: A critical review. *Clinical Psychology Review, 16,* 729–773.

Gibbs, N. A., & Oltmanns, T. F. (1995). The relation between obsessive–compulsive personality traits and subtypes of compulsive behavior. *Journal of Anxiety Disorders, 9,* 397–410.

Gillan, C. M., Papmeyer, M., Morein-Zamir, S., Sahakian, B. J., Fineberg, N. A., Robbins, T. W., et al. (2011). Disruption in the balance between goal-directed behavior and habit learning in obsessive–compulsive disorder. *American Journal of Psychiatry, 168,* 718–726.

Gillan, C. M., & Sahakian, B. J. (2015). Which is the driver, the obsessions or the compulsions, in OCD? *Neuropsychopharmacology, 40,* 247–248.

Gillett, C. B., Bilek, E. L., Hanna, G. L., & Fitzgerald, K. D. (2018). Intolerance of uncertainty in youth with obsessive–compulsive disorder and generalized anxiety disorder: A ransdiagnostic construct with implications for phenomenology and treatment. *Clinical Psychology Review, 60,* 100–106.

Girishchandra, B. G., & Khanna, S. (2001). Phenomenology of obsessive compulsive disorder: A factor analytic approach. *Indian Journal of Psychiatry, 43,* 306–316.

Goetz, A. R., Lee, H.-J., Cougle, J. R., & Turkel, J. E. (2013). Disgust propensity and sensitivity: Differential relationships with obsessive–compulsive symptoms and behavioral approach task performance. *Journal of Obsessive–Compulsive and Related Disorders, 2,* 412–419.

Goldsmith, T., Shapira, N. A., Phillips, K. A., & McElroy, S. L. (1998). Conceptual foundations of obsessive–compulsive spectrum disorders. In R. P. Swinson, M. M. Antony, S. Rachman, & M. A. Richter (Eds.), *Obsessive–compulsive disorder: Theory, research, and treatment* (pp. 397–425). New York: Guilford Press.

Gönner, S., Ecker, W., Leonhart, R., & Limbacher, K. (2010). Multidimensional assessment of OCD: Integration and revision of the Vancouver Obsessional–Compulsive Inventory and the Symmetry Ordering and Arranging Questionnaire. *Journal of Clinical Psychology, 66,* 739–757.

Goodman, W. K., Price, L. H., Rasmussen, S. A., Mazure, C., Delgado, P., Heninger, G. R., et al. (1989). The Yale–Brown Obsessive–Compulsive Scale II: Validity. *Archives of General Psychiatry, 46,* 1012–1016.

Goodman, W. K., Price, L. H., Rasmussen, S. A., Mazure, C., Fleischmann, R. L., Hill, C. L., et al. (1989). The Yale–Brown Obsessive–Compulsive Scale I: Development, use, and reliability. *Archives of General Psychiatry, 46,* 1006–1011.

Gordon, O. M., Salkovskis, P. M., Oldfield, V. B., & Carter, N. (2013). The association between obsessive–compulsive disorder and obsessive–compulsive personality disorders: Prevalence and clinical presentation. *British Journal of Clinical Psychology, 52,* 300–315.

Grabill, K., Merlo, L., Duke, D., Harford, K.-L., Keeley, M. L., Geffken, G. R., et al. (2008). Assessment of obsessive–compulsive disorder: A review. *Journal of Anxiety Disorders, 22,* 1–17.

Grant, J. E., Odlaug, B. L., & Kim, S. W. (2010). A clinical presentation of pathologic skin picking and obsessive–compulsive disorder. *Comprehensive Psychiatry, 51,* 347–352.

Greenberg, D., & Huppert, J. D. (2010). Scrupulosity: A unique subtype of obsessive–compulsive disorder. *Current Psychiatry Reports, 12,* 282–289.

Greenberg, D., & Shefler, G. (2002). Obsessive compulsive disorder in ultra-orthodox Jewish patients: A comparison of religious and non-religious symptoms. *Psychology and Psychotherapy: Theory, Research and Practice, 75,* 123–130.

Greenberg, D., & Witztum, E. (2001). Treatment of strictly religious patients. In M. I. Pato & J. Zobar (Eds.), *Current treatments of obsessive–compulsive disorder* (2nd ed., pp. 173–191). Washington, DC: American Psychiatric Association.

Greenberger, D., & Padesky, C. A. (2016). *Mind over mood: Change how you feel by changing the way you think* (2nd ed.). New York: Guilford Press.

Grenier, S., O'Connor, K. P., & Bélanger, C. (2010). Belief in the obsessional doubt as a real probability and its relation to other obsessive–compulsive beliefs and to the severity of symptomatology. *British Journal of Clinical Psychology, 49,* 67–85.

Grisham, J. R., & Williams, A. D. (2009). Cognitive control of obsessional thoughts. *Behaviour Research and Therapy, 47,* 395–402.

Gross, P. R., & Eifert, G. H. (1990). Components of generalized anxiety: The role of intrusive thought vs. worry. *Behaviour Research and Therapy, 28,* 421–428.

Gruner, P., & Pittenger, C. (2017). Cognitive inflexibility in obsessive–compulsive disorder. *Neuroscience, 345,* 243–255.

Haidt, J., McCauley, C., & Rozin, P. (1994). Individual differences in sensitivity to disgust: A scale sampling seven domains of disgust elicitors. *Personality and Individual Differences, 16,* 701–713.

Hale, M. A., & Clark, D. A. (2013). When good people have bad thoughts: Religiosity and the emotional regulation of guilt-inducing intrusive thoughts. *Journal of Psychology and Theology, 41,* 24–35.

Hall, B. J., Tolin, D. F., Frost, R. O., & Steketee, G. (2013). An exploration of comorbid symptoms and clinical correlates of clinically significant hoarding symptoms. *Depression and Anxiety, 30,* 67–76.

Halldorsson, B., Salkovskis, P. M., Kobori, O., & Pagdin, R. (2016). I do not know what else to do: Caregivers' perspective on reassurance seeking in OCD. *Journal of Obsessive–Compulsive and Related Disorders, 8,* 21–30.

Halvorsen, M., Hagen, R., Hjemdal, O., Eriksen, M. S., Sørli, A. J., Waterloo, K., et al. (2015). Metacognitions and thought control strategies in unipolar major depression: A comparison of currently depressed, previously depressed, and never-depressed individuals. *Cognitive Therapy and Research, 39,* 31–40.

Haslam, N., Williams, B. J., Kyrios, M., McKay, D., & Taylor, S. (2005). Subtyping obsessive–compulsive disorder: A taxometric analysis. *Behavior Therapy, 36*, 381–391.

Hasler, G., Holland LaSalle-Ricci, V., Ronquillo, J. G., Crawley, S. A., Cochran, L. W., Kazuba, D., et al. (2005). Obsessive–compulsive disorder symptom dimensions show specific relationships to psychiatric comorbidity. *Psychiatry Research, 135*, 121–132.

Heinonen, E., Lindfors, O., Härkänen, T., Virtala, E., Jääkeläinen, T., & Knekt, P. (2014). Therapists' professional and personal characteristics as predictors of working alliance in short-term and long-term psychotherapies. *Clinical Psychology and Psychotherapy, 21*, 475–494.

Hermans, D., Engelen, U., Grouwels, L., Joos, E., Lemmens, J., & Pieters, G. (2008). Cognitive confidence in obsessive–compulsive disorder: Distrusting perception, attention and memory. *Behaviour Research and Therapy, 46*, 98–113.

Hersoug, A. G., Høgland, P., Havik, O., von der Lippe, A., & Monsen, J. (2009). Therapist characteristics influencing the quality of alliance in long-term psychotherapy. *Clinical Psychology and Psychotherapy, 16*, 100–110.

Hewitt, P. L., Flett, G. L., & Mikail, S. F. (2017). *Perfectionism: A relational approach to conceptualization, assessment, and treatment.* New York: Guilford Press.

Hezel, D. M., & McNally, R. J. (2016). A theoretical review of cognitive biases and deficits in obsessive–compulsive disorder. *Biological Psychiatry, 121*, 221–232.

Hezel, D. M., Riemann, B. C., & McNally, R. J. (2012). Emotional distress and pain tolerance in obsessive–compulsive disorder. *Journal of Behavior Therapy and Experimental Psychiatry, 43*, 981–987.

Himle, J. A., Muroff, J. R., Taylor, R. J., Baser, R. E., Abelson, J. M., Hanna, G. L., et al. (2008). Obsessive–compulsive disorder among African Americans and blacks of Caribbean descent: Results from the National Survey of American Life. *Depression and Anxiety, 25*, 993–1005.

Hinds, A. L., Woody, E. Z., Drandic, A., Schmidt, L. A., Van Ameringen, M., Coroneos, M., et al. (2010). The psychology of potential threat: Properties of the security motivation system. *Biological Psychology, 85*, 331–337.

Hinds, A. L., Woody, E. Z., Schmidt, L. A., Van Ameringen, M., & Szechtman, H. (2015). In the wake of a possible mistake: Security motivation, checking behavior, and OCD. *Journal of Behavior Therapy and Experimental Psychiatry, 49*, 133–140.

Hinds, A. L., Woody, E. Z., Van Ameringen, M., Schmidt, L. A., & Szechtman, H. (2012). When too much is not enough: Obsessive–compulsive disorder as a pathology of stopping, rather than starting. *PLOS ONE, 7*, e30586.

Hirschtritt, M. E., Lee, P. C., Pauls, D. L., Dion, Y., Grados, M. A., Illmann, C., et al. (2015). Lifetime prevalence, age of risk, and genetic relationships of comorbid psychiatric disorders in Tourette syndrome. *JAMA Psychiatry, 72*, 325–333.

Hjemdal, O., Stiles, T., & Wells, A. (2013). Automatic thoughts and meta-cognition as predictors of depressive or anxious symptoms: A prospective study of two trajectories. *Scandinavian Journal of Psychology, 54*, 59–65.

Hodgson, R. J., & Rachman, S. J. (1972). The effects of contamination and washing in obsessional patients. *Behaviour Research and Therapy, 10,* 111–117.

Hodgson, R. J., & Rachman, S. J. (1977). Obsessional compulsive complaints. *Behaviour Research and Therapy, 15,* 389–395.

Hofmeijer-Sevink, M. K., van Oppen, P., van Megan, H. J., Batelaan, N. M., Cath, D. C., van der Wee, N. J. A., et al. (2013). Clinical relevance of comorbidity in obsessive–compulsive disorder: The Netherlands OCD Association Study. *Journal of Affective Disorders, 150,* 847–854.

Hollander, E. (1996). New developments in impulsivity and compulsivity. *European Neuropsychopharmacology, 6*(Suppl. 3), 91.

Hollon, S. D., & Beck, A. T. (1986). Cognitive and cognitive-behavioral therapies. In S. L. Garfield & A. E. Bergin (Eds.), *Handbook of psychotherapy and behavior change* (3rd ed., pp. 443–481). New York: Wiley.

Holmes, E. A., Arntz, A., & Smucker, M. (2007). Imagery rescripting in cognitive behavior therapy: Images, treatment techniques and outcomes. *Journal of Behavior Therapy and Experimental Psychiatry, 38,* 297–305.

Holzer, J. C., Goodman, W. K., McDougle, C. J., Baer, L., Boyarsky, B. K., Leckman, J. F., et al. (1994). Obsessive–compulsive disorder with and without a chronic tic disorder: A comparison of symptoms in 70 patients. *British Journal of Psychiatry, 164,* 469–473.

Hooper, N., & McHugh, L. (2013). The effects of repeated thought suppression attempts on thought occurrence. *American Journal of Psychology, 126,* 315–322.

Höping, W., & de Jong-Meyer, R. (2003). Differentiating unwanted intrusive thoughts from thought suppression: What does the White Bear Suppression Inventory measure? *Personality and Individual Differences, 34,* 1049–1055.

Horowitz, M. J. (1975). Intrusive and repetitive thoughts after experimental stress: A summary. *Archives of General Psychiatry, 32,* 1457–1463.

Horvath, A. O., Del Re, A. C., Flückiger, C., & Symonds, D. (2011). Alliance in psychotherapy. *Psychotherapy, 48,* 9–16.

Horvath, A. O., & Greenberg, L. S. (1989). Development and validation of the Working Alliance Inventory. *Journal of Counseling Psychology, 36,* 223–233.

Huang, L.-C., Tsai, K.-J., Wang, H.-K., Sung, P.-S., Wu, M.-H., Hung, K.-W., et al. (2014). Prevalence, incidence, and comorbidity of clinically diagnosed obsessive–compulsive disorder in Taiwan: A national population-based study. *Psychiatry Research, 220,* 335–341.

Huppert, J. D., Simpson, H. B., Nissenson, K. J., Liebowitz, M. R., & Foa, E. B. (2009). Quality of life and functional impairment in obsessive–compulsive disorder: A comparison of patients with and without comorbidity, patients in remission, and health controls. *Depression and Anxiety, 26,* 39–45.

Huppert, J. D., Walther, M. R., Hajcak, G., Yadin, E., Foa, E. B., Simpson, H. B., et al. (2007). The OCI-R: Validation of the subscales in a clinical sample. *Journal of Anxiety Disorders, 21,* 394–406.

Ingram, I. M. (1961a). Obsessional illness in mental health patients. *Journal of Mental Science, 197,* 382–402.

Ingram, I. M. (1961b). The obsessional personality and obsessional illness. *American Journal of Psychiatry, 117,* 1016–1019.

Inozu, M., Clark, D. A., & Eremsoy, C. (2015). *An experimental investigation of*

Middle Eastern and Western differences in disgust propensity: Implications for cognitive theories of OCD. Manuscript in preparation.

Inozu, M., Clark, D. A., & Karanci, A. N. (2012). Scrupulosity in Islam: A comparison of highly religious Turkish and Canadian samples. *Behavior Therapy, 43*, 190–202.

Inozu, M., Karanci, A. N., & Clark, D. A. (2012). Why are religious individuals more obsessional?: The role of mental control beliefs and guilt in Muslims and Christians. *Journal of Behavior Therapy and Experimental Psychiatry, 43*, 959–966.

Inozu, M., Ulukut, F. O., Ergun, G., & Alcolado, G. M. (2014). The mediating role of disgust sensitivity and thought–action fusion between religiosity and obsessive compulsive symptoms. *International Journal of Psychology, 49*, 334–341.

Insel, T. R., & Akiskal, H. S. (1986). Obsessive–compulsive disorder with psychotic features: A phenomenologic analysis. *American Journal of Psychiatry, 143*, 1527–1533.

Ishikawa, R., Kobori, O., Ikota, D., & Shimizu, E. (2014). Development and validation of the Japanese version of Responsibility Attitude Scale and Responsibility Interpretations Questionnaire. *International Journal of Culture and Mental Health, 8*, 231–243.

Izard, C. E. (1971). *The face of emotion*. New York: Appleton-Century-Crofts.

Jacobsen, P., Freeman, D., & Salkovskis, P. (2012). Reasoning bias and belief conviction in obsessive–compulsive disorder and delusions: Jumping to conclusions across disorders? *British Journal of Clinical Psychology, 51*, 84–99.

Jacoby, R. J., & Abramowitz, J. S. (2016). Inhibitory learning approaches to exposure therapy: A critical review and translation to obsessive–compulsive disorder. *Clinical Psychology Review, 49*, 28–40.

Jacoby, R. J., Fabricant, L. E., Leonard, R. C., Riemann, B. C., & Abramowitz, J. S. (2013). Just to be certain: Confirming the factor structure of the Intolerance of Uncertainty Scale in patients with obsessive–compulsive disorder. *Journal of Anxiety Disorders, 27*, 535–542.

Jakes, I. (1996). *Theoretical approaches to obsessive–compulsive disorder*. Cambridge, UK: Cambridge University Press.

Jakubovski, E., Pittenger, C., Torres, A. R., Fontenelle, L. F., do Rosario, M. C., Ferrão, Y. A., et al. (2011). Dimensional correlates of poor insight in obsessive–compulsive disorder. *Progress in Neuro-Psychopharmacology and Biological Psychiatry, 35*, 1677–1681.

Janeck, A. S., & Calamari, J. E. (1999). Thought suppression in obsessive–compulsive disorder. *Cognitive Therapy and Research, 23*, 497–509.

Janeck, A. S., Calamari, J. E., Riemann, B. C., & Heffelfinger, S. K. (2003). Too much thinking about thinking?: Metacognitive differences in obsessive–compulsive disorder. *Journal of Anxiety Disorders, 17*, 181–195.

Janet, P. (1903). *Les obsessions et la psychasthénie* (Vols. 1 & 3, 2nd ed.). Paris: Alcan.

Jaspers, K. (1963). *General psychopathology* (J. Hoenig & M. W. Hamilton, Trans.). Chicago: University of Chicago Press.

Jennings, K. D., Ross, S., Popper, S., & Elmore, M. (1999). Thoughts of harming infants in depressed and nondepressed mothers. *Journal of Affective Disorders, 54*, 21–28.

Joiner, T. E., & Metalsky, G. I. (2001). Excessive reassurance seeking: Delineating a risk factor involved in the development of depressive symptoms. *Psychological Science, 12,* 371–378.

Jones, M. K., & Menzies, R. G. (1997). Danger ideation reduction therapy (DIRT): Preliminary findings with three obsessive–compulsive washers. *Behaviour Research and Therapy, 35,* 955–960.

Jones, M. K., & Menzies, R. G. (1998). Danger ideation reduction therapy (DIRT) for obsessive–compulsive washers: A controlled trial. *Behaviour Research and Therapy, 36,* 959–970.

Julien, D., O'Connor, K. P., & Aardema, F. (2007). Intrusive thoughts, obsessions, and appraisals in obsessive–compulsive disorder: A critical review. *Clinical Psychology Review, 27,* 366–383.

Julien, D., O'Connor, K. P., & Aardema, F. (2009). Intrusions related to obsessive–compulsive disorder: A question of content or context? *Journal of Clinical Psychology, 65,* 709–722.

Julien, D., O'Connor, K. P., Aardema, F., & Todorov, C. (2006). The specificity of belief domains in obsessive–compulsive symptom subtypes. *Personality and Individual Differences, 41,* 1205–1216.

Kane, M. J., Brown, L. H., McVay, J. C., Silvia, P. J., Myin-Germeys, I., & Kwapil, T. R. (2007). For whom the mind wanders, and when: An experience-sampling study of working memory and executive control in daily life. *Psychological Science, 18,* 614–621.

Karadağ, F., Oguzhanoglu, N K., Özdel, O., Ateşci, F. C., & Amuk, T. (2006). OCD symptoms in a sample of Turkish patients: A phenomenological picture. *Depression and Anxiety, 23,* 145–152.

Karno, M., & Golding, J. M. (1991). Obsessive compulsive disorder. In L. N. Robins & D. A. Regier (Eds.), *Psychiatric disorders in America: The Epidemiologic Catchment Area Study* (pp. 204–219). New York: Free Press.

Karno, M., Golding, J. M., Sorenson, S. B., & Burnam, A. (1988). The epidemiology of obsessive–compulsive disorder in five US communities. *Archives of General Psychiatry, 45,* 1094–1099.

Kashyap, H., Kumar, J. K., Kandavel, T., & Reddy, Y. C. J. (2017). Relationships between neuropsychological variables and factor-analysed symptom dimensions in obsessive–compulsive disorder. *Psychiatry Research, 249,* 58–64.

Kazantzis, N., Dattilio, F. M., & Dobson, K. S. (2017). *The therapeutic relationship in cognitive-behavioral therapy: A clinician's guide.* New York: Guilford Press.

Kazantzis, N., Tee, J. M., Dattilio, F. M., & Dobson, K. S. (2013). How to develop collaborative empiricism in cognitive behavior therapy: Conclusions from the C & BP special series. *Cognitive and Behavioral Practice, 20,* 455–460.

Keeley, M. L., Storch, E. A., Merlo, L. J., & Geffken, G. R. (2008). Clinical predictors of response to cognitive-behavioral therapy for obsessive–compulsive disorder. *Clinical Psychology Review, 28,* 118–130.

Kendell, R. E., & Discipio, W. J. (1970). Obsessional symptoms and obsessional personality traits in patients with depressive illness. *Psychological Medicine, 1,* 65–72.

Kennedy, S. M., Grossman, R. A., & Ehrenreich-May, J. (2016). Revisiting the factor structure of the White Bear Suppression Inventory in adolescents: An exploratory structural equation modeling approach. *Personality and Individual Differences, 92,* 186–190.

Key, B., & Bieling, P. J. (2015). Beyond DSM diagnosis: The pros and cons of cognitive case formulation. In G. P. Brown & D. A. Clark (Eds.), *Assessment in cognitive therapy* (pp. 221–239). New York: Guilford Press.

Kichuk, S. A., Torres, A. R., Fontenelle, L. F., Rosário, M. C., Shavitt, R. G., Miguel, E. C., et al. (2013). Symptom dimensions are associated with age of onset and clinical course of obsessive–compulsive disorder. *Progress in Neuro-Psychopharmacology and Biological Psychiatry, 44,* 233–239.

Kikul, J., van Allen, T. S., & Exner, C. (2012). Underlying mechanisms of verbal memory deficits in obsessive–compulsive disorder and major depression: The role of cognitive self-consciousness. *Journal of Behavior Therapy and Experimental Psychiatry, 43,* 863–870.

Killingsworth, M. A., & Gilbert, D. T. (2010). A wandering mind is an unhappy mind. *Science, 330,* 932.

Kim, S.-K., McKay, D., Taylor, S., Tolin, D., Olatunji, B., Timpano, K., et al. (2016). The structure of obsessive compulsive symptoms and beliefs: A correspondence and biplot analysis. *Journal of Anxiety Disorders, 38,* 79–87.

Kitis, A., Akdede, B. B. K., Alptekin, K., Akvardar, Y., Arkar, H., Erol, A., et al. (2007). Cognitive dysfunctions in patients with obsessive–compulsive compared to the patients with schizophrenia patients: Relation to overvalued ideas. *Progress in Neuro-Psychopharmacology and Biological Psychiatry, 31,* 254–262.

Kline, P. (1968). Obsessional traits, obsessional symptoms and anal eroticism. *British Journal of Medical Psychology, 41,* 299–304.

Knopp, J., Knowles, S., Bee, P., Lovell, K., & Bower, P. (2013). A systematic review of predictors and moderators of response to psychological theories in OCD: Do we have enough empirical evidence to target treatment? *Clinical Psychology Review, 33,* 1967–1081.

Kobori, O., & Salkovskis, P. M. (2013). Patterns of reassurance seeking and reassurance–related behaviours in OCD and anxiety disorders. *Behavioural and Cognitive Psychotherapy, 41,* 1–23.

Kobori, O., Salkovskis, P. M., Read, J., Lounes, N., & Wong, V. (2012). A qualitative study of the investigation of reassurance seeking in obsessive–compulsive disorder. *Journal of Obsessive–Compulsive and Related Disorders, 1,* 25–32.

Kobori, O., Sawamiya, Y., Iyo, M., & Shimizu, E. (2015). A comparison of manifestations and impact of reassurance seeking among Japanese individuals with OCD and depression. *Behavioural and Cognitive Psychotherapy, 43,* 623–634.

Koch, J., & Exner, C. (2015). Selective attention deficits in obsessive–compulsive disorder: The role of metacognitive processes. *Psychiatry Research, 225,* 550–555.

Koob, G. F., & Le Moal, M. (2005). Plasticity of reward neurocircuitry and the "dark side" of drug addiction. *Nature Neuroscience, 8,* 1442–1444.

Kozak, M. J., & Foa, E. B. (1994). Obsessions, overvalued ideas, and delusions in obsessive–compulsive disorder. *Behaviour Research and Therapy, 32,* 343–353.

Kozak, M. J., & Foa, E. B. (1997). *Mastery of obsessive–compulsive disorder: A cognitive-behavioral approach—therapist guide.* San Antonio, TX: Graywind.

Krans, J., de Bree, J., & Moulds, M. L. (2015). Involuntary cognitions in everyday life: Exploration of type, quality, content, and function. *Frontiers in Psychiatry, 6*(Article No. 7), 1–11.

Kringlen, E., Torgersen, S., & Cramer, V. (2001). A Norwegian psychiatric epidemiological study. *American Journal of Psychiatry, 158,* 1091–1098.

Krochmalik, A., Jones, M. K., & Menzies, R. G. (2001). Danger ideation reduction therapy (DIRT) for treatment-resistant compulsive washing. *Behaviour Research and Therapy, 39,* 897–912.

Krochmalik, A., Jones, M. K., Menzies, R. G., & Kirkby, K. (2004). The superiority of danger ideation reduction therapy (DIRT) over exposure and response prevention (ERP) in treating compulsive washing. *Behaviour Change, 21,* 252–268.

Kühn, S., Vanderhasselt, M.-A., De Raedt, R., & Gallinat, J. (2014). The neural basis of unwanted thoughts during resting state. *Social Cognitive and Affective Neuroscience, 9,* 1320–1324.

Kusunoki, T., Sato, C., Taga, T., Yoshida, K., Komori, T., Narita, S., et al. (2000). Low novelty-seeking differentiates obsessive–compulsive disorder from major depression. *Acta Psychiatrica Scandinavica, 101,* 403–405.

Ladouceur, R., Freeston, M. H., Rhéaume, J., Dugas, M. J., Gagnon, F., Thibodeau, N., et al. (2000). Strategies used with intrusive thoughts: A comparison of OCD patients with anxious and community controls. *Journal of Abnormal Psychology, 109,* 179–187.

Langlois, F., Freeston, M. H., & Ladouceur, R. (2000a). Differences and similarities between obsessive intrusive thoughts and worry in a non-clinical population: Study 1. *Behaviour Research and Therapy, 38,* 157–173.

Langlois, F., Freeston, M. H., & Ladouceur, R. (2000b). Differences and similarities between obsessive intrusive thoughts and worry in a non-clinical population: Study 2. *Behaviour Research and Therapy, 38,* 175–189.

Laposa, J. M., Collimore, K. C., Hawley, L. L., & Rector, N. A. (2015). Distress tolerance in OCD and anxiety disorders, and its relationship with anxiety sensitivity and intolerance of uncertainty. *Journal of Anxiety Disorders, 33,* 8–14.

Lázaro, L., Calvo, A., Ortiz, A. G., Ortiz, A. E., Morer, A., Moreno, E., et al. (2014). Microstructural brain abnormalities and symptom dimensions in child and adolescent patients with obsessive–compulsive disorder: A diffusion tensor imaging study. *Depression and Anxiety, 31,* 1007–1017.

Lazarov, A., Dar, R., Oded, Y., & Liberman, N. (2010). Are obsessive–compulsive tendencies related to reliance on external proxies for internal states?: Evidence from biofeedback-aided relaxation studies. *Behaviour Research and Therapy, 48,* 561–523.

Leahy, R. L. (2001). *Overcoming resistance in cognitive therapy.* New York: Guilford Press.

Leahy, R. L. (2018). *The jealousy cure: Learn to trust, overcome possessiveness, and save your relationship.* Oakland, CA: New Harbinger.

Leckman, J. F. (1993). Tourette's syndrome. In E. Hollander (Ed.), *Obsessive–compulsive-related disorders* (pp. 113–137). Washington, DC: American Psychiatric Association.

Leckman, J. F., Denys, D., Simpson, H. B., Mataix-Cols, D., Hollander, E., Saxena, S., et al. (2010). Obsessive–compulsive disorder: A review of the diagnostic criteria and possible subtypes and dimensional specifiers for DSM-V. *Depression and Anxiety, 27*, 507–527.

Leckman, J. F., Grice, D. E., Boardman, J., Zhang, H., Vitale, A., Bondi, C., et al. (1997). Symptoms of obsessive–compulsive disorder. *American Journal of Psychiatry, 154*, 911–917.

Leckman, J. F., McDougle, C. J., Pauls, D. L., Peterson, B. S., Grice, D. E., King, R. A., et al. (2000). Tic-related versus non-tic-related obsessive–compulsive disorder. In W. K. Goodman, M. V. Rudorfer, & J. D. Maser (Eds.), *Obsessive–compulsive disorder: Contemporary issues in treatment* (pp. 43–68). Mahwah, NJ: Erlbaum.

Lee, H.-J., & Kwon, S.-M. (2003). Two different types of obsession: Autogenous obsessions and reactive obsessions. *Behaviour Research and Therapy, 41*, 11–29.

Lee, H.-J., Kwon, S.-M., Kwon, J. S., & Telch, M. J. (2005). Testing the autogenous–reactive model of obsessions. *Depression and Anxiety, 21*, 118–129.

Lee, H.-J., Lee, S.-H., Kim, H. S., Kwon, S.-M., & Telch, M. J. (2005). A comparison of autogenous/reactive obsessions and worry in a nonclinical population: A test of the continuum hypothesis. *Behaviour Research and Therapy, 43*, 999–1010.

Lelliott, P. T., Noshirvani, H. F., Basoglu, M., Marks, I. M., & Monteiro, W. O. (1988). Obsessive–compulsive beliefs and treatment outcome. *Psychological Medicine, 18*, 697–702.

Lemmens, L. H. J. M., Galindo-Garre, F., Arntz, A., Peeters, F., Hollon, S. D., DeRubeis, R. J., et al. (2017). Exploring mechanisms of change in cognitive therapy and interpersonal psychotherapy for adult depression. *Behaviour Research and Therapy, 94*, 81–92.

Lensi, P., Cassano, G. B., Correddu, G., Ravagli, S., Kunovac, J. L., & Akiskal, H. S. (1996). Obsessive–compulsive disorder: Familial-developmental history, symptomatology, comorbidity and course with special reference to gender-related differences. *British Journal of Psychiatry, 169*, 101–107.

Leonard, H. L., Goldberger, E. L., Rapoport, J. L., Cheslow, D. L., & Swedo, S. E. (1990). Childhood rituals: Normal development or obsessive–compulsive symptoms? *Journal of the American Academy of Child and Adolescent Psychiatry, 29*, 17–23.

Leonard, R. C., & Riemann, B. C. (2012). The co-occurrence of obsessions and compulsions in OCD. *Journal of Obsessive–Compulsive and Related Disorders, 1*, 211–215.

Levine, A. Z., & Warman, D. M. (2016). Appraisals of and recommendations for managing intrusive thoughts: An empirical investigation. *Psychiatry Research, 245*, 207–216.

Lewis, A. (1936). Problems of obsessional illness. *Proceedings of the Royal Society of Medicine, 24*, 13–24.

Leyro, T. M., Zvolensky, M. J., & Bernstein, A. (2010). Distress tolerance and psychopathological symptoms and disorders: A review of the empirical literature among adults. *Psychological Bulletin, 136,* 576–600.

Li, Y., Marques, L., Hinton, D. E., Wang, Y., & Xiao, Z.-P. (2009). Symptom dimensions in Chinese patients with obsessive–compulsive disorder. *CNS Neuroscience and Therapeutics, 15,* 276–282.

Lo, W. H. (1967). A follow-up of obsessional neurotics in Hong Kong Chinese. *British Journal of Psychiatry, 113,* 823–832.

Lochner, C., Fineberg, N. A., Zohar, J., van Ameringen, M., Juven-Wetzler, A., Carlo, A., et al. (2014). Comorbidity in obsessive–compulsive disorder (OCD): A report from the International College of Obsessive–Compulsive Spectrum Disorders (ICOCS). *Comprehensive Psychiatry, 55,* 1513–1519.

Lochner, C., Grant, J. E., Odlaug, B. L., Woods, D. W., Keuthen, N. J., & Stein, D. J. (2012). DSM-5 field survey: Hair-pulling disorder (trichotillomania). *Depression and Anxiety, 29,* 1011–1025.

Lopatka, C., & Rachman, S. (1995). Perceived responsibility and compulsive checking: An experimental analysis. *Behaviour Research and Therapy, 33,* 673–684.

López-Solà, C., Fontenelle, L. F., Verhulst, B., Neale, M. C., Menchón, J. M., Alonso, P., et al. (2016). Distinct etiological influences on obsessive–compulsive symptom dimensions: A multivariate twin study. *Depression and Anxiety, 33,* 179–191.

Lorenzo-Luaces, L., DeRubeis, R. J., & Webb, C. A. (2014). Client characteristics as moderators of the relation between the therapeutic alliance and outcome in cognitive therapy for depression. *Journal of Consulting and Clinical Psychology, 82,* 368–373.

Ludvik, D., Boschen, M. J., & Neumann, D. L. (2015). Effective behavioural strategies for reducing disgust in contamination-related OCD: A review. *Clinical Psychology Review, 42,* 116–129.

Lynch, T. R., Schneider, K. G., Rosenthal, M. Z., & Cheavens, J. S. (2007). A mediational model of trait negativity affectivity, dispositional thought suppression, and intrusive thoughts following laboratory stressors. *Behaviour Research and Therapy, 45,* 749–761.

Lyon, A. R., Connors, E., Jenssen-Doss, A., Landes, S. J., Lewsi, C. C., McLeod, B. D., et al. (2017). Intentional research design in implementation science: Implications for the use of nomothetic and idiographic assessment. *Translational Behavioral Medicine, 7,* 567–580.

Macatee, R. J., Allan, N. P., Gajewska, A., Norr, A. M., Raines, A. M., Albanese, B. J., et al. (2016). Shared and distinct cognitive/affective mechanisms in intrusive cognition: An examination of worry and obsessions. *Cognitive Therapy and Research, 40,* 80–91.

Macatee, R. J., Capron, D. W., Schmidt, N. B., & Cougle, J. R. (2013). An examination of low distress tolerance and life stressors as factors underlying obsessions. *Journal of Psychiatric Research, 47,* 1462–1468.

Macatee, R. J., & Cougle, J. R. (2015). Development and evaluation of a computerized intervention for low distress tolerance and its effect on performance on a neutralization task. *Journal of Behavior Therapy and Experimental Psychiatry, 48,* 33–39.

MacLeod, C. (1993). Cognition in clinical psychology: Measures, methods or models? *Behaviour Change, 10,* 169–195.

Magee, J. C., Harden, K. P., & Teachman, B. A. (2012). Psychopathology and thought suppression: A quantitative review. *Clinical Psychology Review, 32,* 189–201.

Magee, J. C., & Teachman, B. A. (2007). Why did the white bear return?: Obsessive–compulsive symptoms and attributions for unsuccessful thought suppression. *Behaviour Research and Therapy, 45,* 2884–2898.

Mancini, F., Gangemi, A., Perdighe, C., & Marini, C. (2008). Not just right experience: Is it influenced by feelings of guilt? *Journal of Behavior Therapy and Experimental Psychiatry, 39,* 162–176.

Mancini, F., Gragnani, A., & D'Olimpio, F. (2001). The connection between disgust and obsessions and compulsions in a non-clinical sample. *Personality and Individual Differences, 31,* 1173–1180.

Mantz, S. C., & Abbott, M. J. (2017). The relationship between responsibility beliefs and symptoms and processes in obsessive compulsive disorder: A systematic review. *Journal of Obsessive–Compulsive and Related Disorders, 14,* 13–26.

March, J. S., & Mulle, K. (1998). *OCD in children and adolescents: A cognitive-behavioral treatment manual.* New York: Guilford Press.

Marcks, B. A., & Woods, D. W. (2007). Role of thought-related beliefs and coping strategies in the escalation of intrusive thoughts: An analog to obsessive-compulsive disorder. *Behaviour Research and Therapy, 45,* 2640–2651.

Marker, C. D., Calamari, J. E., Woodward, J. L., & Riemann, B. C. (2006). Cognitive self-consciousness, implicit learning and obsessive–compulsive disorder. *Journal of Anxiety Disorders, 20,* 389–407.

Marks, I. M., O'Dwyer, A. M., Meehan, O., Greist, J., Baer, L., & McGuire, P. (2000). Subjective imagery in obsessive–compulsive disorder before and after exposure therapy. *British Journal of Psychiatry, 176,* 387–391.

Martinelli, M., Chasson, G. S., Wetterneck, C. T., Hart, J. M., & Björgvinsson, T. (2014). Perfectionism dimensions as predictors of symptom dimensions of obsessive–compulsive disorder. *Bulletin of the Menninger Clinic, 78,* 140–159.

Mason, M. F., Norton, M. I., Van Horn, J. D., Wegner, D. M., Grafton, S. T., & Macrae, C. N. (2007). Wandering minds: The default network and stimulus-independent thought. *Science, 315,* 393–395.

Mataix-Cols, D., do Rosario-Campos, M., & Leckman, J. F. (2005). A multidimensional model of obsessive–compulsive disorder. *American Journal of Psychiatry, 162,* 228–238.

Mataix-Cols, D., Marks, I. M., Greist, J. H., Kobak, K. A., & Baer, L. (2002). Obsessive–compulsive symptom dimensions as predictors of compliance with and response to behavior therapy: Results from a controlled trial. *Psychotherapy and Psychosomatics, 71,* 255–262.

Mataix-Cols, D., Pertusa, A., & Leckman, J. F. (2007). Issues for DSM-V: How should obsessive–compulsive and related disorders be classified? *American Journal of Psychiatry, 164,* 1313–1314.

Mathews, A. (1990). Why worry?: The cognitive function of worry. *Behaviour Research and Therapy, 28,* 455–468.

Matsunaga, H., Hayashida, K., Kiriike, N., Maebayashi, K., & Stein, D. J. (2010). The clinical utility of symptom dimensions in obsessive–compulsive disorder. *Psychiatry Research, 180,* 25–29.

McCarty, R. J., Guzick, A. G., Swan, L. K., & McNamara, J. P. H. (2017). Stigma and recognition of different types of symptoms in OCD. *Journal of Obsessive–Compulsive and Related Disorders, 12,* 64–70.

McFall, M. E., & Wollersheim, J. P. (1979). Obsessive–compulsive neurosis: A cognitive-behavioral formulation and approach to treatment. *Cognitive Therapy and Research, 3,* 333–348.

McHugh, R. K., & Barlow, D. H. (2010). The dissemination and implementation of evidenced-based psychological treatments: A review of current affairs. *American Psychologist, 65,* 73–84.

McKay, D. (2006). Treating disgust reactions in contamination-based obsessive–compulsive disorder. *Journal of Behavior Therapy and Experimental Psychiatry, 37,* 53–59.

McKay, D., Abramowitz, J. S., Calamari, J. E., Kyrios, M., Radomsky, A., Sookman, D., et al. (2004). A critical evaluation of obsessive–compulsive disorder subtypes: Symptoms versus mechanisms. *Clinical Psychology Review, 24,* 282–313.

McKay, D., Sookman, D., Neziroglu, F., Wilhelm, S., Stein, D. J., Kyrios, M., et al. (2015). Efficacy of cognitive-behavioral therapy for obsessive–compulsive disorder. *Psychiatry Research, 225,* 236–246.

McNally, R. J. (2001). On the scientific status of cognitive appraisal models of anxiety disorder. *Behaviour Research and Therapy, 39,* 513–521.

McNally, R. J., Mair, P., Mugno, B. L., & Riemann, B. C. (2017). Co-morbid obsessive–compulsive disorder and depression: A Bayesian network approach. *Psychological Medicine, 47,* 1204–1214.

Meier, S. M., Mattheisen, M., Mors, O., Schendel, D. E., Mortensen, P. B., & Kerstin, J. P. (2016). Mortality among persons with obsessive–compulsive disorder in Denmark. *JAMA Psychiatry, 73,* 268–274.

Meiran, N., Diamond, G. M., Toder, D., & Nemets, B. (2011). Cognitive rigidity in unipolar depression and obsessive compulsive disorder: Examination of task switching, Stroop, working memory updating and post-conflict adaptation. *Psychiatry Research, 185,* 149–156.

Melca, I. A., Yücel, M., Mendlowicz, M. V., de Oliveira-Souza, R., & Fontenelle, L. F. (2015). The correlates of obsessive–compulsive, schizotypal, and borderline personality disorders in obsessive–compulsive disorder. *Journal of Anxiety Disorders, 33,* 15–24.

Melli, G., Aardema, F., & Moulding, R. (2016). Fear of self and unacceptable thoughts in obsessive–compulsive disorder. *Clinical Psychology and Psychotherapy, 23,* 226–235.

Melli, G., Avallone, E., Moulding, R., Pinto, A., Micheli, E., & Carraresi, C. (2015). Validation of the Italian version of the Yale–Brown Obsessive–Compulsive Scale— Second Edition (Y-BOCS-II) in a clinical sample. *Comprehensive Psychiatry, 60,* 86–92.

Melli, G., Bulli, F., Carraresi, C., & Stopani, E. (2014). Disgust propensity and contamination-related OCD symptoms: The mediating role of mental contamination. *Journal of Obsessive–Compulsive and Related Disorders, 3,* 77–82.

Melli, G., Gremigni, P., Elwood, L. S., Stopani, E., Bulli, F., & Carraresi, C. (2015). The relationship between trait guilt, disgust propensity, and contamination fear. *International Journal of Cognitive Therapy, 8,* 193–205.

Meyer, J. F., & Brown, T. A. (2012). Psychometric evaluation of the Thought–Action Fusion Scale in a large clinical sample. *Assessment, 20,* 764–775.

Meyer, V. (1966). Modifications of expectations in cases with obsessional rituals. *Behaviour Research and Therapy, 4,* 273–280.

Meyer, V., Levy, R., & Schnurer, A. (1974). The behavioural treatment of obsessive-compulsive disorders. In H. R. Beech (Ed.), *Obsessional states* (pp. 233–258). London: Methuen.

Michael, T., Ehlers, A., Halligan, S. L., & Clark, D. M. (2005). Unwanted memories of assault: What intrusion characteristics are associated with PTSD? *Behaviour Research and Therapy, 43,* 613–628.

Michel, N. M., Rowa, K., Young, L., & McCabe, R. E. (2016). Emotional distress tolerance across anxiety disorders. *Journal of Anxiety Disorders, 40,* 94–103.

Michl, L. C., McLaughlin, K. A., Shepherd, K., & Nolen-Hoeksema, S. (2013). Rumination as a mechanism linking stressful life events to symptoms of depression and anxiety: Longitudinal evidence in early adolescents and adults. *Journal of Abnormal Psychology, 122,* 339–352.

Miller, E. S., Hoxha, D., Wisner, K. L., & Gossett, D. R. (2015). Obsessions and compulsions in postpartum women without obsessive compulsive disorder. *Journal of Women's Health, 24,* 825–830.

Miller, P. R. (2002). Inpatient diagnostic assessments: 3. Causes and effects of diagnostic imprecision. *Psychiatry Research, 111,* 191–197.

Miller, P. R., Dasher, R., Collins, R., Griffiths, P., & Brown, F. (2001). Inpatient diagnostic assessments: 1. Accuracy of structured vs. unstructured interviews. *Psychiatry Research, 105,* 255–264.

Miller, W. S., & Rollnick, S. (2013). *Motivational interviewing: Helping people change* (3rd ed.). New York: Guilford Press.

Monzani, B., Rijsdijk, F., Harris, J., & Mataix-Cols, D. (2014). The structure of genetic and environmental risk factors for dimensional representations of *DSM-5* obsessive–compulsive spectrum disorders. *JAMA Psychiatry, 71,* 182–189.

Moretz, M. W., & McKay, D. (2008). Disgust sensitivity as a predictor of obsessive-compulsive contamination symptoms and associated cognitions. *Journal of Anxiety Disorders, 22,* 707–715.

Moretz, M. W., & McKay, D. (2009). The role of perfectionism in obsessive-compulsive symptoms: "Not just right" experiences and checking symptoms. *Journal of Anxiety Disorders, 23,* 640–644.

Morewedge, C. K., Giblin, C. E., & Norton, M. I. (2014). The (perceived) meaning of spontaneous thoughts. *Journal of Experimental Psychology: General, 143,* 1742–1754.

Morillo, C., Belloch, A., & García-Soriano, G. (2007). Clinical obsessions in obsessive–compulsive patients and obsession-relevant intrusive thoughts in non-clinical, depressed and anxious subjects: Where are the differences? *Behaviour Research and Therapy, 45,* 1319–1333.

Morina, N., Sulaj, V., Schnyder, U., Klaghofer, R., Müller, J., Martin-Sölch, C., et al. (2016). Obsessive–compulsive and posttraumatic stress symptoms among civilian survivors of war. *BMC Psychiatry, 16,* 115.

Moritz, S., Purdon, C., Jelinek. L., Chiang, B., & Hauschildt, M. (2017). If it is absurd, then why do you do it?: The richer the obsessional experience, the more compelling the compulsion. *Clinical Psychology and Psychotherapy, 25,* 210–216.

Moulding, R., Aardema, F., & O'Connor, K. P. (2014). Repugnant obsessions: A review of the phenomenology, theoretical models, and treatment of sexual and aggressive obsessional themes in OCD. *Journal of Obsessive–Compulsive and Related Disorders, 3,* 161–168.

Moulding, R., Anglim, J., Nedeljkovic, M., Doron, G., Kyrios, M., & Ayalon, A. (2011). The Obsessive Beliefs Questionnaire (OBQ): Examination in nonclinical samples and development of a short version. *Assessment, 18,* 357–374.

Moulding, R., Kyrios, M., Doron, G., & Nedeljkovic, M. (2007). Autogenous and reactive obsessions: Further evidence for a two-factor model of obsessions. *Journal of Anxiety Disorders, 21,* 677–690.

Mowrer, O. H. (1939). A stimulus–response analysis of anxiety and its role as a reinforcing agent. *Psychological Review, 46,* 553–565.

Mowrer, O. H. (1953). Neurosis, psychotherapy, and two-factor learning theory. In O. H. Mowrer (Ed.), *Psychotherapy theory and research* (pp. 140–149). New York: Ronald Press.

Mowrer, O. H. (1960). *Learning theory and behavior.* New York: Wiley.

Muris, P., Merckelbach, H., & Clavan, M. (1997). Abnormal and normal compulsions. *Behaviour Research and Therapy, 35,* 249–252.

Muris, P., Merckelbach, H., & Horselenberg, R. (1996). Individual differences on thought suppression: The White Bear Suppression Inventory—factor structure, reliability, validity and correlates. *Behaviour Research and Therapy, 34,* 501–513.

Myers, S. G., Fisher, P. L., & Wells, A. (2008). Belief domains of the Obsessive Beliefs Questionnaire–44 (OBQ-44) and their specific relationship with obsessive–compulsive symptoms. *Journal of Anxiety Disorders, 22,* 475–484.

Myers, S. G., Grøtte, T., Haseth, S., Guzey, I. C., Hansen, B., Vogel, P. A., et al. (2017). The role of metacognitive beliefs about thoughts and rituals: A test of the metacognitive model of obsessive–compulsive disorder in a clinical sample. *Journal of Obsessive–Compulsive and Related Disorders, 13,* 1–6.

Najmi, S., Reese, H., Wilhelm, S., Fama, J., Beck, C., & Wegner, D. M. (2010). Learning the futility of the thought suppression enterprise in normal experience and in obsessive compulsive disorder. *Behavioural and Cognitive Psychotherapy, 38,* 1–14.

Najmi, S., Riemann, B. C., & Wegner, D. M. (2009). Managing unwanted intrusive thoughts in obsessive–compulsive disorder: Relative effectiveness of suppression, focused attention, and acceptance. *Behaviour Research and Therapy, 47,* 494–503.

Najmi, S., & Wegner, D. M. (2008). The gravity of unwanted thoughts: Asymmetric priming effects in thought suppression. *Consciousness and Cognition, 17,* 114–124.

Nakagawa, A., Marks, I. M., Takei, N., De Araujo, L. A., & Ito, L. M. (1996). Comparisons among the Yale–Brown Obsessive–Compulsive Scale, Compulsion Checklist, and other measures of obsessive–compulsive disorder. *British Journal of Psychiatry, 169,* 108–112.

National Institute of Health Care and Excellence. (2005). Obsessive–compulsive disorder and body dysmorphic disorder: Treatment. Clinical guideline [CG31].

Retrieved June 7, 2018, from *www.nice.org.uk/guidance/CG31/chapter/1-Guidance#steps-35-treatment-options-for-people-with-ocd-or-bdd*.

Nestadt, G., Samuels, J. F., Romanoski, A. J., Folstein, M. F., & McHugh, P. R. (1994). Obsessions and compulsions in the community. *Acta Psychiatrica Scandinavica, 89,* 219–224.

Newby, J. M., & Moulds, M. L. (2011). Do negative appraisals and avoidance of intrusive memories predict depression at six months? *International Journal of Cognitive Therapy, 4,* 178–186.

Newth, S., & Rachman, S. (2001). The concealment of obsessions. *Behaviour Research and Therapy, 39,* 457–464.

Neziroglu, F., Anemone, R., & Yaryura-Tobias, J. A. (1992). Onset of obsessive–compulsive disorder in pregnancy. *American Journal of Psychiatry, 149,* 947–950.

Neziroglu, F., McKay, D., Yaryura-Tobias, J. A., Stevens, K. P., & Todaro, J. (1999). The overvalued ideas scale: Development, reliability and validity in obsessive–compulsive disorder. *Behaviour Research and Therapy, 37,* 881–902.

Neziroglu, F., & Stevens, K. P. (2002). Insight: Its conceptualization and assessment. In R. O. Frost & G. Steketee (Eds.), *Cognitive approaches to obsessions and compulsions: Theory, assessment and treatment* (pp. 183–193). Oxford, UK: Elsevier.

Neziroglu, F., Stevens, K. P., McKay, D., & Yaryura-Tobia, J. A. (2001). Predictive validity of the Overvalued Ideas Scale: Outcome in obsessive–compulsive and body dysmorphic disorders. *Behaviour Research and Therapy, 39,* 745–756.

Nicholson, E., & Barnes-Holmes, D. (2012). Developing an implicit measure of disgust propensity and disgust sensitivity: Examining the role of implicit disgust propensity and sensitivity in obsessive–compulsive tendencies. *Journal of Behavior Therapy and Experimental Psychiatry, 43,* 922–930.

Nikodijevic, A., Moulding, R., Anglim, J., Aardema, F., & Nedeljkovic, M. (2015). Fear of self, doubt and obsessive compulsive symptoms. *Journal of Behavior Therapy and Experimental Psychiatry, 49,* 164–172.

Nolen-Hoeksema, S. (1991). Responses to depression and their effects on the duration of depressive episodes. *Journal of Abnormal Psychology, 100,* 569–582.

Nolen-Hoeksema, S. (2000). The role of rumination in depressive disorders and mixed anxiety/depressive symptoms. *Journal of Abnormal Psychology, 109,* 504–511.

Nolen-Hoeksema, S., Parker, L. E., & Larson, J. (1994). Ruminative coping with depressed mood following loss. *Journal of Personality and Social Psychology, 67,* 92–104.

Norcross, J. C., & Wampold, B. E. (2011). Evidenced-based therapy relationships: Research conclusions and clinical practices. *Psychotherapy, 48,* 98–102.

Nota, J. A., Schubert, J. R., & Coles, M. E. (2016). Sleep disruption is related to poor response inhibition in individuals with obsessive–compulsive and repetitive negative thought symptoms. *Journal of Behavior Therapy and Experimental Psychiatry, 50,* 23–32.

Obsessive Compulsive Cognitions Working Group. (1997). Cognitive assessment of obsessive–compulsive disorder. *Behaviour Research and Therapy, 35,* 667–681.

Obsessive Compulsive Cognitions Working Group. (2001). Development and ini-

tial validation of the Obsessive Beliefs Questionnaire and the Interpretation of Intrusions Inventory. *Behaviour Research and Therapy, 39,* 987–1006.
Obsessive Compulsive Cognitions Working Group. (2003). Psychometric validation of the Obsessive Beliefs Questionnaire and the Interpretation of Intrusions Inventory: Part 1. *Behaviour Research and Therapy, 41,* 863–878.
Obsessive Compulsive Cognitions Working Group. (2005). Psychometric validation of the obsessive beliefs questionnaire and the interpretation of intrusions inventory: Part 2. Factor analyses and testing of a brief version. *Behaviour Research and Therapy, 43,* 1527–1542.
O'Connor, K. (2002). Intrusions and inferences in obsessive compulsive disorder. *Clinical Psychology and Psychotherapy, 9,* 38–46.
O'Connor, K. (2009). Book review of *DIRT—danger ideation reduction therapy for obsessive–compulsive washers: A comprehensive guide to treatment. Clinical Psychology and Psychotherapy, 16,* 463–465.
O'Connor, K., & Aardema, F. (2012). *Clinician's handbook for obsessive compulsive disorder.* Chichester, UK: Wiley-Blackwell.
O'Connor, K., Aardema, F., & Pélissier, M.-C. (2005). *Beyond reasonable doubt: Reasoning in obsessive–compulsive disorder and related disorders.* Chichester, UK: Wiley.
O'Connor, K., Freeston, M. H., Gareau, D., Careau, Y., Dufour, M. J., Aardema, R., et al. (2005). Group versus individual treatment in obsessions without compulsions. *Clinical Psychology and Psychotherapy, 12,* 87–96.
O'Connor, K. P., & Robillard, S. (1995). Inference processes in obsessive–compulsive disorder: Some clinical observations. *Behaviour Research and Therapy, 33,* 887–896.
O'Connor, K. P., & Robillard, S. (1999). A cognitive approach to the treatment of primary inferences in obsessive–compulsive disorder. *Journal of Cognitive Psychotherapy: An International Quarterly, 13,* 359–375.
O'Dwyer, A.-M., & Marks, I. (2000). Obsessive–compulsive disorder and delusions revisited. *British Journal of Psychiatry, 176,* 281–284.
Okasha, A., Saad, A., Khalil, A. H., Dawla, S. E., & Yehia, N. (1994). Phenomenology of obsessive–compulsive disorder: A transcultural study. *Comprehensive Psychiatry, 25,* 191–197.
Ólafsson, R. P., Emmelkamp, P. M. G., Gunnarsdóttir, E. R., Snaebjörnsson, T., Ólason, D. T., & Kristjánsson, Á. (2013). Suppressing disgust-related thoughts and performance on a subsequent behavioural avoidance task: Implications for OCD. *Behaviour Research and Therapy, 51,* 152–160.
Ólafsson, R. P., Snorrason, Í., Bjarnason, R. K., Emmelkamp, P. M. G., Ólason, D. T., & Kristjánsson, Á. (2014). Replacing intrusive thoughts: Investigating thought control in relation to OCD symptoms. *Journal of Behavior Therapy and Experimental Psychiatry, 45,* 506–515.
Olatunji, B. O. (2010). Changes in disgust correspond with changes in symptoms of contamination-based OCD: A prospective examination of specificity. *Journal of Anxiety Disorders, 24,* 313–317.
Olatunji, B. O., Cisler, J. M., Deacon, B. J., Connolly, K., & Lohr, J. M. (2007). The Disgust Propensity and Sensitivity Scale—Revised: Psychometric properties and specificity in relation to anxiety disorder symptoms. *Journal of Anxiety Disorders, 21,* 918–930.

Olatunji, B. O., Davis, M. L., Powers, M. B., & Smits, J. A. J. (2013). Cognitive-behavioral therapy for obsessive–compulsive disorder: A meta-analysis of treatment outcome and moderators. *Journal of Psychiatric Research, 47,* 33–41.

Olatunji, B. O., Ebesutani, C., & Abramowitz, J. S. (2017). Examination of a bifactor model of obsessive–compulsive symptom dimensions. *Assessment, 24,* 45–59.

Olatunji, B. O., Tart, C. D., Ciesielski, B. G., McGrath, P. B., & Smits, J. A. J. (2011). Specificity of disgust vulnerability in the distinction and treatment of OCD. *Journal of Psychiatric Research, 45,* 1236–1242.

Olatunji, B. O., Williams, N. L., Tolin, D. F., Abramowitz, J. S., Sawchuk, C. N., Lohr, J. M., et al. (2007). The Disgust Scale: Item analysis, factor structure, and suggestions for refinement. *Psychological Assessment, 19,* 281–297.

Olatunji, B. O., Wolitzky-Taylor, K. B., Willems, J., Lohr, J. M., & Armstrong, T. (2009). Differential habituation of fear and disgust during repeated exposure to threat-relevant stimuli in contamination-based OCD: An analogue study. *Journal of Anxiety Disorders, 23,* 118–123.

O'Neill, M. L., Nenzel, M. E., & Caldwell, W. (2009). Intrusive thoughts and psychopathology in a student and incarcerated sample. *Journal of Behavior Therapy and Experimental Psychiatry, 40,* 147–157.

Öst, L.-G., Havnen, A., Hansen, B., & Kvale, G. (2015). Cognitive behavioral treatments of obsessive–compulsive disorder: A systematic review and meta-analysis of studies published 1993–2014. *Clinical Psychology Review, 40,* 156–169.

Overduin, M. K., & Furnham, A. (2012). Assessing obsessive–compulsive disorder (OCD): A review of self-report measures. *Journal of Obsessive–Compulsive and Related Disorders, 1,* 312–324.

Padesky, C. A., & Greenberger, D. (1995). *Clinician's guide to Mind Over Mood.* New York: Guilford Press.

Parkinson, L., & Rachman, S. J. (1981a). Part II: The nature of intrusive thoughts. *Advances in Behaviour Research and Therapy, 3,* 101–110.

Parkinson, L., & Rachman, S. J. (1981b). Part III: Intrusive thoughts: The effects of an uncontrived stress. *Advances in Behaviour Research and Therapy, 3,* 111–118.

Parrish, C. L., & Radomsky, A. S. (2010). Why do people seek reassurance and check repeatedly?: An investigation of factors involved in compulsive behavior in OCD and depression. *Journal of Anxiety Disorders, 24,* 211–222.

Pélissier, M.-C., O'Connor, K. P., & Dupuis, G. (2009). When doubting begins: Exploring inductive reasoning in obsessive–compulsive disorder. *Journal of Behavior Therapy and Experimental Psychiatry, 40,* 39–49.

Persons, J. B. (2008). *The case formulation approach to cognitive-behavior therapy.* New York: Guilford Press.

Phillips, K. A., Stein, D. J., Rauch, S. L., Hollander, E., Fallon, B. A., Barsky, A., et al. (2010). Should an obsessive–compulsive spectrum grouping of disorders be included in DSM-V? *Depression and Anxiety, 27,* 528–555.

Pietrefesa, A. S., & Coles, M. E. (2008). Moving beyond an exclusive focus on harm avoidance in obsessive compulsive disorder: Considering the role of incompleteness. *Behavior Therapy, 39,* 224–231.

Pietrefesa, A. S., & Coles, M. E. (2009). Moving beyond an exclusive focus on harm avoidance in obsessive compulsive disorder: Behavioral validation for the separability of harm avoidance and incompleteness. *Behavior Therapy, 40*, 251–259.

Pinto, A., Greenberg, B. D., Grados, M. A., Bienvenu, O. J., Samuels, J. F., Murphy, D. L., et al. (2008). Further development of YBOCS dimensions in the OCD Collaborative Genetics Study: Symptoms vs. categories. *Psychiatry Research, 160*, 83–93.

Pinto, A., Mancebo, M. C., Eisen, J. L., Pagano, M. E., & Rasmussen, S. A. (2006). The Brown Longitudinal Obsessive Compulsive Study: Clinical features and symptoms of the sample at intake. *Journal of Clinical Psychiatry, 67*, 703–711.

Poerio, G. L., Totterdell, P., & Miles, E. (2013). Mind-wandering and negative mood: Does one thing really lead to another? *Consciousness and Cognition, 22*, 1412–1421.

Pollak, J. M. (1979). Obsessive–compulsive personality: A review. *Psychological Bulletin, 86*, 225–241.

Pollard, C. A., Henderson, J. G., Frank, M., & Margolis, R. B. (1989). Help-seeking patterns of anxiety-disordered individuals in the general population. *Journal of Anxiety Disorders, 3*, 131–138.

Pollitt, J. (1957). Natural history of obsessional states: A study of 150 cases. *British Medical Journal, 1*, 194–198.

Power, M., & Dalgleish, T. (1997). *Cognition and emotion: From order to disorder*. East Sussex, UK: Psychology Press.

Pozza, A., & D[eaccent]ttore, D. (2014). Are inflated responsibility beliefs specific to OCD?: Meta-analysis of the relations of responsibility to OCD, anxiety disorders, and depressive symptoms. *Clinical Neuropsychiatry: Journal of Treatment Evaluation, 11*, 170–181.

Purdon, C. (1999). Thoughts suppression and psychopathology. *Behaviour Research and Therapy, 37*, 1029–1054.

Purdon, C. L. (2001). Appraisal of obsessional thought recurrences: Impact on anxiety and mood state. *Behavior Therapy, 32*, 47–64.

Purdon, C. L. (2004a). Cognitive-behavioral treatment of repugnant obsessions. *Journal of Clinical Psychology, In Session, 60*, 1169–1180.

Purdon, C. L. (2004b). Empirical investigation of thought suppression in OCD. *Journal of Behavior Therapy and Experimental Psychiatry, 35*, 121–136.

Purdon, C. L. (2017, September). *An anatomy of compulsions*. Invited plenary session for the annual convention of the European Association of Behavioural and Cognitive Therapies, Ljubljana, Slovenia.

Purdon, C. L., & Clark, D. A. (1993). Obsessive intrusive thoughts in nonclinical subjects: Part I. Content and relation with depressive, anxious and obsessional symptoms. *Behaviour Research and Therapy, 31*, 713–720.

Purdon, C. L., & Clark, D. A. (1994a). Obsessive intrusive thoughts in nonclinical subjects: Part II. Cognitive appraisal, emotional response and thought control strategies. *Behaviour Research and Therapy, 32*, 403–410.

Purdon, C. L., & Clark, D. A. (1994b). Perceived control and appraisal of obsessional intrusive thoughts: A replication and extension. *Behavioural and Cognitive Psychotherapy, 22*, 269–285.

Purdon, C. L., & Clark, D. A. (1999). Metacognition and obsessions. *Clinical Psychology and Psychotherapy, 6,* 102–110.

Purdon, C. L., & Clark, D. A. (2000). White bears and other elusive intrusions: Assessing the relevance of thought suppression for obsessional phenomena. *Behavior Modification, 24,* 425–453.

Purdon, C. L., & Clark, D. A. (2001). Suppression of obsession-like thoughts in nonclinical individuals: Part I. Impact on thought frequency, appraisal and mood state. *Behaviour Research and Therapy, 39,* 1163–1181.

Purdon, C. L., Cripps, E., Faull, M., Joseph, S., & Rowa, K. (2007). Development of a measure of egodystonicity. *Journal of Cognitive Psychotherapy: An International Quarterly, 21,* 198–216.

Purdon, C. L., Gifford, S., McCabe, R., & Antony, M. M. (2011). Thought dismissibility in obsessive–compulsive disorder versus panic disorder. *Behaviour Research and Therapy, 49,* 646–653.

Purdon, C. L., Rowa, K., & Antony, M. M. (2005). Thought suppression and its effects on thought frequency, appraisal and mood state in individuals with obsessive–compulsive disorder. *Behaviour Research and Therapy, 43,* 93–108.

Purdon, C. L., Rowa, K., & Antony, M. M. (2007). Diary records of thought suppression by individuals with obsessive–compulsive disorder. *Behavioural and Cognitive Psychotherapy, 35,* 47–59.

Rabavilas, A. D., & Boulougouris, J. C. (1974). Physiological accompaniments of ruminations, flooding and thought-stopping in obsessive patients. *Behaviour Research and Therapy, 12,* 239–243.

Rachman, S. J. (1971). Obsessional ruminations. *Behaviour Research and Therapy, 9,* 229–235.

Rachman, S. J. (1974). Primary obsessional slowness. *Behaviour Research and Therapy, 12,* 9–18.

Rachman, S. J. (1976). The modification of obsessions: A new formulation. *Behaviour Research and Therapy, 14,* 437–443.

Rachman, S. J. (1978). An anatomy of obsessions. *Behavioural Analysis and Modification, 2,* 253–278.

Rachman, S. J. (1980). Emotional processing. *Behaviour Research and Therapy, 18,* 51–60.

Rachman, S. J. (1981). Part I: Unwanted intrusive cognitions. *Advances in Behaviour Research and Therapy, 3,* 89–99.

Rachman, S. J. (1983). Obstacles to the successful treatment of obsessions. In E. B. Foa & P. M. G. Emmelkamp (Eds.), *Failures in behavior therapy* (pp. 35–57). New York: Wiley.

Rachman, S. J. (1985). An overview of clinical and research issues in obsessional–compulsive disorders. In M. Mavissakalian, S. M. Turner, & L. Michelson (Eds.), *Obsessive–compulsive disorder: Psychological and pharmacological treatment* (pp. 1–47). New York: Plenum Press.

Rachman, S. J. (1997). A cognitive theory of obsessions. *Behaviour Research and Therapy, 35,* 793–802.

Rachman, S. J. (1998). A cognitive theory of obsessions: Elaborations. *Behaviour Research and Therapy, 36,* 385–401.

Rachman, S. J. (2002). A cognitive theory of compulsive checking. *Behaviour Research and Therapy, 40,* 625–639.

Rachman, S. J. (2003). *The treatment of obsessions*. Oxford, UK: Oxford University Press.

Rachman, S. J. (2004). Fear of contamination. *Behaviour Research and Therapy, 42*, 1227–1255.

Rachman, S. J. (2006). *Fear of contamination: Assessment and treatment*. Oxford, UK: Oxford University Press.

Rachman, S. J. (2007). Unwanted intrusive images in obsessive compulsive disorder. *Journal of Behavior Therapy and Experimental Psychiatry, 38*, 402–410.

Rachman, S. J., Coughtrey, A., Shafran, R., & Radomsky, A. (2015). *Oxford guide to the treatment of mental contamination*. Oxford, UK: Oxford University Press.

Rachman, S. J., & de Silva, P. (1978). Abnormal and normal obsessions. *Behaviour Research and Therapy, 16*, 233–248.

Rachman, S. J., & Hodgson, R. J. (1980). *Obsessions and compulsions*. Englewood Cliffs, NJ: Prentice-Hall.

Rachman, S. J., Hodgson, R., & Marks, I. M. (1971). The treatment of chronic obsessive–compulsive neurosis. *Behaviour Research and Therapy, 9*, 237–247.

Rachman, S. J., Marks, I. M., & Hodgson, R. (1973). The treatment of obsessive-compulsive neurotics by modelling and flooding in vivo. *Behaviour Research and Therapy, 11*, 463–471.

Rachman, S. J., Radomsky, A. S., Elliott, C. M., & Zysk, E. (2012). Mental contamination: The perpetrator effect. *Journal of Behavior Therapy and Experimental Psychiatry, 43*, 587–593.

Rachman, S. J., Radomsky, A. S., & Shafran, R. (2008). Safety behaviour: A reconsideration. *Behaviour Research and Therapy, 46*, 163–173.

Rachman, S. J., & Shafran, R. (1998). Cognitive and behavioral features of obsessive–compulsive disorder. In R. P. Swinson, M. M. Antony, S. J. Rachman, & M. A. Richter (Eds.), *Obsessive–compulsive disorder: Theory, research, and treatment* (pp. 51–78). New York: Guilford Press.

Rachman, S. J., Shafran, R., Mitchell, D., Trant, J., & Teachman, B. (1996). How to remain neutral: An experimental analysis of neutralization. *Behaviour Research and Therapy, 34*, 889–898.

Radomsky, A. S. (2014, June). *Cognitive frontiers in the treatment of OCD: A kinder, gentler CBT*. Keynote address, Congress of the International Association of Cognitive Psychotherapy, Hong Kong.

Radomsky, A. S., Alcolado, G. M., Abramowitz, J. S., Alonso, P., Belloch, A., Bouvard, M., et al. (2014). Part 1: You can run but you can't hide: Intrusive thoughts on six continents. *Journal of Obsessive–Compulsive and Related Disorders, 3*, 269–279.

Radomsky, A. S., Asbaugh, A. R., Gelfand, L. A., & Dugas, M. J. (2008). Doubting and compulsive checking. In J. S. Abramowitz, D. McKay, & S. Taylor (Eds.), *Obsessive–compulsive disorder: Subtypes and spectrum conditions* (pp. 19–35). Amsterdam: Elsevier.

Radomsky, A. S., Coughtrey, A., Shafran, R., & Rachman, S. (2018). Abnormal and normal mental contamination. *Journal of Obsessive–Compulsive and Related Disorders, 17*, 46–51.

Radomsky, A. S., Dugas, M. J., Alcolado, G. M., & Lavoie, S. L. (2014). When

more is less: Doubt, repetition, memory, metamemory, and compulsive checking in OCD. *Behaviour Research and Therapy, 59,* 30–39.
Radomsky, A. S., & Elliott, C. M. (2009). Analyses of mental contamination: Part II. Individual differences. *Behaviour Research and Therapy, 47,* 1004–1011.
Radomsky, A. S., Gilchrist, P. T., & Dussault, D. (2006). Repeated checking really does cause memory distrust. *Behaviour Research and Therapy, 44,* 305–316.
Radomsky, A. S., Ouimet, A. J., Ashbaugh, A. R., Lavoie, S. L., Parrish, C. L., & O'Connor, K. P. (2006). Psychometric properties of the French and English version of the Vancouver Obsessional–Compulsive Inventory and the Symmetry Ordering and Arranging Questionnaire. *Cognitive Behaviour Therapy, 35,* 164–173.
Radomsky, A. S., & Rachman, S. (2004). Symmetry, ordering and arranging compulsive behavior. *Behaviour Research and Therapy, 42,* 893–913.
Radomsky, A. S., Rachman, S., & Hammond, D. (2001). Memory bias, confidence and responsibility in compulsive checking. *Behaviour Research and Therapy, 39,* 813–822.
Radomsky, A. S., Rachman, S., Shafran, R., Coughtrey, A. E., & Barber, K. C. (2014). The nature and assessment of mental contamination: A psychometric analysis. *Journal of Obsessive–Compulsive and Related Disorders, 3,* 181–187.
Radomsky, A. S., & Taylor, S. (2005). Subtyping OCD: Prospects and problems. *Behavior Therapy, 36,* 371–379.
Rafnsson, F. D., & Smári, J. (2001). Chronic thought suppression and obsessionality: The relationships between the White Bear Inventory and two inventories of obsessive–compulsive symptoms. *Personality and Individual Differences, 30,* 159–165.
Raines, A. M., Oglesby, M. E., Allan, N. P., Mathes, B. M., Sutton, C. A., & Schmidt, N. B. (2018). Examining the role of sex differences in obsessive-compulsive symptom dimensions. *Psychiatry Research, 259,* 265–269.
Rasmussen, S. A., & Eisen, J. L. (1992). The epidemiology and clinical features of obsessive compulsive disorder. *Psychiatric Clinics of North America, 15,* 743–758.
Rasmussen, S. A., & Eisen, J. L. (1998). The epidemiology and clinical features of obsessive–compulsive disorder. In M. A. Jenike & W. E. Minichiello (Eds.), *Obsessive–compulsive disorders: Practical management* (pp. 12–43). St. Louis, MO: Mosby.
Rasmussen, S. A., & Tsuang, M. T. (1986). Clinical characteristics and family history in DSM-III obsessive–compulsive disorder. *American Journal of Psychiatry, 143,* 317–322.
Rassin, E. (2005). *Thought suppression.* Amsterdam: Elsevier.
Rassin, E., Cougle, J. R., & Muris, P. (2007). Content differences between normal and abnormal obsessions. *Behaviour Research and Therapy, 45,* 2800–2803.
Rassin, E., Diepstraten, P., Merckelbach, H., & Muris, P. (2001). Thought–action fusion and thought suppression in obsessive–compulsive disorder. *Behaviour Research and Therapy, 39,* 757–764.
Rassin, E., & Koster, E. (2003). The correlation between thought–action fusion and religiosity in a normal sample. *Behaviour Research and Therapy, 41,* 361–368.

Rassin, E., Merckelbach, H., Muris, P., & Schmidt, H. (2001). The Thought–Action Fusion Scale: Further evidence for its reliability and validity. *Behaviour Research and Therapy, 39,* 537–544.

Rassin, E., Merckelbach, H., Muris, P., & Stapert, S. (1999). Suppression and ritualistic behaviour in normal participants. *British Journal of Clinical Psychology, 38,* 195–201.

Rassin, E., & Muris, P. (2006). Abnormal and normal obsessions: A reconsideration. *Behaviour Research and Therapy, 45,* 1065–1070.

Rassin, E., Muris, P., Schmidt, H., & Merckelbach, H. (2000). Relationships between thought–action fusion, thought suppression and obsessive-compulsive symptoms: A structural equation modeling approach. *Behaviour Research and Therapy, 38,* 889–897.

Rector, N. A., Kamkar, K., Cassin, S. E., Ayearst, L. E., & Laposa, J. M. (2011). Assessing excessive reassurance seeking in the anxiety disorders. *Journal of Anxiety Disorders, 25,* 911–917.

Ree, M. J. (2010). The Thought Control Questionnaire in an inpatient psychiatric setting: Psychometric properties and predictive capacity. *Behaviour Change, 27,* 212–226.

Rego, S. A. (2016). *Treatment plans and interventions for obsessive–compulsive disorder.* New York: Guilford Press.

Rettew, D. C., Swedo, S. E., Leonard, H. L., Lenane, M. C., & Rapoport, J. L. (1992). Obsessions and compulsions across time in 79 children and adolescents with obsessive–compulsive disorder. *Journal of the American Academy of Child and Adolescent Psychiatry, 31,* 1050–1056.

Reuven, D., Kahn, D. T., & Carmeli, R. (2012). The relationship between sensory processing, childhood rituals and obsessive–compulsive symptoms. *Journal of Behavior Therapy and Experimental Psychiatry, 43,* 679–684.

Reynolds, M., & Salkovskis, P. M. (1992). Comparison of positive and negative intrusive thoughts and experimental investigation of the differential effects of mood. *Behaviour Research and Therapy, 30,* 273–281.

Reynolds, M., & Wells, A. (1999). The Thought Control Questionnaire: Psychometric properties in a clinical sample, and relationships with PTSD and depression. *Psychological Medicine, 29,* 1089–1099.

Rhéaume, J., Freeston, M. H., Dugas, M. J., Letartte, H., & Ladouceur, R. (1995). Perfectionism, responsibility and obsessive–compulsive symptoms. *Behaviour Research and Therapy, 33,* 785–794.

Rhéaume, J., Freeston, M. H., Léger, E., & Ladouceur, R. (1998). Bad luck: An underestimated factor in the development of obsessive–compulsive disorder. *Clinical Psychology and Psychotherapy, 5,* 1–12.

Ricciardi, J. N., & McNally, R. J. (1995). Depressed mood is related to obsessions, but not to compulsions in obsessive–compulsive disorder. *Journal of Anxiety Disorders, 9,* 249–256.

Richards, H. C. (1995, July). *The cognitive phenomenology of OCD repeated rituals.* Poster presented at the World Congress of Behavioural and Cognitive Therapies, Copenhagen, Denmark.

Richter, M. A., Cox, B. J., & Direnfeld, D. M. (1994). A comparison of three assessment instruments for obsessive–compulsive symptoms. *Journal of Behavior Therapy and Experimental Psychiatry, 25,* 143–147.

Rickelt, J., Viechtbauer, W., Lieverse, R., Overbeek, T., van Balkom, A. J., van Oppen, P., et al. (2016). The relation between depressive and obsessive–compulsive symptoms in obsessive–compulsive disorder: Results from a large, naturalistic follow-up study. *Journal of Affective Disorders, 203*, 241–247.

Riso, L. P., du Toit, P. L., Blandino, J. A., Penna, S., Dacey, S., Duin, J. S., et al. (2003). Cognitive aspects of depression. *Journal of Abnormal Psychology, 112*, 72–80.

Robichaud, M., & Dugas, M. J. (2006). A cognitive-behavioral treatment targeting intolerance of uncertainty. In G. C. L. Davey & A. Wells (Eds.), *Worry and its psychological disorders: Theory, assessment and treatment* (pp. 289–304). Chichester, UK: Wiley.

Robins, E., & Guze, S. B. (1970). Establishment of diagnostic validity in psychiatric illness: Its application to schizophrenia. *American Journal of Psychiatry, 126*, 983–986.

Rodgers, S., Ajdacic-Gross, V., Kawohl, W., Müller, M., Rössler, W., Hengartner, M. P., et al. (2015). Comparing two basic subtypes in OCD across three large community samples: A pure compulsive versus a mixed obsessive–compulsive subtype. *European Archives of Psychiatry and Clinical Neuroscience, 265*, 719–734.

Roh, D., Kim, K., Chang, J.-G., Kim, S. I., & Kim, C.-H. (2013). Development and validation of a computer-based measure of symmetry and arranging behavior in obsessive–compulsive disorder: A preliminary study. *Comprehensive Psychiatry, 54*, 885–892.

Romanelli, R. J., Wu, F. M., Gamba, R., Mojtabai, R., & Segal, J. B. (2014). Beahvioral therapy and serotonin reuptake inhibitor pharmacotherapy in the treatment of obsessive–compulsive disorder: A systematic review and meta-analysis of head-to-head randomized controlled trials. *Depression and Anxiety, 31*, 641–652.

Romero-Sanchiz, P., Nogueira-Arjona, R., Godoy-Ávila, A., Gavino-Lázaro, & Freeston, M. H. (2017). Differences in clinical intrusive thoughts between obsessive–compulsive disorder, generalized anxiety disorder, and hypochondria. *Clinical Psychology and Psychotherapy, 24*, 1464–1473.

Roper, G., & Rachman, S. J. (1976). Obsessional–compulsive checking: Experimental replication and development. *Behaviour Research and Therapy, 14*, 25–32.

Roper, G., Rachman, S. J., & Hodgson, R. (1973). An experiment on obsessional checking. *Behaviour Research and Therapy, 11*, 271–277.

Roper, G., Rachman, S., & Marks, I. M. (1975). Passive and participant modelling in exposure treatment of obsessive–compulsive neurotics. *Behaviour Research and Therapy, 13*, 271–279.

Rosenberg, C. M. (1968). Obsessional neurosis. *Australian and New Zealand Journal of Psychiatry, 2*, 33–38.

Rosenfeld, R., Dar, R., Anderson, D., Kobak, K. A., & Greist, J. H. (1992). A computer-administered version of the Yale–Brown Obsessive–Compulsive Scale. *Psychological Assessment, 4*, 329–332.

Rosso, G., Albert, U., Asinari, G. F., Bogetto, F., & Maina, G. (2012). Stressful life events and obsessive–compulsive disorder: Clinical features and symptom dimensions. *Psychiatry Research, 197*, 259–264.

Rowa, K., & Purdon, C. (2003). Why are certain intrusive thoughts more upsetting than others? *Behavioural and Cognitive Psychotherapy, 31,* 1–11.
Rowa, K., Purdon, C., Summerfeldt, L. J., & Antony, M. M. (2005). Why are some obsessions more upsetting than others? *Behaviour Research and Therapy, 43,* 1453–1465.
Rowsell, M., & Francis, S. E. (2015). OCD subtypes: Which, if any, are valid? *Clinical Psychology: Science and Practice, 22,* 414–435.
Rozin, P., & Fallon, A. E. (1987). A perspective on disgust. *Psychological Review, 94,* 23–41.
Rozin, P., Haidt, J., & McCauley, C. R. (2008). Disgust. In M. Lewis, J. M. Haviland-Jones, & L. Feldman Barrett (Eds.), *Handbook of emotions* (3rd ed., pp. 757–776). New York: Guilford Press.
Rubel, J. A., Rosenbaum, D., & Lutz, W. (2017). Patients' in-session experiences and symptom change: Session-to-session effects on a within- and between-patient level. *Behaviour Research and Therapy, 90,* 58–66.
Ruscio, A. M., Stein, D. J., Chiu, W. T., & Kessler, R. C. (2010). The epidemiology of obsessive–compulsive disorder in the National Comorbidity Survey Replication. *Molecular Psychiatry, 15,* 53–63.
Salkovskis, P. M. (1985). Obsessional–compulsive problems: A cognitive-behavioural analysis. *Behaviour Research and Therapy, 23,* 571–583.
Salkovskis, P. M. (1989a). Cognitive-behavioural factors and the persistence of intrusive thoughts in obsessional problems. *Behaviour Research and Therapy, 27,* 677–682.
Salkovskis, P. M. (1989b). Obsessions and compulsions. In J. Scott, J. Mark, G. Williams, & A. T. Beck (Eds.), *Cognitive therapy in clinical practice: An illustrative casebook* (pp. 50–77). New York: Routledge.
Salkovskis, P. M. (1996). The cognitive approach to anxiety: Threat beliefs, safety-seeking behavior, and the special case of health anxiety and obsessions. In P. M. Salkovskis (Ed.), *Frontiers of cognitive therapy* (pp. 48–74). New York: Guilford Press.
Salkovskis, P. M. (1998). Psychological approaches to the understanding of obsessional problems. In R. P. Swinson, M. M. Antony, S. Rachman, & M. A. Richter (Eds.), *Obsessive–compulsive disorder: Theory, research, and treatment* (pp. 33–50). New York: Guilford Press.
Salkovskis, P. M. (1999). Understanding and treating obsessive–compulsive disorder. *Behaviour Research and Therapy, 37,* S29–S52.
Salkovskis, P. M., Forrester, E., & Richards, C. (1998). Cognitive-behavioural approach to understanding obsessional thinking. *British Journal of Psychiatry, 173,* 53–63.
Salkovskis, P. M., & Freeston, M. H. (2001). Obsessions, compulsions, motivation, and responsibility for harm. *Australian Journal of Psychology, 53,* 1–6.
Salkovskis, P. M., & Harrison, J. (1984). Abnormal and normal obsessions: A replication. *Behaviour Research and Therapy, 22,* 1–4.
Salkovskis, P. M., & Kobori, O. (2015). Reassuringly calm?: Self-reported patterns to reassurance seeking in obsessive compulsive disorder. *Journal of Behavior Therapy and Experimental Psychiatry, 49,* 203–208.
Salkovskis, P. M., & Millar, J. F. A. (2016). Still cognitive after all these years?:

Perspectives for a cognitive behavioural theory of obsessions and where we are 30 years later. *Australian Psychologist, 51*, 3–13.

Salkovskis, P. M., Millar, J., Gregory, J. D., & Wahl, K. (2017). The termination of checking and the role of just right feelings: A study of obsessional checkers compared with anxious and non-clinical controls. *Behavioural and Cognitive Psychotherapy, 45*, 139–155.

Salkovskis, P. M., Richards, H. C., & Forrester, E. (1995). The relationship between obsessional problems and intrusive thoughts. *Behavioural and Cognitive Psychotherapy, 23*, 281–299.

Salkovskis, P. M., Thorpe, S. J., Wahl, K., Wroe, A. L., & Forrester, E. (2003). Neutralizing increases discomfort associated with obsessional thoughts: An experimental study with obsessional patients. *Journal of Abnormal Psychology, 112*, 709–715.

Salkovskis, P. M., & Wahl, K. (2003). Treating obsessional problems using cognitive-behavioural therapy. In M. Reinecke & D. A. Clark (Eds.), *Cognitive therapy across the lifespan: Theory, research and practice* (138–171). Cambridge, UK: Cambridge University Press.

Salkovskis, P. M., & Warwick, H. M. C. (1985). Cognitive therapy of obsessive–compulsive disorder: Treating treatment failures. *Behavioural Psychotherapy, 13*, 243–255.

Salkovskis, P. M., & Westbrook, D. (1989). Behaviour therapy and obsessional ruminations: Can failure be turned into success? *Behaviour Research and Therapy, 27*, 149–160.

Salkovskis, P. M., Westbrook, D., Davis, J., Jeavons, A., & Gledhill, A. (1997). Effects of neutralizing on intrusive thoughts: An experiment investigating the etiology of obsessive–compulsive disorder. *Behaviour Research and Therapy, 35*, 211–219.

Salkovskis, P. M., Wroe, A. L., Gledhill, A., Morrison, N., Forrester, E., Richards, C., et al. (2000). Responsibility attitudes and interpretations are characteristic of obsessive compulsive disorder. *Behaviour Research and Therapy, 38*, 347–372.

Samuels, J. F., Bienvenu, O. J., Gardos, M. A., Cullen, B., Riddle, M. A., Liang, K.-Y., et al. (2008). Prevalence and correlates of hoarding behavior in a community-based sample. *Behaviour Research and Therapy, 46*, 836–844.

Samuels, J., Nestadt, G., Bienvenu, O. J., Costa, P. T., Riddle, M. A., Liang, K.-Y., et al. (2000). Personality disorders and normal personality dimensions in obsessive–compulsive disorder. *British Journal of Psychiatry, 177*, 457–462.

Sandler, J., & Hazari, A. (1960). The "obsessional": On the psychological classification of obsessional character traits and symptoms. *British Journal of Medical Psychology, 33*, 113–122.

Sasson, Y., Zohar, J., Chopra, M., Lustig, M., Lancu, I. J., & Hendler, T. (1997). Epidemiology of obsessive–compulsive disorder: A world view. *Journal of Clinical Psychiatry, 58*(Suppl.), 7–10.

Scherer, K. R. (1999). Appraisal theory. In T. Dalgleish & M. Power (Eds.), *Handbook of cognition and emotion* (pp. 637–663). Chichester, UK: Wiley.

Schmidt, R. E., Gay, P., Courvoisier, D., Jermann, F., Ceschi, G., David, M., et al. (2009). Anatomy of the White Bear Suppression Inventory (WBSI): A review of previous findings and a new approach. *Journal of Personality Assessment, 91,* 323–330.

Schulze, D., Kathmann, N., & Reuter, B. (2018). Getting it just right: A reevaluation of OCD symptom dimensions integrating traditional and Bayesian approaches. *Journal of Anxiety Disorders, 56,* 63–73.

Schut, A. J., Castonguay, L. G., & Borkovec, T. D. (2001). Compulsive checking behaviors in generalized anxiety disorders. *Journal of Clinical Psychology, 57,* 705–715.

Schwartz, R. A. (2018). Treating incompleteness in obsessive–compulsive disorder: A meta-analytic review. *Journal of Obsessive–Compulsive and Related Disorders, 19,* 50–60.

Segerstrom, S. C., Stanton, A. L., Alden, L. E., & Shortridge, B. E. (2003). A multidimensional structure for repetitive thought: What's on your mind, and how, and how much? *Journal of Personality and Social Psychology, 85,* 909–921.

Segerstrom, S. C., Tsao, J. C. I., Alden, L. E., & Craske, M. G. (2000). Worry and ruminiation: Repetitive thought as a concomitant and predictor of negative mood. *Cognitive Therapy and Research, 24,* 671–688.

Seli, P., Risko, E. F., Purdon, C., & Smilek, D. (2017). Intrusive thoughts: Linking spontaneous mind wandering and OCD symptomatology. *Psychological Research, 81,* 392–398.

Seo, J.-W., & Kwon, S.-M. (2013). Autogenous/reactive obsessions and their relationship with negative self-inferences. *Journal of Obsessive–Compulsive and Related Disorders, 2,* 316–321.

Shafran, R. (1997). The manipulation of responsibility in obsessive–compulsive disorder. *British Journal of Clinical Psychology, 36,* 397–407.

Shafran, R., Egan, S., & Wade, T. (2010). *Overcoming perfectionism: A self-help guide using cognitive behavioural techniques.* London: Robinson.

Shafran, R., & Rachman, S. (2004). Thought–action fusion: A review. *Journal of Behavior Therapy and Experimental Psychiatry, 35,* 87–107.

Shafran, R., Radomsky, A. S., Coughtrey, A. E., & Rachman, S. (2013). Advances in the cognitive-behavioural treatment of obsessive compulsive disorder. *Cognitive Behaviour Therapy, 42,* 265–274.

Shafran, R., Thordarson, D. S., & Rachman, S. J. (1996). Thought–action fusion in obsessive compulsive disorder. *Journal of Anxiety Disorders, 10,* 379–391.

Shapiro, D. (1965). *Neurotic styles.* New York: Basic Books.

Shavitt, R. G., de Mathis, M. A., Oki, F., Ferrao, Y. A., Fontenelle, L. F., Torres, A. R., et al. (2014). Phenomenology of OCD: Lessons from a large multicenter study and implications for ICD-11. *Journal of Psychiatric Research, 57,* 141–148.

Shimshoni, Y., Reuven, O., Dar, R., & Hermesh, H. (2011). Insight in obsessive–compulsive disorder: A comparative study of insight measures in an Israeli clinical sample. *Journal of Behavior Therapy and Experimental Psychiatry, 42,* 389–396.

Sibrava, N. J., Boisseau, C. L., Eisen, J. L., Mancebo, M. C., & Rasmussen, S. A. (2016). An empirical investigation of incompleteness in a large clinical sample of obsessive compulsive disorder. *Journal of Anxiety Disorders, 42,* 45–51.

Sibrava, N. J., Boisseau, C. L., Mancebo, M. C., Eisen, J. L., & Rasmussen, S.

A. (2011). Prevalence and clinical characteristics of mental rituals in a longitudinal clinical sample of obsessive–compulsive disorder. *Depression and Anxiety, 28*, 892–898.

Sica, C., Bottesi, G., Orsucci, A., Pieraccioli, C., Sighinolfi, C., & Ghisi, M. (2015). "Not just right experiences" are specific to obsessive–compulsive disorder: Further evidence from Italian clinical samples. *Journal of Anxiety Disorders, 31*, 73–83.

Sica, C., Coradeschi, D., Sanavio, E., Dorz, S., Manchisi, D., & Novara, C. (2004). A study of the psychometric properties of the Obsessive Beliefs Inventory and Interpretations of Intrusions Inventory on clinical Italian individuals. *Journal of Anxiety Disorders, 18*, 291–307.

Sica, C., Ghisi, M., Altoè, G., Chiri, L. R., Franceschini, S., Coradeschi, D., et al. (2009). The Italian version of the Obsessive Compulsive Inventory: Its psychometric properties on community and clinical samples. *Journal of Anxiety Disorders, 23*, 204–211.

Sica, C., Novara, C., & Sanavio, E. (2002). Religiousness and obsessive–compulsive cognitions and symptoms in an Italian population. *Behaviour Research and Therapy, 40*, 813–823.

Siev, J., Chambless, D. L., & Huppert, J. D. (2010). Moral thought–action fusion and OCD symptoms: The moderating role of religious affiliation. *Journal of Anxiety Disorders, 24*, 309–312.

Siev, J., Steketee, G., Fama, J. M., & Wilhelm, S. (2011). Cognitive and clinical characteristics of sexual and religious obsessions. *Journal of Cognitive Psychotherapy: An International Quarterly, 25*, 167–176.

Simons, J. S., & Gaher, R. M. (2005). The Distress Tolerance Scale: Development and validation of a self-report measure. *Motivation and Emotion, 29*, 83–102.

Simpson, H. B., Maher, M. J., Wang, Y., Bao, Y., Foa, E. B., & Franklin, M. (2011). Patient adherence predicts outcome from cognitive behavioral therapy in obsessive–compulsive disorder. *Journal of Consulting and Clinical Psychology, 79*, 247–252.

Simpson, J., Cove, J., Fineberg, N., Msetfi, R. M., & Ball, L. J. (2007). Reasoning in people with obsessive–compulsive disorder. *British Journal of Clinical Psychology, 46*, 397–411.

Singh, N. N., Wahler, R. G., Winton, A. S., & Adkins, A. (2004). A mindfulness-based treatment of obsessive–compulsive disorder. *Clinical Case Studies, 3*, 275–287.

Skoog, G., & Skoog, I. (1999). A 40-year follow-up of patients with obsessive–compulsive disorder. *Archives of General Psychiatry, 56*, 121–127.

Smallwood, J. (2013). Distinguishing how from why the mind wanders: A process-outcome framework for self-generated mental activity. *Psychological Bulletin, 139*, 519–535.

Smallwood, J., & Schooler, J. W. (2015). The science of mind wandering: Empirically navigating the stream of consciousness. *Annual Review of Psychology, 66*, 487–518.

Smári, J., & Hólmsteinsson, H. E. (2001). Intrusive thoughts, responsibility attitudes, thought–action fusion, and chronic thought suppression in relation to obsessive–compulsive symptoms. *Behavioural and Cognitive Psychotherapy, 29*, 13–20.

Smits, J. A. J., Telch, M. J., & Randall, P. K. (2002). An examination of the decline in fear and disgust during exposure-based treatment. *Behaviour Research and Therapy, 40,* 1243–1253.

Sookman, D., Abramowitz, J. S., Calamari, J. E., Wilhelm, S., & McKay, D. (2005). Subtypes of obsessive–compulsive disorder: Implications for specialized cognitive behavior therapy. *Behavior Therapy, 36,* 393–400.

Spasojević, J., & Alloy, L. B. (2001). Rumination as a common mechanism relating depressive risk factors to depression. *Emotion, 1,* 25–37.

Speckens, A. E. M., Hackmann, A., Ehlers, A., & Cuthbert, B. (2007). Imagery special issue: Intrusive images and memories of earlier adverse events in patients with obsessive compulsive disorder. *Journal of Behavior Therapy and Experimental Psychiatry, 38,* 411–422.

St. Clare, T., Menzies, R. G., & Jones, M. K. (2008). *Danger ideation reduction therapy (DIRT) for obsessive–compulsive washers: A comprehensive guide to treatment.* Queensland: Australian Academic Press.

Stanley, M. A., & Turner, S. M. (1995). Current status of pharmacological and behavioral treatment of obsessive–compulsive disorder. *Behavior Therapy, 26,* 163–186.

Starcevic, V., Berle, D., Brakoulias, V., Sammut, P., Moses, K., Milicevic, D., et al. (2011). Foundations of compulsions in obsessive–compulsive disorder. *Australian and New Zealand Journal of Psychiatry, 45,* 449–457.

Starcevic, V., & Brakoulias, V. (2008). Symptom subtypes of obsessive–compulsive disorder: Are they relevant for treatment? *Australian and New Zealand Journal of Psychiatry, 42,* 651–661.

Stein, D. J., Fineberg, N. A., Bienvenu, O. J., Denys, D., Lochner, C., Nestadt, G., et al. (2010). Should OCD be classified as an anxiety disorder in DSM-V? *Depression and Anxiety, 27,* 495–506.

Stein, D. J., & Hollander, E. (1993). The spectrum of obsessive–compulsive-related disorders. In E. Hollander (Ed.), *Obsessive–compulsive-related disorders* (pp. 241–271). Washington, DC: American Psychiatric Association.

Stein, D. J., Kogan, C. S., Atmaca, M., Fineberg, N. A., Fontenelle, L. F., Grant, J. E., et al. (2016). The classification of Obsessive–Compulsive and Related Disorders in the ICD-11. *Journal of Affective Disorders, 190,* 663–674.

Stein, M. B., Forde, D. R., Anderson, G., & Walker, J. R. (1997). Obsessive–compulsive disorder in the community: An epidemiologic survey with clinical reappraisal. *American Journal of Psychiatry, 154,* 1120–1126.

Steketee, G. S. (1993). *Treatment of obsessive compulsive disorder.* New York: Guilford Press.

Steketee, G. S. (1994). Behavioral assessment and treatment planning with obsessive compulsive disorder: A review emphasizing clinical application. *Behavior Therapy, 25,* 613–633.

Steketee, G. S. (1999). *Overcoming obsessive–compulsive disorder: A behavioral and cognitive protocol for the treatment of OCD.* Oakland, CA: New Harbinger.

Steketee, G. S., & Barlow, D. H. (2002). Obsessive–compulsive disorder. In D. H. Barlow, *Anxiety and its disorders: The nature and treatment of anxiety and panic* (2nd ed., pp. 516–550). New York: Guilford Press.

Steketee, G. S., Frost, R. O., & Bogart, K. (1996). The Yale–Brown Obsessive–

Compulsive Scale: Interview versus self-report. *Behaviour Research and Therapy, 34,* 675–684.

Steketee, G., Frost, R. O., Rhéaume, J., & Wilhelm, S. (1998). Cognitive theory and treatment of obsessive–compulsive disorder. In M. A. Jenike, L. Baer, & W. E. Minichiello (Eds.), *Obsessive–compulsive disorders: Practical management* (3rd ed., pp. 368–399). St. Louis, MO: Mosby.

Steketee, G. S., Grayson, J. B., & Foa, E. B. (1985). Obsessive–compulsive disorder: Differences between washers and checkers. *Behaviour Research and Therapy, 23,* 197–201.

Steketee, G. S., Grayson, J. B., & Foa, E. B. (1987). A comparison of characteristics of obsessive–compulsive disorder and other anxiety disorders. *Journal of Anxiety Disorders, 1,* 325–335.

Steketee, G., Quay, S., & White, K. (1991). Religion and guilt in OCD patients. *Journal of Anxiety Disorders, 5,* 359–367.

Steketee, G., & Shapiro, L. J. (1995). Predicting behavioral treatment outcome for agoraphobia and obsessive compulsive disorder. *Clinical Psychology Review, 15,* 317–346.

Stengel, E. (1945). A study on some clinical aspects of the relationship between obsessional neurosis and psychotic reaction types. *Journal of Mental Science, 91,* 166–187.

Stern, R. S., & Cobb, J. P. (1978). Phenomenology of obsessive–compulsive neurosis. *British Journal of Psychiatry, 132,* 233–239.

Storch, E. A., Abramowitz, J., & Goodman, W. K. (2008). Where does obsessive–compulsive disorder belong in DSM-V? *Depression and Anxiety, 25,* 336–347.

Storch, E. A., Bagner, D., Merlo, L. J., Shapira, N. A., Geffken, G. R., Murphy, T. K., et al. (2007). Florida Obsessive–Compulsive Inventory: Development, reliability, and validity. *Journal of Clinical Psychology, 63,* 851–859.

Storch, E. A., Rasmussen, S. A., Price, L. H., Larson, M. J., Murphy, T. K., & Goodman, W. K. (2010). Development and psychometric evaluation of the Yale–Brown Obsessive–Compulsive Scale—Second Edition. *Psychological Assessment, 22,* 223–232.

Strauss, A. Y., Huppert, J. D., Simpson, H. B., & Foa, E. B. (2018). What matters more?: Common or specific factors in cognitive behavioral therapy for OCD—therapeutic alliance and expectations as predictors of treatment outcome. *Behaviour Research and Therapy, 105,* 43–51.

Strunk, D. R., Brotman, M. A., & DeRubeis, R. J. (2010). The process of change in cognitive therapy for depression: Predictors of early inter-session symptom gains. *Behaviour Research and Therapy, 48,* 599–606.

Subramanian, M., Abdin, E., Vaingankar, J. A., & Chong, S. A. (2012). Obsessive–compulsive disorder: Prevalence, correlates, help-seeking and quality of life in a multiracial Asian population. *Social Psychiatry and Psychiatric Epidemiology, 47,* 2035–2043.

Summerfeldt, L. J. (2001). Obsessive–compulsive disorder: A brief overview and guide to assessment. In M. M. Antony, S. M. Orsillo, & L. Roemer (Eds.), *Practitioner's guide to empirically based measures of anxiety* (pp. 211–217). New York: Kluwer Academic/Plenum.

Summerfeldt, L. J. (2004). Understanding and treating incompleteness in obsessive–compulsive disorder. *Journal of Clinical Psychology, 60,* 1155–1168.

Summerfeldt, L. J., Gilbert, S. J., & Reynolds, M. (2015). Incompleteness, aesthetic sensitivity, and the obsessive–compulsive need for symmetry. *Journal of Behavior Therapy and Experimental Psychiatry, 49,* 141–149.

Summerfeldt, L. J., Huta, V., & Swinson, R. P. (1998). Personality and obsessive–compulsive disorder. In R. P. Swinson, M. M. Antony, S. Rachman, & M. A. Richter (Eds.), *Obsessive–compulsive disorder: Theory, research, and treatment* (pp. 79–119). New York: Guilford Press.

Summerfeldt, L. J., Kloosterman, P. H., Antony, M. M., & Swinson, R. P. (2014). Examining an obsessive–compulsive core dimensions model: Structural validity of harm avoidance and incompleteness. *Journal of Obsessive–Compulsive and Related Disorders, 3,* 83–94.

Summerfeldt, L. J., Richter, M. A., Antony, M. M., & Swinson, R. P. (1999). Symptom structure in obsessive–compulsive disorder: A confirmatory factor-analytic study. *Behaviour Research and Therapy, 37,* 297–311.

Szechtman, H., & Woody, E. (2004). Obsessive–compulsive disorder as a disturbance of security motivation. *Psychological Review, 111,* 111–127.

Szkodny, L. E., Newman, M. G., & Goldfried, M. R. (2014). Clinical experiences in conducting empirically supported treatments for generalized anxiety disorder. *Behavior Therapy, 45,* 7–20.

Tallis, F., & Eysenck, M. W. (1994). Worry: Mechanisms and modulating influences. *Behavioural and Cognitive Psychotherapy, 22,* 37–56.

Tallis, F., Rosen, K., & Shafran, R. (1996). Investigation into the relationship between personality traits and OCD: A replication employing a clinical population. *Behaviour Research and Therapy, 34,* 649–653.

Taylor, J., & Purdon, C. (2016). Responsibility and hand washing behavior. *Journal of Behavior Therapy and Experimental Psychiatry, 51,* 43–50.

Taylor, S. (1995). Assessment of obsessions and compulsions: Reliability, validity, and sensitivity to treatment effects. *Clinical Psychology Review, 15,* 261–296.

Taylor, S. (1998). Assessment of obsessive–compulsive disorder. In R. P. Swinson, M. M. Antony, S. Rachman, & M. A. Richter (Eds.), *Obsessive–compulsive disorder: Theory, research, and treatment* (pp. 229–257). New York: Guilford Press.

Taylor, S. (2002) Cognition in obsessive–compulsive disorder: An overview. In R. O. Frost & G. Steketee (Eds.), *Cognitive approaches to obsessions and compulsions: Theory, assessment and treatment* (pp. 1–12). Oxford, UK: Elsevier.

Taylor, S. (2011). Early versus late onset obsessive–compulsive disorder: Evidence for distinct subtypes. *Clinical Psychology Review, 31,* 1083–1100.

Taylor, S., Abramowitz, J. S., McKay, D., Calamari, J. E., Sookman, D., Kyrios, M., et al. (2006). Do dysfunctional beliefs play a role in all types of obsessive–compulsive disorder? *Journal of Anxiety Disorders, 20,* 85–97.

Taylor, S., Kyrios, M., Thordarson, D. S., Steketee, G., & Frost, R. O. (2002). Development and validation of instruments for measuring intrusions and beliefs in obsessive–compulsive disorder. In R. O. Frost & G. Steketee (Eds.), *Cognitive approaches to obsessions and compulsions: Theory, assessment, and treatment* (pp. 117–138). Amsterdam: Elsevier.

Taylor, S., McKay, D., Crowe, K. B., Abramowitz, J. S., Conelea, C. A., Calamari, J. E., et al. (2014). The sense of incompleteness as a motivator of obsessive–compulsive symptoms: An empirical analysis of concepts and correlates. *Behavior Therapy, 45*, 254–262.

Taylor, S., Thordarson, D. S., & Söchting, I. (2002). Obsessive–compulsive disorder. In M. M. Antony & D. H. Barlow (Eds.), *Handbook of assessment and treatment planning for psychological disorders* (pp. 182–214). New York: Guilford Press.

Teasdale, J. D. (1974). Learning models of obsessional–compulsive disorder. In H. R. Beech (Ed.), *Obsessional states* (pp. 197–229). London: Methuen.

Tee, J., & Kazantzis, N. (2011). Collaborative empiricism in cognitive therapy: A definition and theory for the relationship construct. *Clinical Psychology: Science and Practice, 18*, 47–61.

Tek, C., & Ulug, B. (2001). Religiosity and religious obsessions in obsessive–compulsive disorder. *Psychiatry Research, 104*, 99–108.

Thiel, N., Hertenstein, E., Nissen, C., Herbst, N., Külz, A. K., & Voderholzer, U. (2013). The effect of personality disorders on treatment outcomes in patients with obsessive–compulsive disorders. *Journal of Personality Disorders, 27*, 697–715.

Thomsen, P. H. (1995). Obsessive–compulsive disorder in children and adolescents: Predictors in childhood for long-term phenomenological course. *Acta Psychiatrica Scandinavica, 92*, 255–259.

Thordarson, D. S., Radomsky, A. S., Rachman, S., Shafran, R., Sawchuk, C. N., & Hakstian, A. R. (2004). The Vancouver Obsessional Compulsive Inventory (VOCI). *Behaviour Research and Therapy, 42*, 1289–1314.

Thordarson, D. S., & Shafran, R. (2002). Importance of thoughts. In R. O. Frost & G. Steketee (Eds.), *Cognitive approaches to obsessions and compulsions: Theory, assessment, and treatment* (pp. 16–28). Amsterdam: Elsevier Science.

Timmons, K. A., & Joiner, T. E. (2008). Reassurance seeking and negative feedback seeking. In K. S. Dobson & D. J. A. Dozois (Eds.), *Risk factors in depression* (pp. 429–446). Amsterdam: Elsevier.

Tisher, R., Allen, J. S., & Crouch, W. (2014). The Self-Ambivalence Measure: A psychometric investigation. *Australian Journal of Psychology, 66*, 197–206.

Toffolo, M. B. J., van den Hout, M. A., Engelhard, I. M., Hooge, I. T. C., & Cath, D. C. (2014). Uncertainty, checking, and intolerance of uncertainty in subclinical obsessive compulsive disorder: An extended replication. *Journal of Obsessive–Compulsive and Related Disorders, 3*, 338–344.

Toffolo, M. B. J., van den Hout, M. A., Hooge, I. T. C., Engelhard, I. M., & Cath, D. C. (2013). Mild uncertainty promotes checking behavior in subclinical obsessive–compulsive disorder. *Clinical Psychological Science, 1*, 103–109.

Toftdahl, N. G., Nordentoft, M., & Hjorthøj, C. (2016). Prevalence of substance use disorders in psychiatric patients: A nationwide Danish population-based study. *Social Psychiatry and Epidemiology, 51*, 129–140.

Tolin, D. F., Abramowitz, J. S., Brigidi, B. D., & Foa, E. B. (2003). Intolerance of uncertainty in obsessive–compulsive disorder. *Journal of Anxiety Disorders, 17*, 233–242.

Tolin, D. F., Abramowitz, J. S., Hamlin, C., Foa, E. B., & Synodi, D. S. (2002).

Attributions for thought suppression failure in obsessive–compulsive disorder. *Cognitive Therapy and Research, 26,* 505–517.

Tolin, D. F., Abramowitz, J. S., Kozak, M. J., & Foa, E. B. (2001). Fixity of belief, perceptual aberration, and magical ideation in obsessive–compulsive disorder. *Journal of Anxiety Disorders, 15,* 501–510.

Tolin, D. F., Abramowitz, J. S., Przeworski, A., & Foa, E. B. (2002). Thought suppression in obsessive–compulsive disorder. *Behaviour Research and Therapy, 40,* 1255–1274.

Tolin, D. F., Brady, R. F., & Hannan, S. (2008). Obsessional beliefs and symptoms of obsessive–compulsive disorder in a clinical sample. *Journal of Psychopathology and Behavioral Assessment, 30,* 31–42.

Tolin, D. F., Worhunsky, P., & Maltby, N. (2006). Are "obsessive" beliefs specific to OCD?: A comparison across anxiety disorders. *Behaviour Research and Therapy, 44,* 469–480.

Torres, A. R., Fontenelle, L. F., Shavitt, R. G., Ferrão, Y. A., do Rosário, M. C., Storch, E. A., et al. (2016). Comorbidity variation in patients with obsessive–compulsive disorder according to symptom dimensions: Results from a large multicenter clinical sample. *Journal of Affective Disorders, 190,* 508–516.

Torres, A. R., Prince, M. J., Bebbington, P. E., Bhugra, D., Brugha, T. S., Farrell, M., et al. (2006). Obsessive–compulsive disorder: Prevalence, comorbidity, impact, and help-seeking in the British National Psychiatric Morbidity Survey of 2000. *American Journal of Psychiatry, 163,* 1978–1985.

Torres, A. R., Ramos-Cerqueria, A. T., Fontenelle, L. F., do Rosário, M. C., & Miguel, E. C. (2011). Suicidality in obsessive–compulsive disorder: Prevalence and relation to symptom dimensions and comorbid conditions. *Journal of Clinical Psychiatry, 72,* 17–26.

Tuna, T., Tekan, A. I., & Topçuoğvlu, V. (2005). Memory and metamemory in obsessive–compulsive disorder. *Behaviour Research and Therapy, 43,* 15–27.

Türksoy, N., Tükel, R., Özdemir, Ö., & Karali, A. (2002). Comparison of clinical characteristics in good and poor insight obsessive–compulsive disorder. *Journal of Anxiety Disorders, 16,* 413–423.

Turner, S. M., Beidel, D. C., & Stanley, M. A. (1992). Are obsessional thoughts and worry different cognitive phenomena? *Clinical Psychology Review, 12,* 257–270.

Twohig, M. P., Hayes, S. C., & Masuda, A. (2006). Increasing willingness to experience obsessions: Acceptance and commitment therapy as a treatment for obsessive–compulsive disorder. *Beahvior Therapy, 37,* 3–13.

Van Ameringen, M., Patterson, B., & Simpson, W. (2014). DSM-5 obsessive–compulsive and related disorders: Clinical implications of new criteria. *Depression and Anxiety, 31,* 487–493.

van Balkom, A. J. L. M., van Oppen, P., Vermeulen, A. W. A., van Dyck, R., Nauta, M. C. E., & Vorst, H. C. M. (1994). A meta-analysis on the treatment of obsessive compulsive disorder: A comparison of antidepressants, behavior, and cognitive therapy. *Clinical Psychology Review, 14,* 359–381.

van den Hout, M., & Kindt, M. (2003a). Phenomenological validity of an OCD-memory model and the remember/know distinction. *Behaviour Research and Therapy, 41,* 369–378.

van den Hout, M., & Kindt, M. (2003b). Repeated checking causes memory distrust. *Behaviour Research and Therapy, 41*, 301–316.
van den Hout, M., Kindt, M., Weiland, T., & Peters, M. (2002). Instructed neutralization, spontaneous neutralization and prevented neutralization after an obsession-like thought. *Journal of Behavior Therapy and Experimental Psychiatry, 33*, 177–189.
van den Hout, M., van Pol, M., & Peters, M. (2001). On becoming neutral: Effects of experimental neutralizing reconsidered. *Behaviour Research and Therapy, 39*, 1439–1448.
van Oppen, P., & Arntz, A. (1994). Cognitive therapy for obsessive–compulsive disorder. *Behaviour Research and Therapy, 32*, 79–87.
van Oppen, P., Hoekstra, R. J., & Emmelkamp, P. M. G. (1995). The structure of obsessive–compulsive symptoms. *Behaviour Research and Therapy, 33*, 15–23.
van Overveld, W. J. M., de Jong, P. J., Peters, M. L., Cavanagh, K., & Davey, G. C. L. (2006). Disgust propensity and disgust sensitivity: Separate constructs that are differentially related to specific fears. *Personality and Individual Differences, 41*, 1241–1252.
van Overveld, W. J. M., de Jong, P. J., Peters, M. L., & Schouten, E. (2011). The Disgust Scale–R: A valid and reliable index to investigate separate disgust domains? *Personality and Individual Differences, 51*, 325–330.
van Rijsoort, S., Emmelkamp, P., & Vervaeke, G. (2001). Assessment of worry and OCD: How are they related? *Personality and Individual Differences, 31*, 247–258.
van Schie, K., Wanmaker, S., Yocarini, I., & Bouwmeester, S. (2016). Psychometric qualities of the Thought Suppression Inventory—Revised in different age groups. *Personality and Individual Differences, 91*, 89–97.
Veale, D. (2002). Over-valued ideas: A conceptual analysis. *Behaviour Research and Therapy, 40*, 383–400.
Viar, M. A., Bilsky, S. A., Armstrong, T., & Olatunji, B. O. (2011). Obsessive beliefs and dimensions of obsessive–compulsive disorder: An examination of specific associations. *Cognitive Therapy and Research, 35*, 108–117.
Vogel, P. A., Hansen, B., Stiles, T. C., & Götetam, G. (2006). Treatment motivation, treatment expectancy, and helping alliance as predictors of outcome in cognitive behavioral treatment of OCD. *Journal of Behavior Therapy and Experimental Psychiatry, 37*, 247–255.
Volans, P. J. (1976). Styles of decision-making and probability appraisal in selected obsessional and phobic patients. *British Journal of Social and Clinical Psychology, 15*, 305–317.
Wahl, K., Salkovskis, P. M., & Cotter, I. (2008). "I wash until it feels right": The phenomenology of stopping criteria in obsessive–compulsive washing. *Journal of Anxiety Disorders, 22*, 143–161.
Wahl, K., Schönfeld, S., Hissbach, J., Küsel, S., Zurowski, B., Moritz, S., et al. (2011). Differences and similarities between obsessive and ruminative thoughts in obsessive–compulsive and depressed patients: A comparative study. *Journal of Behavior Therapy and Experimental Psychiatry, 42*, 454–461.
Waller, K., & Boschen, M. J. (2015). Evoking and reducing mental contamination

in female perpetrators of an imagined non-consensual kiss. *Journal of Behavior Therapy and Experimental Psychiatry, 49,* 195–202.

Warnock-Parkes, E., Salkovskis, P. M., & Rachman, J. (2012). When the problem is beneath the surface in OCD: The cognitive treatment of a case of pure mental contamination. *Behavioural and Cognitive Psychotherapy, 40,* 383–399.

Watkins, E. R. (2008). Constructive and unconstructive repetitive thought. *Psychological Bulletin, 134,* 163–206.

Watkins, E. R. (2016). *Rumination-focused cognitive-behavioral therapy for depression.* New York: Guilford Press.

Watkins, E. R., Moulds, M., & Mackintosh, B. (2005). Comparisons between rumination and worry in a non-clinical population. *Behaviour Research and Therapy, 43,* 1577–1585.

Weber, F., Hauke, W., Jahn, I., Stengler, K., Himmerich, H., Zaudig, M., et al. (2014). Does "thinking about thinking" interfere with memory?: An experimental memory study in obsessive–compulsive disorder. *Journal of Anxiety Disorders, 28,* 679–686.

Wegner, D. M. (1994a). Ironic processes of mental control. *Psychological Review, 101,* 34–52.

Wegner, D. M. (1994b). *White bears and other unwanted thoughts: Suppression, obsession, and the psychology of mental control.* New York: Guilford Press.

Wegner, D. M., Schneider, D. J., Carter, S. R., & White, T. L. (1987). Paradoxical effects of thought suppression. *Journal of Personality and Social Psychology, 53,* 5–13.

Wegner, D. M., & Zanakos, S. (1994). Chronic thought suppression. *Journal of Personality, 62,* 615–640.

Weisman, J. S., & Rodebaugh, T. L. (2018). Exposure therapy augmentation: A review and extension of techniques by an inhibitory learning approach. *Clinical Psychology Review, 59,* 41–51.

Weisner, W. M., & Riffel, A. (1960). Scrupulosity: Religion and obsessive compulsive behavior in children. *American Journal of Psychiatry, 117,* 314–318.

Weissman, M. M., Bland, R. C., Canino, G. J., Greenwald, S., Hwu, H.-G., Lee, C. K., et al. (1994). The cross national epidemiology of obsessive compulsive disorder. *Journal of Clinical Psychiatry, 3*(Suppl.), 5–10.

Welkowitz, L. A., Struening, E. L., Pittman, J., Guardino, M., & Welkowitz, J. (2000). Obsessive–compulsive disorder and comorbid anxiety problems in a National Anxiety Screening sample. *Journal of Anxiety Disorders, 14,* 471–482.

Wells, A. (2005). Worry, intrusive thoughts and generalized anxiety disorder: The metacognitive theory and treatment. In D. A. Clark (Ed.), *Intrusive thoughts in clinical disorders: Theory, research, and treatment* (pp. 119–144). New York: Guilford Press.

Wells, A., & Cartwright-Hatton, S. (2004). A short form of the metacognitions questionnaire: Properties of the MCQ-30. *Behaviour Research and Therapy, 42,* 385–396.

Wells, A., & Davies, M. I. (1994). The Thought Control Questionnaire: A measure of individual differences in the control of unwanted thoughts. *Behaviour Research and Therapy, 32,* 871–878.

Wells, A., & Matthews, G. (1994). *Attention and emotion: A clinical perspective.* Hove, UK: Erlbaum.

Wells, A., & Morrison, A. P. (1994). Qualitative dimensions of normal worry and normal obsessions: A comparative study. *Behaviour Research and Therapy, 32,* 867–870.

Welner, A., Reich, T., Robins, E., Fishman, R., & van Doren, T. (1976). Obsessive–compulsive neurosis: Record, follow-up, and family studies: I. Inpatient record study. *Comprehensive Psychiatry, 17,* 527–539.

Westra, H. A., & Norouzian, N. (2017). Using motivational interviewing to manage process markers of ambivalence and resistance in cognitive behavior therapy. *Cognitive Therapy and Research, 42,* 193–203.

Wheaton, M. G., Abramowitz, J. S., Berman, N. C., Riemann, B. C., & Hale, L. R. (2010). The relationship between obsessive beliefs and symptom dimensions in obsessive–compulsive disorder. *Behaviour Research and Therapy, 48,* 949–954.

Wheaton, M. G., Huppert, J. D., Foa, E. B., & Simpson, H. B. (2016). How important is the therapeutic alliance in treating obsessive–compulsive disorder with exposure and response prevention?: An empirical report. *Clinical Neuropsychiatry, 13,* 88–93.

Whitaker, K. L., Watson, M., & Brewin, C. R. (2009). Intrusive cognitions and their appraisal in anxious cancer patients. *Psycho-Oncology, 18,* 1145–1155.

Whittal, M. L., & McLean, P. D. (1999). CBT for OCD: The rationale, protocol, and challenges. *Cognitive and Behavioral Practice, 6,* 383–396.

Whittal, M. L., & McLean, P. D. (2002). Group cognitive behavioral therapy for obsessive compulsive disorder. In R. O. Frost & G. Steketee (Eds.), *Cognitive approaches to obsessions and compulsions: Theory, assessment, and treatment* (pp. 417–433). Amsterdam: Elsevier Science.

Whittal, M. L., Woody, S. R., McLean, P. D., Rachman, S. J., & Robichaud, M. (2010). Treatment of obsessions: A randomized controlled trial. *Behaviour Research and Therapy, 48,* 295–303.

Whitton, A. E., Henry, J. D., & Grisham, J. R. (2014). Moral rigidity in obsessive–compulsive disorder: Do abnormalities in inhibitory control, cognitive flexibility and disgust play a role? *Journal of Behavior Therapy and Experimental Psychiatry, 45,* 152–159.

Wilhelm, S., Berman, N. C., Keshaviah, A., & Schwartz, R. A. (2015). Mechanisms of change in cognitive therapy for obsessive compulsive disorder: Role of maladaptive beliefs and schemas. *Behaviour Research and Therapy, 65,* 5–10.

Wilhelm, S., & Steketee, G. S. (2006). *Cognitive therapy for obsessive–compulsive disorder: A guide for professionals.* Oakland, CA: New Harbinger.

Wilkinson-Tough, M., Bocci, L., Thorne, K., & Herlihy, J. (2010). Is mindfulness-based therapy an effective intervention for obsessive-intrusive thoughts?: A case series. *Clinical Psychology and Psychotherapy, 17,* 250–268.

Williams, A. D., Lau, G., & Grisham, J. R. (2013). Thought–action fusion as a mediator of religiosity and obsessive–compulsive symptoms. *Journal of Behavior Therapy and Experimental Psychiatry, 44,* 207–212.

Williams, J. B. W., Gibbon, M., First, M. B., Spitzer, R. L., Davies, M., Borus, J., et al. (1992). The Structured Clinical Interview for DSM-III-R (SCID): II. Multisite test–retest reliability. *Archives of General Psychiatry, 49*, 630–636.

Williams, M. T., Crozier, M., & Powers, M. (2011). Treatment of sexual orientation obsessions in obsessive–compulsive disorder using exposure and ritual prevention. *Clinical Case Studies, 10*, 53–66.

Williams, M. T., & Farris, S. G. (2011). Sexual orientation obsessions in obsessive–compulsive disorder: Prevalence and correlates. *Psychiatry Research, 187*, 156–159.

Williams, M. T., Farris, S. G., Turkheimer, E., Franklin, M. E., Simpson, H. B., Liebowitz, M., et al. (2014). The impact of symptom dimensions on outcome for exposure and ritual prevention therapy in obsessive–compulsive disorder. *Journal of Anxiety Disorders, 28*, 553–558.

Williams, M. T., Farris, S. G., Turkheimer, E., Pinto, A., Ozanick, K., Franklin, M. F., et al. (2011). Myth of the pure obsessional type in obsessive–compulsive disorder. *Depression and Anxiety, 28*, 495–500.

Williams, M. T., Mugano, B., Franklin, M., & Faber, S. (2013). Symptom dimensions in obsessive–compulsive disorder: Phenomenology and treatment outcomes with exposure and ritual prevention. *Psychopathology, 46*, 365–376.

Wilson, C., & Hall, M. (2012). Thought control strategies in adolescents: Links with OCD symptoms and meta-cognitive beliefs. *Behavioural and Cognitive Psychotherapy, 40*, 438–451.

Witzif, T. F., & Pollard, C. A. (2013). Obsessional beliefs, religious beliefs, and scrupulosity among fundamental Protestant Christians. *Journal of Obsessive–Compulsive and Related Disorders, 2*, 331–337.

Woods, C. M., Tolin, D. F., & Abramowitz, J. S. (2004). Dimensionality of the Obsessive Beliefs Questionnaire (OBQ). *Journal of Psychopathology and Behavioral Assessment, 26*, 113–125.

Woody, S. R., Steketee, G., & Chambless, D. L. (1995). Reliability and validity of the Yale–Brown Obsessive–Compulsive Scale. *Behaviour Research and Therapy, 33*, 597–605.

Woody, S. R., & Tolin, D. F. (2002). The relationship between disgust sensitivity and avoidant behavior: Studies of clinical and nonclinical samples. *Journal of Anxiety Disorders, 16*, 543–559.

Woody, S. R., Whittal, M. L., & McLean, P. D. (2011). Mechanisms of symptom reduction in treatment for obsessions. *Journal of Consulting and Clinical Psychology, 79*, 653–664.

Wootton, B. M., Diefenbach, G. J., Bragdon, L. B., Steketee, G., Frost, R. O., & Tolin, D. F. (2015). A contemporary psychometric evaluation of the Obsessive–Compulsive Inventory—Revised (OCI-R). *Psychological Assessment, 27*, 874–882.

Wroe, A. L., Salkovskis, P. M., & Richards, H. C. (2000). "Now I know it could happen, I have to prevent it": A clinical study of the specificity of intrusive thoughts and the decision to prevent harm. *Behavioural and Cognitive Psychotherapy, 28*, 63–70.

Wu, K. D., & Cortesi, G. T. (2009). Relations between perfectionism and obsessive–compulsive symptoms: Examination of specificity among the dimensions. *Journal of Anxiety Disorders, 23*, 393–400.

Wu, M. S., McGuire, J. F., Hong, B., & Storch, E. A. (2016). Further psychometric properties of the Yale–Brown Obsessive Compulsive Scale—Second Edition. *Comprehensive Psychiatry, 66,* 96–103.

Wu, M. S., McGuire, J. F., Martino, C., Phares, V., Selles, R. R., & Storch, E. A. (2016). A meta-analysis of family accommodation and OCD symptom severity. *Clinical Psychology Review, 45,* 34–44.

Yaryura-Tobias, J. A., Grunes, M. S., Todaro, J., McKay, D., Neziroglu, F. A., & Stockman, R. (2000). Nosological insertion of Axis I disorders in the etiology of obsessive–compulsive disorder. *Journal of Anxiety Disorders, 14,* 19–30.

Yorulmaz, O., Karanci, A. N., Bastug, B., Kisa, C., & Goka, E. (2008). Responsibility, thought–action fusion and thought suppression in Turkish patients with obsessive–compulsive disorder. *Journal of Clinical Psychology, 64,* 308–317.

Zhang, X., Liu, J., Cui, J., & Liu, C. (2013). Study of symptom differences and clinical characteristics in Chinese patients with OCD. *Journal of Affective Disorders, 151,* 868–874.

Zhong, C.-B., & Lijenquist, K. (2006). Washing away your sins: Threatened morality and physical cleansing. *Science, 313,* 1451–1452.

Zvolensky, M. J., Vujanovic, A. A., Bernstein, A., & Leyro, T. (2010). Distress tolerance: Theory, measurement, and relations to psychopathology. *Current Directions in Psychological Science, 19,* 406–410.

Zysk, E., Shafran, R., Williams, T. I., & Melli, G. (2015). Development and validation of the Morphing Fear Questionnaire (MFQ). *Clinical Psychology and Psychotherapy, 22,* 1–10.

Index

Note. Page numbers that appear in *italic* indicate a figure or a table.

Acceptance and commitment therapy (ACT), 280
Adaptive worry, 44
ADIS-IV. *See* Anxiety Disorders Interview Schedule for DSM-IV
Age, OCD and, 9
Alcohol use disorder, 20, 21
Alternate control days exercise, *234*, 244–245
Alternate Days Worksheet (Form 9.3), *242–243*, 253
Alternative interpretations/narratives, 222–224
The Alternative Perspective (Handout 8.4), *222*, 230–231
Ambivalence, therapeutic relationship and, 150–152
Ambivalent self, 317, 319
Anal personality, 21
Anxiety
  intolerance of uncertainty and, 63
  misinterpretation of, 113
  relationship to OCD, 4
Anxiety comparison task, *235*, 248–249
Anxiety disorders
  co-occurrence with OCD, 14, 16–17
  relationship to OCD, 6, 7–8
Anxiety Disorders Interview Schedule for DSM-IV (ADIS-IV), 172–173
Anxiety monitoring exercise, *235*, 248

Anxiety prediction exercise, *235*, 249
Anxiety reduction, 59–60
Anxiety reduction hypothesis, 77, 78–79, 80
Anxiety survey, *235*, 248
Anxiety tolerance, 100
Anxious Thoughts Workbook, The (Clark), 201, 203
Appraisals. *See* Beliefs and appraisals; Faulty appraisals and beliefs; Responsibility appraisals
Appraisal self-monitoring, 207–208, 224
Arranging obsessions. *See* Symmetry, ordering, and arranging
Artificial importance task, *233*, 241–242
Assessment. *See* Clinical assessment; Cognitive assessment
Assessment anxiety, 166
Attentive days task, *234*, 242–243
Atypical exposure, *233*, 238
Autogenous intrusions, 320, 321, 322–324
Avoidance
  concealment as a form of, 155
  description of, 57
  implications for assessment, 168
Avoidance learning, 79
Avoidant personality disorder, 22, 156

BDD. *See* Body dysmorphic disorder
"Behavioral addiction," 21

Behavioral compulsions, 51–53
Behavioral experiments/interventions
  for inflated responsibility, 240
  for intolerance of anxiety/distress, 248–249
  for intolerance of uncertainty, 245–246
  for mental contamination, 273
  for mental control, 243–245
  for overestimated threat, 236–238
  for overimportance of thought, 240–243
  overview and summary, 232–235
  for perfectionism, 246–248
  for TAF bias, 239–240
Behavioral observation, of symptom provocation, 185
Behavioral theory of OCD
  anxiety reduction hypothesis, 77, 78–79, *80*
  emotional processing theory, 80–82
  inhibitory learning theory, 82–83, *84*. *See also* Inhibitory learning theory
  introduction, 77–78
Belief domains
  clinical implications, 115–116
  in OCD, 114–115
Beliefs and appraisals, normative measures of, 179–184
Best Person Ever–Worst Person Ever continuum, 213
BINGS. *See* Brown Incompleteness Scale
Body dysmorphic disorder (BDD), 7, 18–19
Borderline personality disorder, 22
Brown Assessment of Beliefs Scale, 41
Brown Incompleteness Scale (BINGS), 344, 353

Case formulation. *See* CBT case formulation; Cognitive case formulation
CBOCI. *See* Clark–Beck Obsessive–Compulsive Inventory
CBT case formulation
  case illustration, 196–197, *198*
  delineation of associated negative cognitions, 188
  delineation of faulty appraisals and beliefs, 187–188
  delineation of mental control strategies, 188
  implications from understanding compulsions and neutralization, 69–70
  implications from understanding obsessions, 48–49
  importance of, 162, 189
  key aspects of, 186
  with repugnant obsessions, 327–333
  with SOA, 352–355
  treatment goal setting and, 197–200
  See also Cognitive Case Formulation Profile
CBT for OCD
  behavioral experiments. *See* Behavioral experiments/interventions
  case formulation. *See* CBT case formulation
  case illustration, 196–197, *198*
  clinical assessment. *See also* Clinical assessment
    cognitive assessment of OCD, 179–185
    diagnostic and symptom measures, 172–179
    importance of, 162
    special assessment problems in OCD, 163–172
  cognitive interventions
    appraisal self-monitoring, 207–208, 224
    cognitive restructuring, 208–222, 224. *See also* Cognitive restructuring
    generating alternative interpretations, 222–224
    reasons for starting treatment with, 195–196
  psychoeducation, 200–207, 224
  strategies to improve feared self in pathological doubt, 305
  therapeutic relationship. *See* Therapeutic relationship
  treatment components, overview of, 224
  treatment considerations
    with compulsive checking, 283, 290, 307, 308
    with contamination OCD. *See* Contamination OCD, treatment considerations
    with pathological doubt, 307
    with religiosity, 318
    with repugnant obsessions, 333–337, 338
    with SOA, 355–359, 360
  treatment goal setting, 197–200, 224
  See also Generic CBT model of OCD

CBT models
  of compulsive checking, 295–301, 308
  of contamination OCD, 274–277
  of repugnant obsessions, 320–327
  of SOA, 347–351, 360
  See also Generic CBT model of OCD
Certainty, pathological doubt and, 287
Certainty manipulation, *234*, 236
Certainty survey, *234*, 235
Change, therapeutic relationship and, 154
Checking compulsion by proxy, 55
Checking rituals. *See* Compulsive checking
Checklist of Neutralization Strategies Associated with OCD (Form 3.2), 58–59, 72, 188
Childhood ritualistic behavior, SOA and, 347–348, 349
CIQ. *See* Cognitive Intrusions Inventory
Clark–Beck Obsessive–Compulsive Inventory (CBOCI), 176–177, 178
Cleaning compulsions. *See* Washing and cleaning compulsions
Client feedback, therapeutic relationship and, *140*
Client goals
  with exposure and response prevention, 87–92
  goal consensus and the therapeutic relationship, *140*
  treatment goal setting in CBT for OCD and, 197–200
Clinical assessment
  cognitive assessment, 179–185. *See also* Cognitive assessment
  as continuous, 172
  determining an individual's stop rules, 66
  diagnostic and symptom measures
    Clark–Beck Obsessive–Compulsive Inventory, 176–177
    diagnostic interviews, 172–173
    Obsessive–Compulsive Inventory, 175–176
    overview and summary, 172, 178–179
    Vancouver Obsessional Compulsive Inventory, 177–178
    Yale–Brown Obsessive–Compulsive Scale, 173–175
  importance of, 162, 189
  special assessment problems in OCD
    disorder-related problems, 163–165
    overview, 163, *164*
    response style problems, *164*, 166–168
    strategies to improve compliance, 168–172

Clinical Compulsions Checklist (Form 3.1), *52*, 53, 71
Clinical interviews, 172–173
Clinician's Handbook for Obsessive Compulsive Disorder (O'Connor & Aardema), 304
Cognitive Appraisal Worksheet (Form 8.1), 207–208, 225
Cognitive assessment
  idiographic, 184–185
  normative measures of beliefs and appraisals, 179–184
  of SOA, 352–355
Cognitive-behavioral therapy (CBT)
  foundational models on OCD
    inflated responsibility appraisals, 110–112
    mental control, 116–117
    misinterpretation of personal significance, 112–114
    schema vulnerability, 114–116
  notion of normal obsessions and, 38
  See also CBT for OCD; Generic CBT model of OCD
Cognitive-Behavioral Treatment of Perfectionism (Egan et al.), 151
Cognitive case formulation
  case illustration, 196–197, *198*
  key aspects of, 186
  overview and description of, 187–188, 189
  treatment goal setting and, 197–200
  See also CBT case formulation
Cognitive Case Formulation Profile (Form 7.5)
  employing in cognitive case formulation, 187, 189
  employing with psychoeducation, 201, 202–203, 204
  template, 194
Cognitive compulsions. *See* Mental compulsions
Cognitive interventions
  appraisal self-monitoring, 207–208, 224
  cognitive restructuring, 208–222. *See also* Cognitive restructuring strategies
  generating alternative interpretations, 222–224
  reasons for starting treatment with, 195–196
Cognitive Intrusions Inventory (CIQ), 184

Index

Cognitive restructuring strategies
    for inflated responsibility, 214–217
    for intolerance of anxiety/distress, 221–222
    for intolerance of uncertainty and perfectionism, 219–220
    for mental contamination, 273
    for overestimated threat, 209–211
    for overimportance and control of thoughts, 217–219
    reasons for using to treat OCD, 208–209, 224
    for repugnant obsessions, 335–336
    for TAF bias, 212–214
Cognitive risk exercise, 233, 240
Cognitive self-consciousness, 321–322
Cognitive theory
    danger ideation reduction therapy, 279–280
    historical approaches to OCD, 109–110
    inference-based model of OCD, 290–293. *See also* Inference-based model of OCD
    Rachman's theory of compulsive checking, 289–290, 307–308
Cognitive vulnerability, repugnant obsessions and, 320–327
Collaboration
    defined, 145
    therapeutic relationship and, *140*, 144–147
Collaborative contract, 91–92
Comorbidity
    anxiety disorders, 16–17
    definition and overview, 14
    depression, 15–16
    implications for assessment, 165
    obsessive–compulsive personality disorder, 21–23
    obsessive–compulsive spectrum disorder, 18–19
    psychosis, 20
    substance use disorders, 20–21
    tic disorders, 19
Compensatory rebound, 67
Compulsions
    anxiety reduction hypothesis, 78–79
    avoidance and, 57
    behavioral compulsions, 51–53
    defined and characterized, 5–6, 51
    early research on, 23–24
    empirical evidence for the generic CBT model of OCD, 130–132
    examples of, 50
    excessive reassurance seeking, 55–57
    excessive washing and cleaning, 260–263. *See also* Washing and cleaning compulsions
    functional relationship with obsessions, 53
    in the generic CBT model of OCD, *118*, 119
    habit hypothesis of OCD, 27
    highlights for CBT case formulation, 69–70
    inflated responsibility appraisals and, 111–112
    mental compulsions, 53–55
    misinterpretation of personal significance and, 113–114
    paradox of, 50–51
    psychoeducation with CBT for OCD, 203–205
    role of mental control in, 66–69. *See also* Mental control
    stop rules, 65–66
    See also Neutralizations
Compulsive Activity Checklist, 178
Compulsive checking
    case illustration, 281–282
    CBT model of
        context and uncertainty intrusions, 297
        difficulties with safety and resolving doubt, 300
        faulty appraisals and reasoning, 297–300
        overview and summary of, *296*, 300–301, 308
        pathological doubt, 300
        vulnerability factors, 295–297
    checking compulsion by proxy, 55
    clinical features, 282–283
    differentiated from cleaning rituals, 283
    early research on, 24
    pathological doubt and, 284, *296*, 300
    Rachman's cognitive theory of, 289–290, 307–308
    reduced activation of the security motivation system, 300
    response prevention and, 306–307
    stop rules and, 66
    treatment considerations
        for inflated responsibility, 302–303
        overview and critical components, 283, 290
        for tolerance of uncertainty and distress, 305–306
    treatment efficacy, 307, 308

Compulsive cleaning. *See* Washing and cleaning compulsions
Concealment
  considerations in case formulation for repugnant obsessions, 327, 328–329
  implications for assessment, 164–165
  implications for the therapeutic relationship, 155
Contact contamination
  case illustration, 257–258
  clinical features, 258–260
  cognitive-behavioral model of, 274–277
  disgust and contamination sensitivity, 263–267
  treatment considerations, 277
  washing and cleaning compulsions, 260–263
  See also Contamination OCD
Contamination OCD
  case illustration, 257–258
  clinical features, 258–260, 261, 280
  cognitive-behavioral model of, 274–277
  danger ideation reduction therapy, 279–280
  disgust and contamination sensitivity, 263–267
  mental contamination, 267–274
  treatment considerations
    disgust, 266–267
    mental contamination, 272–274, 277
    overview and discussion of, 260, 277–278, 280
    special considerations, 278
    washing and cleaning compulsions, 263
  washing and cleaning compulsions, 260–263. *See also* Washing and cleaning compulsions
Contamination sensitivity, 266, 267
Contamination Sensitivity Scale (CSS), 266, 278
Contamination Thought–Action Fusion Scale, 278
Contextual analysis, with SOA, 354
Control Strategies Worksheet (Form 7.4), 185, 193, 204
Conventional exposure and response prevention, 82–83
Core disgust, 264
Correctness. *See* Perfectionism
Cost–benefit analysis
  behavioral intervention with perfectionism, 234, 246–247
  ERP clients and, 90, 91, 103
Courtroom role play, 216

Covert compulsions. *See* Mental compulsions
CSS. *See* Contamination Sensitivity Scale
Culture
  influence on obsessions, 31, 33
  influence on symmetry, ordering, and arranging, 342
  repugnant obsessions and, 311–312

Danger ideation reduction therapy (DIRT), 279–280
Definitions of Faulty Appraisals (Handout 8.3), 207, 228–229
Delusions, 42–43
Dependent personality disorder, 22
Depression
  co-occurrence with OCD, 14, 15–16
  excessive reassurance seeking and, 55
Desire for predictability, 63–64
Determinants of Neutralization Rating Scale (Form 3.3), 65, 73, 185, 188
Diagnosis
  DSM-5 diagnosis of OCD, 4, 6–8
  essential features of OCD, 5–6
  of repugnant obsessions, 313
Diagnostic and Statistical Manual of Mental Disorders (DSM-5)
  diagnosis of OCD, 4, 6–8
  obsessive–compulsive spectrum disorder in, 18
Diagnostic and symptom measures
  Clark–Beck Obsessive–Compulsive Inventory, 176–177
  diagnostic interviews, 172–173
  Obsessive–Compulsive Inventory, 175–176
  overview and summary, 172, 178–179
  Vancouver Obsessional Compulsive Inventory, 177–178
  Yale–Brown Obsessive–Compulsive Scale, 173–175
Diagnostic comorbidity, 14. *See also* Comorbidity
Diagnostic interviews, 172–173
Diaries, 221–222
Dimensional Obsessive–Compulsive Scale (DOCS), 26, 178, 353
DIRT. *See* Danger ideation reduction therapy
Dirty kiss paradigm, 271–272
Disgust
  clinical features, 263–265
  cognitive-behavioral model of contamination OCD and, 274
  treatment considerations, 266–267

Disgust propensity (DP), 264–265, 267
Disgust Propensity and Sensitivity Scale (DPSS), 265
Disgust Scale, 265
Disgust Scale—Revised, 265
Disgust sensitivity (DS), 264–265
Distress intolerance. *See* Intolerance of anxiety/distress
Distress reduction, 59–60
Distress tolerance (DT)
  inhibitory learning theory perspective on, 100
  neutralization and, 64–65
  strategies to improve in pathological doubt and compulsive checking, 305–306
DOCS. *See* Dimensional Obsessive–Compulsive Scale
Dose-response sensitivity, 89
Double-standard technique, 216
Doubt
  differences between pathological and normal doubt, 284–288
  implications for assessment, 166–167
  implications for the therapeutic relationship, 156–157
  See also Pathological doubt
Downward arrow technique, 218
DPSS. *See* Disgust Propensity and Sensitivity Scale
DT. *See* Distress tolerance

Early-onset OCD, SOA and, 342
EDQ. *See* Ego-Dystonicity Questionnaire
Educational attainment, 11
Ego dystonicity
  defined, 159
  implications for the therapeutic relationship, 159
  repugnant obsessions and, 325–326, 327, 329–331
Ego-Dystonicity Questionnaire (EDQ), 326
Elevated evidence requirement, 65
Emotional detachment, therapeutic relationship and, 155–156
Emotional processing theory, 80–82
Empathy, *140*
Empirical hypothesis testing, 232–249. *See also* Behavioral experiments/interventions
Empiricism, 147–148
Environmental risk factors, 10

Epidemiology and demography
  ethnicity, marital status, and family involvement, 10–11
  gender, age, and onset, 9–10
  prevalence, 8–9
  quality of life and suicidality, 11–12
ERP. *See* Exposure and response prevention
ERP Cost–Benefit Worksheet (Form 4.2), 90, *91*, 103
ERP lifestyle, 97
ERS. *See* Excessive reassurance seeking
Ethnicity, 10
Exaggerated exposure, 99
Examples of Faulty Appraisals Involved in the Persistence of Obsessions (Handout 8.2), 207, 227
Excessive reassurance seeking (ERS)
  description of, 55–57
  therapeutic relationship and, 152–154
Excessive thought control, 114. *See also* Mental control
Exconsequentia reasoning, 221, 276, 277–278
Excoriation disorder, 7, 18–19
Expectancy Exposure Worksheet (Form 4.6), 98, 107
Expectancy violation, 98–99
Exposure
  atypical exposure, *233*, 238
  complete cessation of neutralization, 99–100
  in ERP, 85–86, 94–96
  exaggerated, 99
  expectancy violation, 98–99
  imaginal exposure, 333–334
  intense exposure, 99
  promotion of anxiety/distress tolerance, 100
  uncertainty exposure exercise, *234*, 246
  variability and surprise, 99
  in vivo exposure, 96
  within-session exposure, 96
  See also Exposure hierarchy
Exposure and response prevention (ERP)
  basic components
    client goals and expectations, 87–92
    exposure hierarchy, 94, *95*
    exposure sessions and homework, 94–96
    overview, 87
    pretreatment assessment, 92
    psychoeducation, 92–94
    relapse prevention, 96–98
    treatment readiness, 87
  beginning treatment with, 195

for compulsive checking and pathological doubt, 307, 308
for contamination OCD, 277, 279, 280
exposure treatment, 85–86
inhibitory learning theory and, 82–83, 84, 98–101
introducing in CBT for OCD, 204–205, 206–207
limitations of, 101
origins and overview, 77, 83, 85–87
practice guidelines, 87
for repugnant obsessions, 337, 338
for SOA, 355–356
Exposure and response prevention (ERP) clients
assessment of treatment readiness, 87
collaborative contract, 91–92
cost-benefit analysis, 90, 91, 103
faulty beliefs about ERP, 89–90
past experiences and knowledge of ERP, 88–89
practical obstacles to commitment, 90
Exposure hierarchy
compulsive cleaning example, 86
in ERP, 94, 95
Exposure Hierarchy Worksheet (Form 4.4), 94, 95, 105
Exposure Worksheet (Form 4.5), 94–95, 98, 106

Family involvement, OCD and, 11
Faulty appraisals and beliefs
compulsive checking and, 296, 297–300
empirical evidence for the generic CBT model of OCD
appraisals of thought control failure, 129–130
causal status of, 125–126
elevated levels in OCD, 122–123
overview, 122
specific association with OCD symptoms, 123–125
implications for assessment, 168
incompleteness and SOA, 348, 350–351
psychoeducation with CBT for OCD, 202–203
repugnant obsessions and, 324–326
self-monitoring, 207–208, 224
strategies to improve assessment compliance, 171–172
Faulty reasoning
compulsive checking and, 297–300
inference-based model of OCD, 290–295

pathological doubt and, 285–286
strategies to improve in pathological doubt, 303–304
Fear
emotional processing theory, 80–82
OCD and, 4
Feared self
compulsive checking and, 295–297
repugnant obsessions and, 319–320, 327, 332–333
strategies to improve in pathological doubt, 304–305
Feared self-narrative, 333
Fear habituation, 81–82
Fear of Self Questionnaire (FSQ), 296–297, 305, 326, 332
Fear tolerance, 83
Feeling of knowing, pathological doubt and, 287
Florida Obsessive–Compulsive Inventory (FOCI), 178–179
Flowchart exercise, 209–211
FOCI. *See* Florida Obsessive–Compulsive Inventory
Focused assessment, 171
Follow-up sessions, with ERP, 97–98
Frost MultiDimensional Perfectionism Scale, 354
FSQ. *See* Fear of Self Questionnaire

GAD. *See* Generalized anxiety disorder
Gender, 9–10
Generalized anxiety disorder (GAD)
co-occurrence with OCD, 16, 17, 44
intolerance of uncertainty and, 63
pathological worry and, 44
Generic CBT model of OCD
compulsive checking, 295–301, 308
conceptual origins, 132–133
contamination OCD, 274–277
criticisms and limitations of, 133–134
empirical evidence
compulsive rituals, 130–132
excessive mental control and its appraisal, 126–130
faulty appraisals and beliefs, 122–126
stop criteria, 132
summary and significance of, 133
universality of unwanted intrusions, 119–121
historical roots of, 109–110
overview, 108, 117–119
See also CBT for OCD
Guided discovery, 148–150

Habit learning hypothesis of OCD, 27, 131–132
Harm obsessions, 309–310. *See also* Repugnant obsessions
HD. *See* Hoarding disorder
Hoarding disorder (HD), 7, 18–19
Homosexual OCD, 310–311
Hypermorality, therapeutic relationship and, 156–157. *See also* Morality
Hypothesis testing. *See* Empirical hypothesis testing

IBT. *See* Inference-based model
ICQ. *See* Inferential Confusion Questionnaire
ICQ-EV. *See* Inferential Confusion Questionnaire—Expanded Version
Ideal self-narrative, 329–331
Idiographic assessment
 of cognition, 184–185
 of SOA, 354–355
III. *See* Interpretations of Intrusions Inventory
ILT. *See* Inhibitory learning theory
Imagery, obsessional, 34
Imagery rescripting
 for inflated responsibility in compulsive checking, 302–303
 for mental contamination, 274
Imaginal exposure, 333–334
Importance/control of thoughts. *See* Mental control; Overimportance of thoughts
Importance manipulation exercise, *233*, 242
Incompleteness
 as a feature of SOA, 343, 344–347, *348*, 350, 360
 key findings on, *346*
 treatment considerations with SOA, 356–357
 See also "Not just right" experience
Indecision
 implications for assessment, 166–167
 implications for the therapeutic relationship, 156–157
Inference-based model (IBT) of OCD
 description of, 290–293
 overview, 308
 treatment of compulsive checking, 302
 treatment of pathological doubt, 293–295, 303–304

Inferential confusion
 compulsive checking and, *296*, 299–300
 defined, 291
 as a feature of pathological doubt, 285–286, 292–293
 in inference-based theory, 291, 292
 strategies to improve in pathological doubt, 303–304
Inferential Confusion Questionnaire (ICQ), 286, 292–293
Inferential Confusion Questionnaire—Expanded Version (ICQ-EV), 286, 292
Inflated responsibility
 behavioral interventions, *233*, 241
 clinical implications, 112
 cognitive restructuring, 214–217
 compulsive checking and, *296*, 298
 definition and description of, 110–112, *115*
 misinterpretation of personal significance and, 113
 strategies to improve in compulsive checking, 302–303
Inflated significance task, *234*, 242
Inhibitory learning theory (ILT)
 ERP and, 82–83, *84*, 98–101
 overview and description of, 82–83
Insight
 into one's obsessions, 40–41
 problem of lack of insight for assessment, 167
Instructed checking exercise, *235*, 248
Intense exposure, 99
Intentional errors exercise, *235*, 247–248
Interpersonal deficiencies, therapeutic relationship and, 155–156
Interpretations of Intrusions Inventory (III), 184
Intolerance of anxiety/distress
 behavioral interventions, *235*, 248–249
 cognitive restructuring, 221–222
Intolerance of uncertainty (IU)
 behavioral interventions, *234*, 245–246
 cognitive restructuring, 219–220
 compulsive checking and, *296*, 298
 defined, *115*
 overview and description of, 63–64
 pathological doubt and, 288
 scrupulosity and, 316–317
Intolerance of Uncertainty Scale (IUS), 181
Intrusion and appraisal questionnaires, 184

Intrusions
  autogenous intrusions, 320, 321, 322–324
  cognitive restructuring, 217–219
  generic CBT model of OCD and, 117–121
  obsessions and unwanted intrusive thoughts, 35, 37–39
  psychoeducation with CBT for OCD, 201–202
  self-report measures, 184
  uncertainty intrusions and context, 297
  See also Obsessions
Intrusions survey, 233, 239
Intrusive perception, SOA and, 348, 349
In vivo exposure, 96
IU. *See* Intolerance of uncertainty
IUS. *See* Intolerance of Uncertainty Scale

Low memory confidence (low cognitive confidence)
  compulsive checking and, 296, 299–300
  implications for the therapeutic relationship, 158
  pathological doubt and, 286–287

Major depression, 15–16
Maladaptive beliefs, pathological doubt and, 287–288
Maladaptive thought control, 129
Marital status, 10–11
MCQ. *See* Metacognitions Questionnaire
Memory, compulsive checking and, 296, 299–300. *See also* Low memory confidence
Mental compulsions, 53–55
Mental contamination
  clinical features and types of, 267–272
  treatment considerations, 272–274, 277
Mental control
  behavioral interventions, 234, 243–245
  in the CBT formulation of obsessions, 116–117
  cognitive-behavioral model of contamination OCD and, 276
  cognitive restructuring of thought control, 217–219
  empirical evidence for the generic CBT model of OCD
    excessive mental control and vulnerability to OCD, 126–128
    faulty appraisal of thought control failure and OCD, 129–130
    maladaptive thought control and OCD, 129

empirical research, 68–69
  facets of, 115
  paradox of, 116–117, 205–206
  psychoeducation with CBT for OCD, 205–206
  Rachman's concept of excessive thought control, 114
  repugnant obsessions and, 320, 321, 324, 326, 327, 332
  theoretical considerations, 66–68
  See also Overimportance of thoughts
Mental control holiday, 234
Mental pollution, 267, 268, 269
Metacognitions Questionnaire (MCQ), 182–183, 321
Metamemory, compulsive checking and, 296, 299–300
Metaphors, 218, 304
MFQ. *See* Morphing Fear Questionnaire
MI. *See* Motivational interviewing
Mindfulness, treatment of contamination OCD, 280
Mind wandering, 120
Mini-rituals, 97
Misinterpretation of personal significance, 112–114
Morality
  considerations in case formulation for repugnant obsessions, 327, 329–331
  moral inflexibility and the therapeutic relationship, 156–157
  repugnant obsessions and, 314–315
Moral Values Survey (Form 9.2), 239–240, 252
Moral violation, 268, 269
Morphing, 269, 270
Morphing Fear Questionnaire (MFQ), 278
Motivational interviewing (MI), 152
Multiple obsessions, 31, 165
Multivariate analysis of symptom dimensions, 25–27

Narrative units, 293–294
Need for control, therapeutic relationship and, 154–155
Negative cognitions/thoughts
  identifying in CBT case formulation, 188
  repetitive, 43–48
  See also Obsessions
Neutralization
  clinical application, 65
  definition and conceptualization of, 50, 57–59

Neutralization *(cont.)*
  determinants of
    anxiety/distress reduction, 59–60
    distress tolerance, 64–65
    intolerance of uncertainty, 63–64
    "not just right" experiences, 61–63
    overview, 59
    perceived responsibility, 61
    safety seeking, 60–61
  empirical evidence for the generic CBT model of OCD, 130–132
  excessive reassurance seeking, 55–57
  excessive washing and cleaning, 260–263
  exposure and, 99–110
  highlights for CBT case formulation, 69–70
  inflated responsibility appraisals and, 111–112
  misinterpretation of personal significance and, 113–114
  prevention in treatment for repugnant obsessions, 334–335
  psychoeducation with CBT for OCD, 203–205
  role of mental control in, 66–69. *See also* Mental control
  See also Compulsions
New parents, harm obsessions and, 312
NJRE. *See* "Not just right" experience
NJRE-QR. *See* Not Just Right Experiences Questionnaire—Revised
Noncompliance
  implications for assessment, 168
  strategies to improve assessment compliance, 168–172
Normal obsessions
  criteria for distinguishing from abnormal obsessions, 39
  unwanted intrusive thoughts versus abnormal obsessions, 37–39
Normative assessment, of SOA, 352–354
"Not just right" experience (NJRE)
  description of, 61–63
  as a feature of SOA, 344–347, *348*, 350, 360
  pathological doubt and, 287, 288
  treatment considerations with SOA, 356–357
  See also Incompleteness
Not Just Right Experiences Questionnaire—Revised (NJRE-QR), 352–353

OBQ. *See* Obsessive Beliefs Questionnaire
"Obsessional–Compulsive Problems" (Salkovskis), 110
Obsessional content
  clinical examples, *32*
  cultural influences on, 31, 33
  multiple obsessions, 31
  obsessional imagery, 34
  temporal instability of, 31
  trauma-related obsessions, 33–34
Obsessional imagery, 34
Obsessional ruminations, 24, 47
Obsessions
  anxiety reduction hypothesis, 78
  avoidance and, 57
  CBT formulation of mental control, 116–117
  cognitive restructuring, 217–219
  content of, 31–34. *See also* Obsessional content
  continuum of insight into, 40–41
  core features of, 34–37
  criteria for distinguishing between normal and abnormal obsessions, 39
  definitions and characterizations of, 5, 30, 34–35
  delusions, 42–43
  differentiating worry and rumination from, 43–48
  functional relationship with compulsions, 53
  in the generic CBT model of OCD, 117–119
  highlights for CBT case formulation, 48–49
  inflated responsibility appraisals, 110–111
  misinterpretation of personal significance, 112–113
  overvalued ideation, 41–42
  role of mental control in, 66–69. *See also* Mental control
  unwanted intrusive thoughts, 37–39
Obsessions and Compulsions (Rachman & Hodgson), 110
Obsessions and Compulsions Experience Form (Form 7.1), 185, 190
Obsessive Beliefs Questionnaire (OBQ), 179–180, 287–288, 298, 332
Obsessive–compulsive and related disorders, 4

Obsessive Compulsive Cognitions Working
    Group (OCCWG), 114–116
Obsessive–Compulsive Core Dimensions
    Questionnaire (OC-CDQ), 344,
    345, 353
Obsessive–compulsive disorder (OCD)
  as a "behavioral addiction," 21
  comorbidity, 14–23. *See also*
      Comorbidity
  course and outcome, 12–14
  diagnosis, 5–8
  epidemiology and demography
    ethnicity, marital status, and family
        involvement, 10–11
    gender, age, and onset, 9–10
    prevalence, 8–9
    quality of life and suicidality, 11–12
  habit learning hypothesis of, 131–132
  hallmarks of, 3–5
  historical roots of the cognitive approach
      to, 109–110
  inference-based model of, 290–295
  perfectionism and, 349
  symptoms. *See* OCD symptoms
  treatment considerations
    challenges for the clinician, 5
    implications from the phenomenology
        of OCD, 28–29
    implications from understanding
        compulsions and neutralization,
        69–70
    implications from understanding
        obsessions, 48–49
    treatment seeking by individuals with
        OCD, 12–13
Obsessive–Compulsive Inventory (OCI),
    175–176, 178
Obsessive–Compulsive Inventory—Revised
    (OCI-R), 175–176, 178, 326
Obsessive–compulsive personality disorder
    (OPCD)
  co-occurrence with OCD, 21–23
  perfectionism and compulsive checking,
      297
Obsessive–compulsive psychosis, 41
Obsessive–compulsive spectrum disorder
    (OCSD), 18–19
Obsessive doubt. *See* Pathological doubt
OC-CDQ. *See* Obsessive–Compulsive Core
    Dimensions Questionnaire
OCCWG. *See* Obsessive Compulsive
    Cognitions Working Group

OCD. *See* Obsessive–compulsive disorder
OCD bubble, 304
OCD Cost–Benefit Worksheet (Form 6.1),
    152, 161
OCD symptoms
  diagnosis of OCD, 4, 6–8
  natural course and outcomes, 13–14
  problems for assessment
    multiplicity, 165
    shared symptoms, 163–164
    symptom heterogeneity, 164
    temporal instability, 165
  subtypes
    alternative subtyping, 27–28
    early research on, 23–24
    multivariate symptom dimensions,
        25–27
    overview, 23
  symptom provocation. *See* Symptom
      induction/provocation
OCD Treatment Goals and Expectations
    Worksheet (Form 4.1), 88, 94, 102
OCI. *See* Obsessive–Compulsive Inventory
OCI-R. *See* Obsessive–Compulsive
    Inventory—Revised
OCSD. *See* Obsessive–compulsive spectrum
    disorder
Onset, 9–10
Ordering and rearranging compulsions. *See*
    Symmetry, ordering, and arranging
Overestimation of threat. *See* Threat
    overestimation
Overimportance of thoughts
  behavioral interventions, *233–234*,
      241–243
  cognitive restructuring, 217–219
  compulsive checking and, *296*, 298
  defined, *115*
  repugnant obsessions and, 324, *327*, 332
  See also Mental control
Overvalued Ideas Scale, 41, 42
Overvalued ideation (OVI)
  definition and description of, 41–42
  differentiating from delusions, 42–43
OVI. *See* Overvalued ideation
*Oxford Guide to the Treatment of Mental
    Contamination* (Rachman et al.),
    272

Padua Inventory, 352
Panic disorder, 16, 17
Paradox of mental control, 116–117, 205–206

Pathological doubt
  case illustration, 281–282
  clinical features and differences from normal doubt, 284–288
  compulsive checking and, 284, *296*, 300
  inference-based model and treatment, 290–295
  relationship OCD, 301–302
  strategies to improve feared self, 304–305
  strategies to improve inferential confusion and faulty reasoning, 303–304
  strategies to improve tolerance of uncertainty and distress, 305
  treatment efficacy, 307, 308
Pathological worry, 44
Penn Inventory of Scrupulosity (PIOS), 316
Perceived responsibility, 61
Perceived uncontrollability of obsessions, 35, 36–37
Perfectionism
  ambivalence toward the therapeutic relationship and, 151
  assessment of, 354
  behavioral interventions, *234–235*, 246–248
  cognitive restructuring, 219–220
  compulsive checking and, 297
  defined, *115*
  implications for assessment, 166
  OCD and, 349
  SOA and, 348–349, 357–359
Perfectionism observation exercise, *235*, 247
Personality disorders, 21–23
Personal responsibility continuum, 216–217
Personal significance, misinterpretation of, 112–114
Pharmacotherapy, with "pure obsessions," 335
Pie charts. *See* Responsibility pie chart
PIOS. *See* Penn Inventory of Scrupulosity
Positive regard, therapeutic relationship and, *140*
Posttraumatic stress disorder, 33–34
Power of thoughts exercise, *233*, 240
Pre-Exposure Worksheet (Form 4.3), 92, 94, 104
Pregnancy, 9–10
Premonitions experiment, *233*, 239
Prevalence, 8–9
Primary obsessional slowness, 167

Psychoeducation
  with CBT for OCD
    definition and overview, 200–201, 224
    excessive mental control, 205–206
    faulty appraisals, 202–203
    neutralization, 203–205
    normalizing unwanted intrusions, 201–202
    stop criteria, 206
    treatment rationale, 206–207
  with ERP, 92–94
  to improve assessment compliance, 169–170
  for mental contamination, 272
Psychological fusion, 180
Psychosis, 20
Pure obsessions ("pure O"), 310, 313

Quality of life, 11–12

Rachman's cognitive theory of compulsive checking, 289–290, 307–308
Rachman's misinterpretation of personal significance, 112–114
Racial/ethnic groups, 10
RAS. *See* Responsibility Attitude Scale
Reactive obsessions, 322–324
Reality sensing, 294–295
Record of Anticipated Consequences (Form 7.3), 185, 192
Record of Triggers for Order and Symmetry (Form 13.1), 354, 361
Relapse prevention
  in ERP, 96–98
  with mental contamination, 274
Relationship obsessive–compulsive disorder (ROCD), 301–302
Relationship Obsessive Compulsive Inventory (ROCI), 301
Religious obsessions (religiosity)
  case illustration, 309–310
  cultural studies on, 33
  implications for the therapeutic relationship, 156–157
  morality and, 314
  pertinent issues in CBT for, *318*
  rumination and, 48
  scrupulosity and clinical features, 315–317
  See also Repugnant obsessions
Repeating and redoing rituals. *See* Compulsive checking
Repetitive negative thoughts, 43–48

Repugnant obsessions
  case illustration, 309–310
  CBT model of
    autogenous intrusions, 322–324
    cognitive vulnerability, 320–322
    faulty appraisals and beliefs, 324–326
    mental control strategies, 326
    overview, 320, *321*
    termination rules, 326–327
  clinical features, 310–312, 338
  cognitive-behavioral case formulation
    concealment, 328–329
    ego dystonicity, 329–331
    feared self, 332–333
    importance/control of thoughts, 332
    overview, *321*, 327
    TAF-morality bias, 331
  cultural differences, 311–312
  diagnosis, 313
  morality, 314–315
  as pure obsessions, 310, 313
  religiosity and scrupulosity, 315–317, *318*
  selfhood, 317, 319–320
  treatment
    cognitive restructuring, 335–336
    imaginal exposure, 333–334
    neutralization prevention, 334–335
    treatment efficacy and other modalities, 336–337, 338
Resistance, to obsessions, *35*, 36
Response prevention (RP)
  in exposure and response prevention, 86–87
  with repugnant obsessions, 334–335
  treatment of compulsive checking and, 306–307
  See also Exposure and response prevention
Responsibility appraisals, 61
Responsibility Attitude Scale (RAS), 181–182
Responsibility bias, 275–276
Responsibility gradient exercise, *233*, 241
Responsibility Interpretations Questionnaire (RIQ), 181, 182
Responsibility manipulation, *233*
Responsibility pie chart, 214–215
Responsibility transfer
  to improve assessment compliance, 170
  to restructure inflated responsibility, 216
Revised Obsessional Intrusions Inventory (ROII), 184
Rigidity and inflexibility, therapeutic relationship and, 154
RIQ. *See* Responsibility Interpretations Questionnaire
Risk assessment exercise, *233*, 236
Ritualizing, implications for assessment, 167
ROCD. *See* Relationship obsessive-compulsive disorder
ROCI. *See* Relationship Obsessive Compulsive Inventory
ROII. *See* Revised Obsessional Intrusions Inventory
RP. *See* Response prevention
Rumination
  defined, 46
  differentiating from obsessions, 43, 46–48
  overview, 43, 46–47

Safety seeking
  exposure and, 99–110
  neutralization and, 60–61
Salkovskis's inflated responsibility concept, 110–112
Schema vulnerability
  belief domains in OCD, 114–115
  clinical implications, 115–116
Schizophrenia, 20, 42
SCID-IV. *See* Structured Clinical Interview for DSM-IV
Scrupulosity, 315–317
Security motivation theory, 66, 262–263, 300
Selected List of Unwanted Intrusive Thoughts (Handout 8.1), 201–202, 226, 239
Self-contamination
  clinical features, 268–269
  cognitive-behavioral model of, 274–275, 276
Self-determination, collaboration and, 145
Self-domains, 319
Selfhood
  morality and, 324–315
  repugnant obsessions and, 317, 319–320
Self-monitoring
  assessment of cognition, 185
  of faulty appraisals and beliefs, 207–208, 224
  with SOA, 354
  treatment of mental contamination, 272–273

Self-narratives
  feared self-narrative, 333
  ideal self-narrative, 329–331
Self-report measures, 179–184
Self-representation
  ambivalence and the therapeutic relationship, 151
  compulsive checking and, 295–297
Semistructured clinical interviews, 172
Separation anxiety disorder, 17
Sexual obsessions, 309–310. *See also* Repugnant obsessions
Sexual orientation fears, 310–311
Significance, misinterpretations of, 112–114
Situation Record and Rating Scales (Form 7.2), 185, 191
Skin-picking disorder (SPD), 7, 18–19
Slowness, implications for assessment, 167
SOA. *See* Symmetry, ordering, and arranging
SOAQ. *See* Symmetry, Ordering, and Arranging Questionnaire
SOA Symptom Induction Ratings (Form 13.2), 355, 362
Social anxiety disorder, 16, 17, 156
Socratic questioning, 148–150
Solution learning, 78–79
SPD. *See* Skin-picking disorder
Specific phobias, 16, 17
Spectrum disorders, 7
Standardized diagnostic interviews, 172–173
Stimulus-independent thought, 119–120
Stop rules/criteria
  cognitive-behavioral model of contamination OCD and, 275, 276–277
  with compulsions, 65–66
  empirical evidence for the generic CBT model of OCD, 132
  with ordering compulsions, 348, 351
  psychoeducation with CBT for OCD, 206
  with repugnant obsessions, 326–327
  with washing and cleaning compulsions, 262, 276, 278
Stress management training, 337
Structured Clinical Interview for DSM-IV (SCID-IV), 172–173
Substance use disorders, 20–21
Subthreshold obsessive–compulsive disorder, 8
Suicidality, 12

Surveys
  anxiety survey, 235, 248
  certainty survey, 234, 235
  intrusions survey, 233, 239
  Moral Values Survey, 239–240, 252
  threat survey, 233, 238
  treatment of mental contamination, 1273
Symmetry, ordering, and arranging (SOA)
  case illustrations, 52–53, 339–340
  CBT model of
    faulty appraisals and beliefs, 348, 350–351
    incompleteness, 348, 350
    intrusive perception, 348, 349
    ordering compulsions and stop criteria, 348, 351
    overview, 347, 348, 360
    vulnerability factors, 347–349
  clinical features, 360
  cognitive assessment and case formulation, 352–355
  distinctiveness of, 344–347
  incompleteness and, 343, 344–347
  "not just right" experiences and, 62
  overview and clinical features, 340–343
  treatment considerations
    incompleteness, 356–357
    overview, 355–356, 360
    perfectionism, 357–359
    personal insignificance of symptoms and symptom normalization, 359
Symmetry, Ordering, and Arranging Questionnaire (SOAQ), 342, 352
Symmetry obsessions. *See* Symmetry, ordering, and arranging
Symptom induction/provocation
  assessment of SOA, 354–355
  idiographic assessment of cognition, 185

TAF bias. *See* Thought–action fusion bias
TAF Scale. *See* Thought–Action Fusion Scale
TCQ. *See* Thought Control Questionnaire
Termination rules. *See* Stop rules/criteria
Therapeutic relationship
  case example, 137–138
  CBT-specific relational elements
    collaboration, 144–147
    empiricism, 147–148
    Socratic questioning, 148–150
  concepts and research, 139–141

importance of, 137–138, 159
OCD threats of
  ambivalence, 150–152
  case example, 137–138
  concealment, 155
  doubt and indecision, 156–157
  ego dystonicity, 159
  empiricist approach to, 148
  excessive reassurance seeking, 152–154
  interpersonal deficiencies and emotional detachment, 155–156
  low confidence in memory, 158
  moral inflexibility and religiosity, 157–158
  need for control, 154–155
  overview, 160
  rigidity and inflexibility, 154
self-reflection on the quality of, *144*
strengthening the critical elements of, *140*
therapist characteristics and competencies, 142–143
working alliance, *140*, 141–143
Therapeutic Relationship in Cognitive-Behavioral Therapy, The (Kazantzis et al.), 138
Thought–action fusion (TAF) bias
  behavioral interventions for, *233*, 239–240
  cognitive-behavioral model of contamination OCD and, 274–275
  cognitive restructuring, 212–214
  compulsive checking and, *296*, 298
  failed mental control and, 116
  misinterpretation of personal significance and, 113
  repugnant obsessions and, 325
  considerations in case formulation, 327, 331
Thought–Action Fusion (TAF) Scale
  Likelihood subscale, 122
  moral inflexibility and, 157, 314
  Moral subscale, 122, 157, 314, 325, 331
  overview and description of, 122–123, 180–181
  using with repugnant obsessions, 325, 331
Thought–Action Fusion Scale—Revised (TAF-R), 180–181
Thought control. *See* Mental control
Thought Control Questionnaire (TCQ), 182

Thought dismissal, 205–206
Thought overimportance. *See* Overimportance of thought
Thought retention, 205
Threat overestimation
  behavioral interventions, *233*
  cognitive restructuring, 209–211
  compulsive checking and, *296*, 298
  defined, 113, *115*
Threat Prediction Form (Form 9.1), 237, 250–251
Threat prediction intervention, *233*, 236–237
Threat survey, *233*, 238
Tic disorder, 6, 19
Tourette syndrome, 19
Transfer of responsibility. *See* Responsibility transfer
Trauma-related obsessions, 33–34
Treatment goals
  goal consensus and the therapeutic relationship, *140*
  goal setting in CBT for OCD, 197–200, 224
Treatment outcome, effects of the working alliance on, 141–142
Treatment rationale, 206–207
Trichotillomania (TTM), 7, 18–19
TTM. *See* Trichotillomania

Unacceptability of obsessions, 35, 36
Uncertainty exposure exercise, *234*, 246
Uncertainty intrusions, compulsive checking and, 297
Uncertainty paralysis, 63–64
Uncertainty tolerance, 305–306
Unstructured clinical interviews, 172
Unwanted intrusive thoughts
  overview and description of, 37–39
  universality of, 119–121
  See also Intrusions; Obsessions

Validation, to improve assessment compliance, 168–169
Vancouver Obsessional Compulsive Inventory (VOCI), 177–178, 278, 353–354
Vicarious reassurance and responsibility, 170
Visual contamination, 269, 270
VOCI. *See* Vancouver Obsessional Compulsive Inventory
Vulnerability self-theme, 294, 304

WAI. *See* Working Alliance Inventory
Washing and cleaning compulsions
  clinical features, 260–263
  differentiated from compulsive checking, 283
  early research on, 23–24
  illustrative exposure hierarchy for, *86*
  mental contamination and, 268
  stop rules and, 262, 276, 278
  treatment considerations, 263
WBSI. *See* White Bear Suppression Inventory
White Bear Suppression Inventory (WBSI), 128, 183–184
White bear thought suppression experiment
  behavioral intervention with excessive mental control, 243–244
  cognitive restructuring of thought control, 218
  description of, 205–206, *234*

Wise mind technique, 218
Within-session exposure, 96
Women, OCD and, 9–10
Working alliance, *140*, 141–143
Working Alliance Inventory (WAI), 141
Worry
  differentiating from obsessions, 43, 44–46
  intolerance of uncertainty and, 63
  overview, 43, 44

Yale–Brown Obsessive–Compulsive Scale (YBOCS)
  overview and description of, 173–175
  self-report YBOCS, 174, 175, 178
  Symptom Checklist, 25, 283, 343
  Y-BOCS-II, 174–175
YBOCS. *See* Yale–Brown Obsessive–Compulsive Scale
Yedasentience, 66
Young adults, OCD and, 9